Ovarian Hyperstimulation Syndrome (OHSS) is a condition that can occur in women undergoing in vitro fertilization, after having follicle stimulating hormone (FSH) injections to stimulate egg growth and maturation. Some patients respond excessively to the drug and dose given. If large numbers of eggs mature, the high hormone levels coming out of the hyperstimulated ovaries, combined with the increased size of the ovaries, can cause extremely serious, and sometimes lethal, side effects. Moderate-to-severe OHSS requires admission to a hospital. Dr. Rizk is one of the world's top experts on managing OHSS.

This is the first published book dedicated to all aspects of OHSS. The pathophysiology, prevention and management of this syndrome have been revolutionized over the past decade, and it is important for reproductive practicioners and infertility specialists to understand the latest findings about this potentially deadly condition. The author reviews in depth the classification, epidemiology, pathophysiology, complications, and prediction, prevention and treatment options for OHSS. This book is intended for infertility specialists, reproductive medicine specialists and assisted reproduction specialists.

Botros R. M. B. Rizk is Professor and Chief, Division of Reproductive Endocrinology and Infertility, Department of Obstetrics and Gynecology at the University of South Alabama School of Medicine. He is also Medical and Scientific Director of the University of South Alabama in vitro fertilization program.

OVARIAN HYPERSTIMULATION SYNDROME

Epidemiology, Pathophysiology, Prevention and Management

BOTROS R. M. B. RIZK

University of South Alabama
School of Medicine

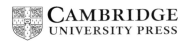

CAMBRIDGE
UNIVERSITY PRESS

32 Avenue of the Americas, New York NY 10013-2473, USA

Cambridge University Press is part of the University of Cambridge.

It furthers the University's mission by disseminating knowledge in the pursuit of education, learning and research at the highest international levels of excellence.

www.cambridge.org
Information on this title: www.cambridge.org/9780521857987

First published 2006

A catalogue record for this publication is available from the British Library

Library of Congress Cataloguing in Publication data

Rizk, Botros.
    Ovarian hyperstimulation syndrome : epidemiology, pathophysiology,
      prevention and management / Botros Rizk.
       p. ; cm.
    Includes bibliographical references and index.
    ISBN-13: 978-0-521-85798-7 (hardback : alk. paper)
    ISBN-10: 0-521-85798-8 (hardback : alk. paper)
    1. Ovaries – Diseases.   2. Human reproductive technology –
      Complications.
    [DNLM: 1. Ovarian Hyperstimulation Syndrome.
    WP 320 R627o 2006] I.
      Title.
    RG441.R59 2006
    618.1'1–dc22

                                     2006001455

ISBN 978-0-521-85798-7 Hardback

This book is dedicated to my very dear and beloved parents, Dr. Isis Mahrous Rofail, my mother, and Mitry Botros Rizk, my father. Their unlimited true love, genuine sacrifice, care and support have filled my life with happiness, fulfilment and gratitude. Their memories, wisdom and thoughts will stay with us forever to guide us.

CONTENTS

FOREWORD

A COMPLICATED COMPLICATION

The subject of this book continues to attract serious medical attention. Ovarian hyperstimulation was a problem from before the days of in vitro fertilization (IVF), when it was noted by an Israeli group among their patients being stimulated for ovulation induction. It also emerged when IVF created the need to apply ovarian stimulation to produce, say, 10 mature oocytes for fertilization in vitro. Today, the condition is well known and heavily researched as it spreads with every practising IVF centre, where there is a constant need to produce a medium number of follicles per patient. Unfortunately, as originally discovered in laboratory animals, there is a very weak correlation between the dose of gonadotrophins and the number of ovulated oocytes, indicating that unknown numbers of follicles may begin their growth and expansion. Numerous attempts have been made to introduce useful therapies for this condition, and these are effective to varying degrees of efficiency.

Botros (Peter) Rizk is highly talented and presents a text that is well balanced between the description of OHSS, its causes and effects, and means of controlling its very serious complications. His own opinions come through very clearly and will help professionals involved in assisted reproduction to keep up-to-date with current therapies. Available therapies are assessed in detail, which is certain to be of help to many clinicians. He gives his own clear opinions on the risks and the means of prevention. Since he writes simply and informatively, it is a pleasure to read the various sections of this book. The clear layout, good illustrations and numerous references in the book should help to clarify the causes of this condition. Every point made in the book has several associated references, providing clear pointers to further reading. The numerous illustrations help to carry the reader through this exhaustive evaluation of the causes of and, hopefully, cures for OHSS. Overall, the text is so clear and authoritative that attention must be given in this Foreword to the aspects of ovarian hyperstimulation covered.

Successive chapters cover the classification of the syndrome, its epidemiology, pathophysiology and genetics. These are followed by chapters on the complications of hyperstimulation, its prediction and patient education to help with this disorder. The book is completed with chapters on the prevention and treatment of hyperstimulation. The layout is very simple and attractive, such as in the opening classification where the objectives of classification are considered, including a description of its first classification by Rabau et al. in 1967, followed by successive modifications (e.g. the division of its symptoms into mild, moderate and severe as successive investigators modified the original protocol), until workers today go into such detail as suspecting hypothyroidism or FSH receptors may be involved. Discussing the epidemiology of ovarian hyperstimulation, the author stresses the effects of IVF on our understanding of ovarian hyperstimulation, the need for milder treatments, the relationships with polycystic ovarian disease and the roles of hyperinsulinism. The accompanying endocrine revolution led to the introduction of human menopausal gonadotrophin (hMG) and then recombinant preparations of gonadotrophins and the introduction of GnRH, its agonists and antagonists. The complex problems of the short luteal phase in relation to the use of ovarian stimulation in cyclic women is discussed in detail and assessed for spontaneous and recurrent situations.

Extensive attention is naturally paid to the pathophysiology of hyperstimulation and its associated massive ovarian enlargement and circulatory disorders. These highly serious conditions have, fortunately, attracted the attention of many investigators who have steadily characterized their successive stages. A glance at the work of Van Beaumont in 1872 introduces the problems of osmoregulation, capillary permeability, the roles of various steroids and the ovarian renin–angiotensin system. This section also stresses the genetic nature of OHSS, with references to the actions of prostaglandins, Von Willebrand factor and of vascular endothelial growth factor (VEGF) as an agent affecting capillary permeability. Its actions in follicular fluid are presented in detail and in relation to the ratio between total and free VEGF. Analyses of the roles of interleukins, selectins and intercellular adhesion molecule (ICAM) follow in succession.

Not surprisingly, the genetics of OHSS occupies the succeeding chapter, opening with descriptions of recent work on the follicle stimulating hormone (FSH) receptor, its mutations and the origin of spontaneous OHSS. Extensive detail is considered in this and the previous chapter, as the slow but certain clarification of the background genetics is assessed. Reaching the molecular level is certain to open new leads, such as the higher sensitivity to human chorionic gonadotrophin (hCG) to specific forms of the FSH receptor mutants. This polymorphic system may determine the severity of many systems reliant on FSH activity and the threshold effects of the various mutants.

The complications of OHSS also attract, quite correctly, the detailed attention of the author. Fatalities are very rare, yet nevertheless have attracted considerable attention ever since the first case was described by Lunenfeld and his colleagues. Cerebrovascular complications include thromboembolic complications and hypercoaguable states, and their early and later effects are assessed. The detailed discussion of these states and their related effects leads to a most authoritative analysis by the author. Family histories, rare vascular complications, myocardial infarction and respiratory complications are all described. The details of these complications are so numerous as to demand a close reading of this chapter. Predicting OHSS is not easy, and is considered in

Chapter VI. Classical appproaches involve estrogen assays, yet their value is still questioned today despite exhaustive studies. The author discusses the value of assessing the rising levels of VEGF from granulosa cells and in blood. Assays for Von Willebrand factor, especially near the time of implantation, and for inhibin are mentioned, together with the use of ultrasound for scoring the sizes of the numerous follicles, measuring ovarian volume and low intravascular ovarian resistance. Risk factors include rapidly rising plasma oestrogen levels and young women with polycystic ovaries with excessive follicular response, especially soon after the hCG injection (early OHSS).

The author clarifies the risks to patient health and provides help to increase awareness of this distressing disorder. 'Ten Commandments' for preventing OHSS initiate Chapter VII, and these are soon doubled. The first set includes the use of low doses of stimulatory gonadotrophins, and ovarian diathermy prior to stimulation. The second list proposes delaying hCG, avoiding it by using GnRH to induce ovulation and progesterone for luteal phase support. Risks of polycystic ovary syndrome (PCOS), the use of metformin and weight reduction are essential reading, although the consequences of changing gonadotrophin levels have always been somewhat unpredictable, while results with metformin, aromatase inhibitors, pentoxyfylline and other formulations require much more analysis. Ovarian drilling and the use of GnRH antagonists are discussed at some length, although more data are clearly needed. Likewise, by using natural cycle IVF, single-embryo transfer may help, although the author concludes that no single protocol has yet proved effective.

Adjusting the effects of ovarian stimulation by "coasting" HCG has been in use for many years now, and the author gives much space to its practice. Summarizing numerous reports, he concludes there is still a paucity of randomized trials, and that coasting risks decreases in oocyte numbers and pregnancy rates. Using GnRH antagonists, and recombinant luteinizing hormone (rLH) does not lead to firm conclusions, although rLH may offer the best alternative. Injecting albumim or starch are of doubtful value, and reducing follicle numbers, or cryopreserving oocytes for a later cycle seem to offer little. The author suggests a combined approach is best, involving decreasing gonadotrophins, coasting, reducing HCG levels to induce ovulation, and giving progesterone for luteal support.

The final chapter deals with treatments for OHSS. This has attracted detailed attention and the author recommends thorough check-up and follow-up. Moderate forms may be treated on an outpatient basis, with ultrasound, blood counts, liver function and coagulation monitoring, and perhaps too with rehydration, culdocentesis and albumin injections. Severe forms involve aspirating ascitic fluid, giving intravenous fluids, hydration, paracentesis, liver function tests, investigating respiratory compromise, anticoagulants to preserve renal function, and also treating many other symptoms. Ascitic fluid and pleural effusions may be aspirated, many clinicians considering this a matter of priority. Abdominal paracentesis has been questioned but is now regarded as essential. The author covers the basics of these studies and concludes by describing novel forms of blocking VEGFR-2.

This book has several very attractive advantages. It is well written and maintains a momentum that carries the reader with the text. It is clearly authoritative and written by a clinician with considerable experience. The detailed references set the scene for further reading, give credit to workers in the field and display the immense amounts of effort put into hyperstimulation research. It will be a very handy tome on a clinician's bookshelf, and should also attract the attention of non-clinical scientists and researchers and those practising IVF. And in the future, it could be updated fairly quickly as the saga of ovarian hyperstimulation enters new fields of scientific awareness.

Professor Robert G. Edwards, C.B.E., Ph.D., D.Sc., F.R.C.O.G., F.R.S.
Emeritus Professor, Cambridge University, Cambridge, England
Editor-in-Chief, Reproductive Biomedicine Online

PREFACE

Ovarian hyperstimulation syndrome (OHSS) presents a unique challenge in the practice of medicine in general and reproductive medicine in particular. There is no other situation where a "healthy" patient seeks medical assistance and may end up with serious medical complications. About 20 years ago, when I was working at Northwick Park Hospital in London, UK, a young patient presented to the emergency department a few days after a Gamete Intra-Fallopian Transfer (GIFT) procedure with severe OHSS, shortly followed by stroke. Amazingly, she completely recovered and delivered a healthy girl. The acute developments in this patient had an extraordinary effect on me, and since then I have dedicated a significant part of my career to this iatrogenic complication.

Worldwide, more than 500 000 in vitro fertilization (IVF) cycles are performed every year, and five to six times this number of superovulation cycles are performed. Therefore, severe OHSS will be encountered in small numbers by individual centers, although large numbers of cases will occur worldwide. This has led to lack of expertise in dealing with the myriad of complications of OHSS, especially because of their multisystem effects. Furthermore, the emphasis has been on how to maximize the success of IVF. This emphasis should shift to how to maximize its safety, and this is the ultimate goal of this book.

Writing this book, I was driven by a desire to provide a clinical guide that will help those practicing in the field of assisted reproduction and infertility. Both clinicians and scientists were in my mind. The infertility specialist will find the book a resource on how to evaluate patients before starting fertility treatment, with keen attention on to how to avoid the development of OHSS by a series of well-chosen decisions. The success of this book should be judged by a decline in the incidence and severity of OHSS seen in IVF centers and by infertility specialists. The scientist reading this book will immediately realize that recent discoveries in receptor mutations emphasize that only systematic scientific research can provide real understanding of the pathophysiology of OHSS and the potential for change. I hope this book boosts their enthusiasm to make further discoveries. The IVF nurse coordinator who is directly involved in ovarian stimulation will find this book helps her understand what is going through the minds of the IVF team during the cycle, and so helps her to serve her patients better.

The structure of the book is simple, with eight chapters covering all important areas. It was essential to start with classification in Chapter I – categorizing patients makes it possible to decide who can be treated as an outpatient and who needs to be admitted to hospital or intensive care. Chapter II on epidemiology emphasizes which groups of patients are at risk, taking into consideration patient characteristics and treatment protocols. The call to establish an international registry should be a priority of the American Society for Reproductive Medicine and the European Society for Human Reproduction and Embryology. The pathophysiology of OHSS is where all the recent research developments have occurred, and in Chapters III and IV in-depth discussion of the molecular biology research over the last decade complements our understanding. These developments should stimulate basic science researchers to advance our knowledge not only of hyperstimulation but also of routine ovulation induction. In Chapter V the detailed discussion of the complications of OHSS should prepare clinicians for difficulties they may encounter. Prediction, prevention and treatment are covered in the final three chapters. There has been an extraordinary effort to prevent OHSS. Eventually, this should mean that we all have extensive experience of prevention and less experience of treatment. Chapter VIII focuses on outpatient and inpatient treatment, as well as intensive care and novel medical therapies that we may see in the next few years.

The work presented in this book has been the result of tremendous research and contributions from clinicians and scientists all over the world. The fight against OHSS has been global, with important contributions from Europe, the USA and the Middle East. While early work is quoted in detail in this book, the recent advances in the last five years are emphasized. The wonderful stimulation, leadership and guidance provided by Bob Edwards has been extraordinary and could have never been replaced. I have also greatly enjoyed my extensive collaboration over the last two decades with Dr. Johan Smitz from Belgium, Dr. Mohamed Aboulghar from Egypt, and Dr. Melanie Davies, Dr. Charles Kingsland and Dr. Sam Abdalla from the UK. I would also like to thank Dr. Bridgett Mason and Professor Howard Jacobs from London and Professor Steve Smith from Cambridge for the magnificent opportunities they gave me in those two great cities in the UK. Working with skilled clinicians, such as Dr. Dudley Mathews from Kent and Dr. Roger Martin and Simon Crocker from Norwich provided great enjoyment. I thank Miss Julie Hazelton for her dedication and assistance in typing the manuscript of this book. I believe that our collaboration with investigators from Spain, Greece and Italy will open the way to more innovations. I have tried my best to present impartially the evidence on every issue that is open for debate, while making my personal views clear. I hope that clinicians will identify much useful experience, and that scientists will maintain their eagerness for research that will enlighten our understanding; and ultimately that our patients will benefit from all our efforts.

Botros Rizk, M.D., M.A., F.R.C.O.G., F.R.C.S.(C.), H.C.L.D., F.A.C.O.G., F.A.C.S.
Alabama 2006

CLASSIFICATION OF OVARIAN HYPERSTIMULATION SYNDROME

Ovarian hyperstimulation syndrome (OHSS) is characterized by bilateral, multiple follicular and thecal lutein ovarian cysts (Figure I.1) and an acute shift in body fluid distribution resulting in ascites (Figure I.2).

THE PURPOSE OF OVARIAN HYPERSTIMULATION SYNDROME CLASSIFICATIONS

The objectives of all OHSS classifications are three-fold (Aboulghar and Mansour, 2003). The first objective is to compare the incidence of OHSS. The second objective is to evaluate the efficacy of the different approaches for prevention of the syndrome. The final objective is to plan the management of OHSS, according to its severity and the presence or absence of complications.

OVERVIEW OF OHSS CLASSIFICATIONS

There has been no unanimity in classifying OHSS, and divergent classifications have made comparisons between studies difficult (Rizk, 1993). Aboulghar and

Fig. I.1: Multiple follicular cysts in the ovaries of a hyperstimulated patient

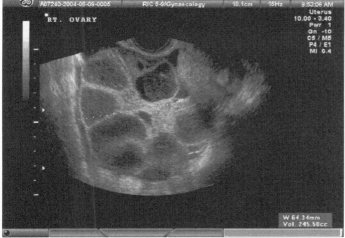

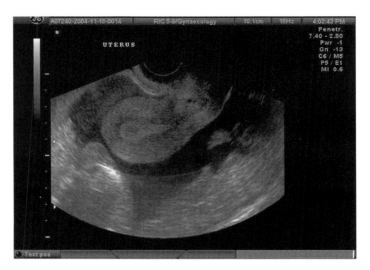

Fig. I.2: Ascites in a hyperstimulated patient

Mansour (2003) have reviewed the classifications used for OHSS over the last four decades (Table I.1).

A group of pioneers in ovulation induction observed what they called adverse events in the first 100 patients undergoing ovulation induction (Rabau et al., 1967). This led them to propose the first classification of OHSS. This was later reorganized by Schenker and Weinstein (1978) into three main clinical categories and six grades. Golan et al. (1989) introduced a new classification of three categories and five grades of OHSS. This was later modified by further dividing the severe form into two subgroups (Navot et al., 1992). The most recent classifications with further modifications were introduced in 1999 by Rizk and Aboulghar (1999).

THE FIRST CLASSIFICATION OF OHSS

Rabau et al. (1967) proposed the first classification of OHSS which combined both laboratory and clinical findings (Table I.2). The authors reported one of the original series of ovulation induction in 110 patients who had undergone 202 courses of treatment. In most instances, hyperstimulation was limited to increased estrogen and pregnanediol urinary excretion values without palpable cysts or enlargement of the ovaries. In seven cases the authors noted ovarian enlargement or cysts, low abdominal pain and/or distention and nausea (Group 3, Table I.3). Five of the seven patients in Group 3 also vomited or complained of diarrhea (Group 4). The authors classified Groups 3 and 4 as mild adverse reactions. They hospitalized these two groups to prevent exacerbation or further complications (Mozes et al., 1965). In seven patients, the clinical presentation was enlargement of the ovaries, distention, cysts, nausea, and diarrhea and ascites. Four of these seven patients also had hydrothorax (Group 5). Three patients

Table 1.1 Classifications of ovarian hyperstimulation syndrome (1967–1999)

Reproduced with permission from Aboulghar and Mansour (2003). Hum Reprod Update 9:275–89

Study	Mild	Moderate	Severe	
Rabau et al. (1967)	*Grade 1:* estrogen >150 μg/24 h and pregnanediol >10 mg/24 h *Grade 2:* + enlarged ovaries and possibly palpable cysts Grade 1 and 2 were not included under the title of mild OHSS	*Grade 3:* grade 2 + confirmed palpable cysts and distended abdomen *Grade 4:* grade 3 + vomiting and possibly diarrhea	*Grade 5:* grade 4 + ascites and possibly hydrothorax	*Grade 6:* grade 5 + changes in blood volume, viscosity and coagulation time
Schenker and Weinstein (1978)	*Grade 1:* estrogen >150 μg/24 h and pregnanediol >10 mg/24 h *Grade 2:* grade 1 + enlarged ovaries, sometimes small cysts	*Grade 3:* grade 2 + abdominal distension *Grade 4:* grade 3 + nausea, vomiting and/or diarrhea	*Grade 5:* grade 4 + large ovarian cysts, ascites and/or hydrothorax	*Grade 6:* marked hemoconcentration + increased blood viscosity and possibly coagulation abnormalities
Golan et al. (1989)	*Grade 1:* abdominal distension and discomfort *Grade 2:* grade 1 + nausea, vomiting and/or diarrhea, enlarged ovaries 5–12 cm	*Grade 3:* grade 2 + ultrasound evidence of ascites	*Grade 4:* grade 3 + clinical evidence of ascites and/or hydrothorax and breathing difficulties	*Grade 5:* grade 4 + hemoconcentration, increased blood viscosity, coagulation abnormality and diminished renal perfusion
Navot et al. (1992)	–		*Severe OHSS:* variable enlarged ovary: massive ascites ± hydrothorax: hemocrit >45%: WBC >15 000; oliguria: creatinine 1.0–1.5; creatinine clearance ≥50 ml/min; liver dysfunction; anasarca	*Critical OHSS:* variable enlarged ovary: tense ascites ± hydrothorax: hemocrit >55%; WBC >25 000; oliguria: creatinine >1.6; creatinine clearance <50 ml/min; renal failure; thromboembolic phenomena; adult respiratory distress syndrome
Rizk and Aboulghar (1999)	–	Discomfort, pain, nausea, distension, ultrasonic evidence of ascites and enlarged ovaries, normal hematological and biological profiles	*Grade A:* dyspnoea, oliguria, nausea, vomiting, diarrhea, abdominal pain, clinical evidence of ascites, marked distension of abdomen or hydrothorax, ultrasound showing large ovaries and marked ascites, normal biochemical profile	*Grade B:* grade A + massive tension ascites, markedly enlarged ovaries, severe dyspnea and marked oliguria, increased hematocrit, elevated serum creatinine and liver dysfunction *Grade C:* complications as respiratory distress syndrome, renal shut-down or venous thrombosis

3

Table I.2 First classification of OHSS
Reproduced with permission from Rabau et al. (1967). Am J Obstet Gynecol
98:*92–8*

| | No reaction[*] | | Adverse reactions | | | |
| | | | Mild[**] | | Severe[†] | |
Laboratory and clinical findings	1	2	3	4	5	6
Estrogens > 150 µg/24 h	+	+	+	+	+	+
Pregnanediol > 10 mg/24 h	+	+	+	+	+	+
Enlarged ovaries		+	+	+	+	+
Palpable cysts		?	+	+	+	+
Distension of abdomen			+	+	+	+
Nausea			+	+	+	+
Vomiting				+	+	+
Diarrhea				?	+	+
Ascites					+	+
Hydrothorax					?	+
Changes in blood volume, viscosity and coagulation time						+

[*] No treatment required
[**] Required observation
[†] Required hospitalization

from Group 5 subsequently showed changes in blood volume, viscosity and hypercoagulability (Group 6). Groups 5 and 6 needed hospitalization and therapeutic control of blood volume viscosity and coagulation time, as well as evacuation of fluid cavities. Rabau et al. (1967) reclassified Groups 5 and 6 as severe adverse reactions and reported the serious complications and management in a much quoted publication (Mozes et al., 1965).

REORGANIZATION OF OHSS CLASSIFICATION

Schenker and Weinstein (1978) reorganized the classification by Rabau et al. (1967) into three main clinical categories and six grades according to the severity of symptoms and signs, and laboratory findings.

(1) **Mild hyperstimulation**
    Grade 1, defined by laboratory findings of estrogen levels above 150 µg/24 h and pregnanediol excretion above 10 mg/24 h
    Grade 2, in addition, includes enlargement of ovaries; sometimes small cysts are present

Table I.3 Mild and severe cases of OHSS
Reproduced with permission from Rabau et al. (1967). Am J Obstet Gynecol **98**:*92–8*

	Mild				Severe			
Diagnosis	*Case*	*Ampules of Pergonal*	*hCG (IU)*	*Remarks*	*Case*	*Ampules of Pergonal*	*hCG (IU)*	*Remarks*
Primary amenorrhea	Ge. E.20/31	25	25 000	Pregnancy	Do. M. 108/199	22	25 000	pregnancy
	Le. R. 63/108	28	26 000	–				
Secondary amenorrhea	Ge. P. 21/32	55	29 000	–	Ge. P. 21/34	73	15 000	–
Secondary amenorrhea; MAP +					Ki. A. 59/149	14	25 000	pregnancy
secondary amenorrhea and galactorrhea	Sh. M. 72/121	28	29 000	–				
Postpartum amenorrhea and galactorrhea	Lo. S. 40/67	19	25 000	Pregnancy	Bi. F. 11/17	3460	21 500	quadruplet abortion
					Ba. A. 13/21		25 000	
Anovulation	Iv. B. 1/1 Hi. E. 89/163	2927	20 000 25 000	–	Be. Z. 19/29	20	10 000	–
Proliferative follicular phase				–	Po. A. 53/90	20	25 000	twin pregnancy

(2) **Moderate hyperstimulation**

Grade 3, in addition to elevated urinary steroid levels and ovarian cysts, abdominal distension is present

Grade 4, nausea, vomiting and/or diarrhea are also observed

(3) **Severe hyperstimulation**

Grade 5, in addition to the above, the ovarian cysts are large and ascites and/or hydrothorax are present

Grade 6, marked hemoconcentration with increased blood viscosity may result in coagulation abnormalities

MODERNIZATION OF THE OHSS CLASSIFICATION

Golan et al. (1989) proposed a new classification in which 24-hour urinary assays of hormones became obsolete, and subsequently estrogen and preg-nanediol assays were also omitted. Nausea, vomiting and abdominal distension were relocated from moderate to mild OHSS, and then moderate OHSS was no longer divided into two different grades as in the previous specification; it mainly added ultrasound evidence of ascites to the features of Grade 2 OHSS. In my opinion, this was an important addition. Severe OHSS was classified into two grades (Grade 4 and 5), which were similar to the previous classification.

(1) **Mild OHSS**

Grade 1, abdominal distension and discomfort

Grade 2, features of grade 1 plus nausea, vomiting and/or diarrhea; ovaries are enlarged from 5 to 12 cm

(2) **Moderate OHSS**

Grade 3, features of mild OHSS plus ultrasonic evidence of ascites

(3) **Severe OHSS**

Grade 4, features of moderate OHSS plus evidence of ascites and/or hydrothorax and breathing difficulties

Grade 5, all of the above, plus change in the blood volume, increased blood viscosity due to hemoconcentration, coagulation abnormality, and diminished renal perfusion and function

DESIGNATION OF CRITICAL OHSS
AS A SPECIAL ENTITY

Navot et al. (1992) suggested making a distinction between severe and life-threatening OHSS by dividing it into two subgroups. Severe OHSS was characterized by variably enlarged ovaries, massive ascites and/or hydrothorax, hematocrit over 45%, WBC > 15 000, oliguria, creatinine of 1.0–1.5 and creatinine clearance of ≥50 ml/min. Furthermore, generalized edema and liver dysfunction were considered to be signs of severe OHSS. Critical OHSS was characterized by enlarged ovaries, tense ascites, hematocrit of over 55%, WBC ≥25 000, oliguria, creatinine ≥1.6 and creatinine clearance <50 ml/min. Renal failure, thromboembolic phenomena and adult respiratory distress syndrome (ARDS) constituted critical OHSS. This subdivision was important from both clinical and prognostic aspects. The group of patients labeled as critical OHSS should be treated under very close supervision in an intensive care setting.

CLINICAL CLASSIFICATION OF OHSS

More recently, Rizk and Aboulghar (1999) classified the syndrome into only two categories, moderate and severe. The purpose of this classification is to categorize patients with OHSS into more-defined clinical groups that correlate with the prognosis of the syndrome. This would be ideal from an epidemiological point of view to set a registry for these cases. Furthermore, treatment could be advised depending on which group the patient belongs to.

The mild category of OHSS, as in previous classifications by Rabau et al. (1967) and Golan et al. (1989), was omitted from our new classification, as this occurs in the majority of cases of ovarian stimulation and does not require special treatment. The great majority of cases of OHSS presenting with symptoms belong to the moderate categories of OHSS. In addition to the presence of ascites on ultrasound, the patients' complaints are usually limited to mild abdominal pain and distension, and their hematological and biochemical profiles are normal.

Finally, how does this classification guide treatment of the syndrome? Our new classification can be correlated with the treatment protocol and prognosis more clearly. Severe OHSS Grade C, which is critical, would be treated in an intensive care setting; whereas severe OHSS Grade B would be treated in an inpatient hospital setting with expert supervision. Severe OHSS Grade A could be treated in an inpatient or outpatient setting, depending on the physician's comfort, the patient's compliance and the medical facility. Moderate OHSS could be treated on an outpatient basis with extreme vigilance.

(1) **Moderate OHSS**

Discomfort, pain, nausea, abdominal distension, no clinical evidence of ascites, but ultrasonic evidence of ascites and enlarged ovaries, normal hematological and biological profiles

(2) **Severe OHSS**

Grade A

Dyspnea, oliguria, nausea, vomiting, diarrhea, abdominal pain

Clinical evidence of ascites plus marked distension of abdomen or hydrothorax

Ultrasound scan showing large ovaries and marked ascites
Normal biochemical profiles

Grade B
All symptoms of grade A, plus:
Massive tension ascites, markedly enlarged ovaries, severe dyspnea and
marked oliguria
Biochemical changes in the form of increased hematocrit, elevated serum
creatinine and liver dysfunction

Grade C
OHSS complicated by respiratory distress syndrome, renal shut-down or
venous thrombosis

EARLY AND LATE OHSS

OHSS in patients undergoing controlled ovarian hyperstimulation has been
observed to occur in two distinct forms: early onset and late onset, with
possibly different predisposing factors. Early OHSS presents 3 to 7 days after
the ovulatory dose of hCG, whereas late OHSS presents 12 to 17 days after
hCG. Early OHSS relates to "excessive" preovulatory response to stimulation,
whereas late OHSS depends on the occurrence of pregnancy, is more likely to
be severe, and is only poorly related to preovulatory events (Dhal-Lyons et al.,
1994; Mathur et al., 2000).

SPONTANEOUS AND IATROGENIC OHSS

Traditionally, it has always been stated that OHSS is the most serious iatrogenic
complication of ovulation induction. Interestingly, over the last decade, a
significant number of reports have been published about spontaneous OHSS
without any pharmacological intervention. Most of these cases have been
observed in multiple pregnancies (Check et al., 2000) or hyaditiform moles
notorious for high hCG values (Ludwig et al., 1998). Some cases were
associated with hypothyroidism and the possibility that the high levels of
TSH could stimulate the ovaries has been raised (Nappi et al., 1998). A series of
cases where recurrent OHSS occurred (Zalel et al., 1995; Olatunbosun et al.,
1996; Di Carlo et al., 1997) have been reported. More recently, mutations
of FSH receptors have been implicated as a cause for spontaneous OHSS
(Vasseur et al., 2003; Smits et al., 2003; Montanelli et al., 2004). Spontaneous
forms of OHSS were generally reported to develop between 8 and 14 weeks of
amenorrhea. In contrast, iatrogenic OHSS usually starts between 3 and 5 weeks
of amenorrhea.

REFERENCES

Aboulghar MA & Mansour RT (2003). Ovarian hyperstimulation syndrome: classifications and critical analysis of preventive measures. *Hum Reprod Update* **9**:275−89.

Check JH, Choe JK & Nazari A (2000). Hyperreactio luteinalis despite the absence of a corpus luteum and suppressed follicle stimulation concentrations in a triplet pregnancy. *Hum Reprod* **15**:1043−5.

Dahl-Lyons CA, Wheeler CA, Frishman GN et al. (1994). Early and late presentation of the ovarian hyperstimulation syndrome: two distinct entities with different risk factors. *Hum Reprod* **9**:792−9.

Di Carlo C, Bruno PA, Cirillo D et al. (1997). Increased concentrations of renin, aldosterone and Ca125 in a case of spontaneous, recurrent, familial, severe ovarian hyper-stimulation syndrome. *Hum Reprod* **12**:2115−17.

Golan A, Ron-El R, Herman A et al. (1989). Ovarian hyperstimulation syndrome: an update review. *Obstet Gynecol Surv* **44**:430−40.

Ludwig M, Gembruch U, Bauer O et al. (1998). Ovarian hyperstimulation syndrome (OHSS) in a spontaneous pregnancy with a fetal and placental triploidy: information about the general pathophysiology of OHSS. *Hum Reprod* **13**:2082−7.

Mathur RS, Akande AV, Keay SD et al. (2000). Distinction between early and late ovarian hyperstimulation syndrome. *Fertil Steril* **73**:901−7.

Montanelli L, Delbaere A, Di Carlo C et al. (2004). A mutation in the follicle-stimulating hormone receptor as a cause of familial spontaneous ovarian hyperstimulation syndrome. *J Clin Endocrinol Metab* **89**:1255−8.

Mozes M, Bogowsky H, Anteby E et al. (1965). Thrombo-embolic phenomena after ovarian stimulation with human menopausal gonadotrophins. *Lancet* **2**:1213−5.

Nappi RG, Di Nero E, D'Aries AP & Nappi I. (1998). Natural pregnancy in hypothyroid woman complicated by spontaneous ovarian hyperstimulation syndrome. *Am J Obstet Gynecol* **178**:610−11.

Navot D, Bergh PA & Laufer N (1992). Ovarian hyperstimulation syndrome in novel reproductive technologies: prevention and treatment. *Fertil Steril* **58**:249−61.

Olatunbosun OA, Gilliland B, Brydon LA et al. (1996). Spontaneous ovarian hyper-stimulation syndrome in four consecutive pregnancies. *Clin Exp Obstet Gynecol* **23**:127−32.

Rabau E, Serr DM, David A et al. (1967). Human menopausal gonadotrophin for anovulation and sterility. *Am J Obstet Gynecol* **98**:92−8.

Rizk B. (1993). Ovarian hyperstimulation syndrome. In (Studd J, Ed.), *Progress in Obstetrics and Gynecology*, Volume 11. Edinburgh: Churchill Livingstone, Chapter 18, pp. 311−49.

Rizk B & Aboulghar MA (1999). Classification, pathophysiology and management of ovarian hyperstimulation syndrome. In (Brinsden P, Ed.), *A Textbook of In-Vitro Fertilization and Assisted Reproduction*, Second Edition, Carnforth, UK: Parthenon, Chapter 9, pp. 131−55.

Schenker JG & Weinstein D (1978). Ovarian hyperstimulation syndrome: a current survey. *Fertil Steril* **30**:255−68.

Smits G, Olatunbosun O, Delbaere A et al. (2003). Ovarian hyperstimulation syndrome due to a mutation in the follicle-stimulating hormone receptor. *N Eng J Med* **349**:760−6.

Vasseur C, Rodien P, Beau I et al. (2003). A chorionic gonadotrophin-sensitive mutation in the follicle-stimulating hormone receptor as a cause of familial gestational spontaneous ovarian hyperstimulation syndrome. *N Engl J Med* **349**:753−9.

Zalel Y, Orvieto RM, Ben-Rafael Z et al. (1995). Recurrent spontaneous ovarian hyperstimulation syndrome associated with polycystic ovary syndrome. *Gynecol Endocrinol* **9**:313−15.

II

EPIDEMIOLOGY OF OVARIAN HYPERSTIMULATION SYNDROME: IATROGENIC AND SPONTANEOUS

Rizk and Smitz (1992), in an analytical study of the factors that influence the incidence of OHSS, found wide variation between different centers. This is partly because of different definitions for the grades of severity and partly because of the adoption of different criteria for prevention. The incidence of OHSS has been estimated at 20–33% for mild cases, moderate cases of OHSS are estimated at 3–6%, and severe cases at 0.1–2% (Rizk, 1993a, b; Serour et al., 1998, Mathur et al., 2000).

THE IMPACT OF IN VITRO FERTILIZATION ON THE DEVELOPMENT OF OHSS

The development of in vitro fertilization (IVF) by Professor Robert Edwards and Dr. Patrick Steptoe was the gateway to modern human reproduction (Steptoe and Edwards, 1978). The impact of IVF on reproductive medicine has been phenomenal. It opened new horizons in every discipline from cell biology to genetics. Robert Edwards is a legend of the twentieth century, and it is always fascinating to see that he had already thought of and debated issues in the 1960s and 1970s that our profession and society are just discovering (Aboulghar et al. 1998a). In relation to ovarian stimulation, Louise Brown was conceived after natural-cycle IVF without gonadotrophins. The use of gonadotrophins became popular in the early 1980s. It is interesting to note that the incidence of OHSS following IVF in the 1980s (Table II.1) was higher than that following ovulation induction in the 1970s without the widespread use of estradiol monitoring or ultrasonography (Table II.2).

Rizk and Smitz (1992) thought this high incidence possibly represents an increase in aggressiveness in stimulation during the 1980s, and secondarily the use of long GnRH agonist protocols. Professor Edwards was among the first *to question the wisdom of aggressive ovarian stimulation* and advocated a gentle approach (Edwards et al., 1996; Fauser et al., 1999). The best example of this very serious epidemic has been clearly demonstrated by Abramov et al. (1999). In a multicenter report of OHSS cases from 16 out of 19 tertiary medical centers in Israel, the authors revealed some shocking findings. While the number of severe cases of OHSS following ovulation induction treatments remained unchanged, the number of cases following IVF increased dramatically from 2 (0.06% of all IVF cases in 1987) to 41 (0.24% of all IVF cases in 1996)(Figures II.1 and II.2). The total number of IVF cycles performed during

Table II.1 Moderate and severe OHSS in relation to the nature of the gonadotrophin releasing hormone (GnRH) agonist used, the protocol for human menopausal gonadotrophins (hMG) therapy, the type of luteal support and the occurrence of pregnancies

Reproduced with permission from Rizk and Smitz (1992). Hum Reprod. 7:320–7

Reference	Study group	Incidence of OHSS (%)	GnRh agonist used	Dose	% OHSS pregnant	HMG regimen	Luteal support
Golan et al. (1988)	143 cycles 117 patients	8.4	D-Trp 6	3.2 mg long-acting	83	started with 3 ampules	2500 IU hCG every 72 h. and adjusted to estradiol
Belaisch-Allart and De Mouzon (1989)	304 embryo transfers	5.9	D-Trp 6 or D-Ser(TBU 6)	NM	NM	NM	2500 IU hCG (151 patients), or placebo (153 patients) randomized
Buvat et al. (1989)	171 embryo transfers	1.8 (moderate)	D-Trp 6	Short-acting	NM	NM	3 × 1500 IU hCG or 400 mg progesterone oral daily
Herman et al. (1990)	36 embryo transfers	14	D-Trp 6	3.2 mg long-acting	80	started with 2 ampules hCG and adjusted to estradiol	2500 IU every third day or placebo (18 patients)
Forman et al. (1990)	413 cycles	1.9 (severe)	D-Trp 6 or D-Ser (TBU) 6	3.75 mg long-acting injection 100 ng/day or nasal spray 500 ng/day	88	started with 2 ampules hCG and adjusted to estradiol	didrogesterone 30 mg/day orally or 2500 IU hCG every 72 h
Smitz et al. (1990)	1673 cycles	0.6 (severe)	D-Ser (TBU) 6	600 ng daily nasal spray	70	started with 2 ampules hCG and adjusted to estradiol	1500 IU every 72 h or progesterone vaginal or intramuscular
Rizk et al. (1992)	1562	1.3 (severe)	D-Ser (TBU) 6	subcutaneous injection 200 µg/day or nasal spray 500 µg g/day	57	started with 2 ampules hCG and adjusted to estradiol	2000 IU on days 2 and 5 or progesterone 200 mg/day vaginal suppository

NM, not mentioned; hCG, human chorionic gonadotropin

Table II.2 Incidence of OHSS in hMG/hCG cycles
Reproduced with permission from Rizk, B. Ovarian hyperstimulation syndrome. In (Studd J, Ed.), Progress in Obstetrics and Gynecology, vol. 11. Churchill-Livingstone, Edinburgh, 1993, Chapter 18, pp. 311–49

Author	Year	Mild (%)	Moderate (%)	Severe (%)
Rabau et al.	1967			3.5
Tyler	1968	23		1.5
Taymor	1968	20		2
Thompson and Hansen	1970			1.2
Goldfarb and Rakoff	1973	10	0.005	0.008
Jewelewicz et al.	1973	20	7	1.8
Hammond and Marshall	1973	21		10
Caspi et al.	1974		6	1.17
Lunenfeld and Insler	1974	8.4		0.8
Schwartz et al.	1980		6.3	1.4

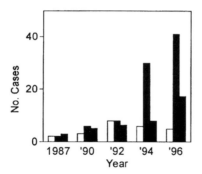

Fig. II.1: OHSS following ovulation induction and IVF and the number of IVF cycles over a decade between January 1987 and December 1996
Reproduced with permission from Abramov et al. (1999). Hum Reprod 14:2181–3

this time also increased from 2890 in 1987 to 17 283 in 1996. The authors explained this epidemic by the over-utilization of high-dose gonadotrophin protocols by assisted reproduction units. These units, in their opinion, seemed to have become more competitive in the last decade, with oocyte and embryo numbers being considered as the main criteria for success. With refinements in embryo cryopreservation allowing repeat embryo transfers, these numbers have become more relevant. Expansion of oocyte donation programs, where high-dose gonadotrophin protocols play a key role in achieving the maximum number of oocytes to be donated, may have also contributed to this problem. Finally, GnRH agonist protocols have been blamed in part for the increase.

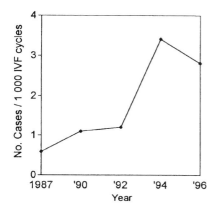

Fig. II.2: The annual incidence of severe OHSS per 1000 IVF cycles between January 1987 and December 1996
*Reproduced with permission from Abramov et al. (1999). Hum Reprod, **14**:2181−3*

CHARACTERIZATION OF PATIENTS AT RISK OF SEVERE OHSS

Several studies have attempted to collect and analyze data in order to characterize the patient population at risk for OHSS (Schenker and Weinstein, 1978; Navot et al., 1988; Golan et al., 1988) and to define risk factors for developing this syndrome (Blankstein et al., 1987; Asch et al., 1991; Rizk et al., 1991a, b; Rizk and Smitz, 1992). More recently, the epidemiology of OHSS has been studied in large series with the same two objectives by three groups of investigators from Belgium, Israel and Egypt. The Belgian study was a retrospective analysis of 128 cases from 13 IVF centers. The series from Israel was a retrospective analysis of 209 cases of severe OHSS after IVF in 16 out of 19 tertiary medical centers in Israel. The Egyptian series consisted of cases of moderate and severe OHSS from a single IVF center study of 3500 consecutive IVF cases (Delvigne et al., 1993a; Delvigne and Rozenberg, 2002; Serour et al., 1998; Abramov et al., 1998, 1999).

FACTORS THAT INFLUENCE THE INCIDENCE OF OHSS

Selection of Patients

Age

It is commonly observed that women suffering from ovarian hyperstimulation are significantly younger (Navot et al., 1988). This does not mean that older women are not at risk for OHSS but it means that *younger women are at higher risk*. Delvigne et al. (1993a) in a large Belgian study including 128 cases of OHSS and 256 controls, observed that the mean age for OHSS patients was 30.2 ± 3.5 versus 32.0 ± 4.5 years in controls. Enskog et al. (1999), in a prospective cohort study of 428 patients undergoing controlled ovarian hyperstimulation, observed that the patients in whom severe, moderate or mild ovarian hyperstimulation syndrome developed were younger than the patients in whom OHSS did not develop. The difference in the mean age between the patients in whom severe OHSS developed and the control group was approximately 2 years. The difference between all patients in whom OHSS developed and the control group was somewhat less. It is interesting to note that the difference in ages is very similar between the Belgian and the Swedish studies; the Belgian study reporting a difference of 1.8 years versus 2 years in the Swedish study, and the age factor seems to be a constant finding in most reports (Delvigne et al., 1993a; Enskog et al., 1999; Rizk and Abdalla, 2006).

Body-Mass Index

Most clinicians have the impression that OHSS is more common in patients with a lower BMI. Navot et al. (1988) described a positive correlation between a lean body mass and OHSS, whereas several other investigators could not confirm such a correlation (Lewis et al., 1990; Delvigne et al., 1993a, b; Enskog et al., 1999).

Etiology of Infertility

OHSS has been observed equally in primary and secondary infertility (Delvigne et al., 2004). The duration of infertility does not influence the occurrence of OHSS (Navot et al., 1988). Most certainly, women who have previously developed OHSS are at increased risk (Delvigne et al., 1993a, b). A significantly higher incidence of OHSS is reported in group II patients (World Health Organization classification; WHO, 1973). Lunenfeld and Insler (1974) found the incidence of mild and severe OHSS in 621 cycles of patients belonging to group I to be 5.5% and 0.6% respectively, compared with 10.8% and 1.2% in 784 cycles in group II. Thompson and Hansen (1970) analyzed 3002 hMG/hCG cycles in 1280 patients and found no cases of hyperstimulation syndrome in patients with primary amenorrhea (group I). Similar observations have been made by world-leading investigators (Caspi et al., 1974; Schenker and Weinstein, 1978; Tulandi et al., 1984).

POLYCYSTIC OVARIAN SYNDROME

Polycystic ovarian syndrome (PCOS) is the most common endocrinopathy affecting 4—12% of women of reproductive age. PCOS is a syndrome of ovarian dysfunction, along with the cardinal features of hyperandrogenism and polycystic ovary (PCO) morphology (Rotterdam ESHRE/ASRM Sponsored PCOS Consensus Workshop Group, 2003). The characteristic appearance of sclerocystic ovaries at laparoscopy or laparotomy is well known to every reproductive surgeon (Figure II.3). Clinically, PCOS is characterized by *hyperandrogenism* and *chronic* anovulation. Approximately 40—60% of

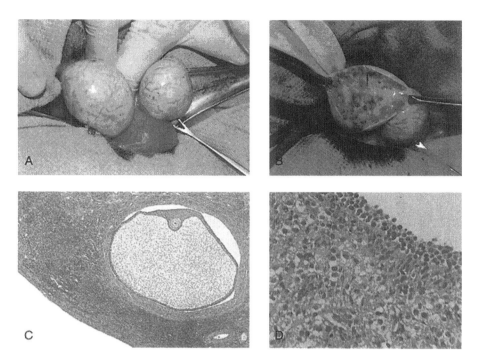

Fig. II.3: The gross and microscopic characteristics of polycystic ovaries
Reproduced with permission from Chang (2004). Polycystic ovary syndrome and hyperandrogenic states. In (Strauss, Barbieri, Eds), Yen and Jaffe's Reproductive Endocrinology: Physiology, Pathophysiology and Clinical Management, 5th edition. Philadelphia: Elsevier, Saunders, Chapter 19, p. 600

women with PCOS are obese and 60% display insulin resistance. The pathophysiology of PCOS has been extensively evaluated over the last two decades (Figure II.4). The clinical picture of patients with PCOS exhibits considerable heterogeneity (Balen et al., 1995). At one end of the spectrum, the polycystic ovary detected by ultrasound is the only finding. At the other end of the spectrum, obesity, menstrual cycle disturbance, hyperandrogenism and infertility may occur either singly or in combination (Balen et al., 1999) (Table II.3).

Rizk and Smitz (1992) found polycystic ovarian syndrome (PCOS) to be the major predisposing factor for OHSS. Schenker and Weinstein (1978) found that 12 out of 25 patients who developed severe OHSS had PCOS as determined by endoscopy. Charbonnel et al. (1987) encountered ovarian hyperstimulation in all 33 cycles in PCOS patients. Bider et al. (1989) found a higher proportion of severe OHSS, 38% in PCOS patients. Smitz et al. (1990) found a hormone profile suggestive of hyperandrogenism in eight out of ten patients who developed severe OHSS. Aboulghar et al. (1992) reported that 15 of 18 patients with severe OHSS had PCOS. Rizk et al. (1991a) found that 13 out of 21 patients with severe OHSS had PCOS confirmed by ultrasound and endocrine criteria. MacDougall et al. (1992, 1993) showed ultrasonically diagnosed PCOS in 63% of severe OHSS cases from the Hallam Medical Center.

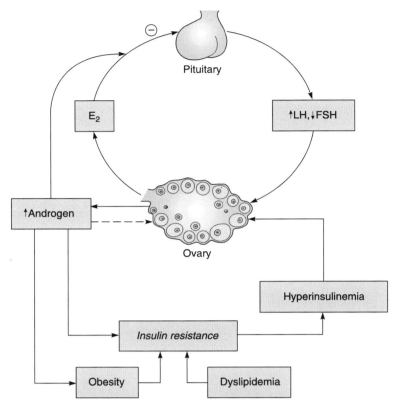

Fig. II.4: Pathophysiologic concept of polycystic ovary syndrome
Reproduced with permission from Chang RJ (2004). Polycystic ovary syndrome and hyperandrogenic states. In (Strauss, Barbieri, Eds), Yen and Jaffe's Reproductive Endocrinology: Physiology, Pathophysiology and Clinical Management, 5th edition. Philadelphia: Elsevier, Saunders, Chapter 19, p. 617

The outcome of IVF was compared in 76 patients with polycystic ovaries diagnosed on ultrasound scan and 76 control patients with normal ovaries, who were matched for age, cause of infertility and stimulation regimen. Of the polycystic ovary patients, 10.5% developed moderate/severe OHSS compared with none of the controls ($p = 0.006$). Delvigne et al. (1993a, b) reported 37% of 128 cases had PCOS, compared with 15% among the 256 controls.

Hyperinsulinism and OHSS

Hyperinsulinemia contributes to hyperandrogenism by increasing ovarian androgen production and suppressing sex-hormone-binding globulin by the liver, thereby increasing free testosterone levels. In PCOS patients, hyperinsulinemia is more profound in obese patients, although the presence of insulin resistance is independent of body weight (Dunaif et al., 1989; Carmina and Lobo, 1999; Rizk and Abdalla, 2006). PCOS patients who have hyperinsulinism were reported to have a higher incidence of OHSS compared with PCOS

Table II.3 Heterogeneity of clinical manifestations of PCOS
Reproduced with permission from Balen et al. In (Brinsden P, Ed.), A Textbook of In-Vitro Fertilization and Assisted Reproduction. Carnforth, UK: Parthenon Publishing, 1999, Chapter 8, pp. 109–30

Symptoms	% patients affected	Associated endocrine manifestations	Possible late sequelae
Obesity	38	elevated androgens (testosterone and androstenedione)	diabetes mellitus (11%)
Menstrual disturbance	66	elevated LH	cardiovascular disease
Hyperandrogenism	48	increased LH:FSH ratio	hyperinsulinemia
Infertility	73% anovulatory infertility	increased serum estrogens	high LDL, low HDL
Asymptomatic	20	elevated fasting insulin	endometrial carcinoma
		elevated prolactin	hypertension
		decreased sex hormone binding globulin	

LH, luteinizing hormone; FSH, follicle stimulating hormone; LDL, low-density lipoprotein; HDL, high-density lipoprotein

patients with normo-insulinism (Fulghesu et al., 1997). A complex interaction between insulin and follicular maturation has been suggested. Granulosa cells play a major role in OHSS development, and insulin increases the aromatase activity of granulosa cells, resulting in a higher ratio of estradiol to androstenedione (Fulghesu et al., 1997). Higher insulin levels alter the ovarian response to FSH and enhance the production of antral follicles as observed in OHSS. The authors hypothesized that hyperinsulinism might play an etiological role in the development of OHSS in PCOS patients. Delvigne et al. (2002) studied the metabolic characteristics of women who developed ovarian hyperstimulation syndrome. The primary purpose of the study was to investigate whether the higher incidence of hyperinsulinism is found in women who developed OHSS, whether or not they were PCOS patients. There were no differences in the distribution of patients with insulin resistance between the OHSS group and the control group. Insulin resistance was found in six women, three women in each group. The results are in agreement with those of Fedorcsak et al. (2001), who found no relation between hyperinsulinemia and IVF outcomes or OHSS rates (Fedorcsak et al., 2001).

ALLERGY

Interestingly, Enskog et al. (1999) observed an increased prevalence of allergy in patients who developed OHSS in a study involving 420 patients undergoing controlled ovarian hyperstimulation during a 6-month period. The authors hypothesized that differences in the immunologic sensitivity of patients are a predictor of OHSS. This was based on their observation that the pathophysiologic changes that occur in the ovary in response to OHSS closely resemble an overactive inflammatory response, with the participation of immunomodulatory cytokines. Therefore, before starting their controlled ovarian hyperstimulation, all 428 patients were questioned about allergy as a sign of a hyperreactive immune system, and disposition to infection as a sign of hyporeactivity. The interesting observation of a significantly higher incidence of allergy in severe OHSS may indicate that general immunologic mechanisms may play a role in the development of an inflammatory response. No previous study has reported this association between allergy and OHSS.

OVARIAN STIMULATION PROTOCOL

Gonadotrophins

The development of gonadotrophins (Figure II.5) is one of the most significant advances in the treatment of infertility in the 20th century (Rizk, 1993a, b). Gonadotrophins have been used worldwide since the 1930s. Animal extracts from the urine of mares, and later of pigs, were used for 30 years. During the 1950s two extraction processes were pursued in parallel: to obtain human gonadotrophins from the human cadaver pituitary glands or from the urine of postmenopausal women. Postmenopausal urine had the advantage of a relatively high concentration of gonadotrophins resulting from the hypergonadotropic status of postmenopausal women. In the late 1950s, researchers

Fig. II.5: The evolution of gonadotrophins
Reproduced with permission from Edwards RG, Risquez F (Eds) (2003). Modern Assisted Conception. Cambridge, UK: Reprod Biomed Online, Reproductive Health Care Ltd, p. 93

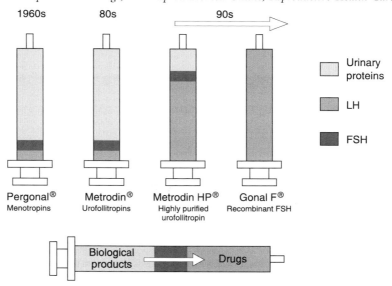

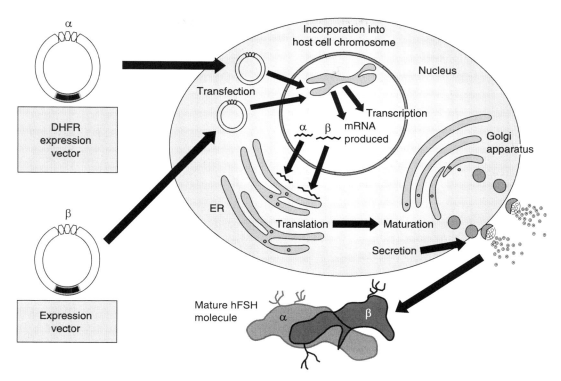

Fig. II.6: Expression of rFSH in Chinese hamster ovarian cells
Reproduced with permission from Howles (1996). Hum Reprod Update 2:172–91

working on pituitary gonadotrophins were the first to achieve success in terms of ovulation and pregnancy (Gemzell et al., 1958). A few years later, human menopausal gonadotrophin was developed from urine. Urine extraction was scaled up by the pharmaceutical industry and superseded pituitary extraction, which continued to be used by only a small number of state agencies in Australia (Loumaye and Howles, 1999). As stated by Loumaye and Howles, extensive use of urine-derived gonadotrophin was fortunate because it avoided the sad story of Creutzfeldt–Jakob disease (CJD) transmitted by pituitary-derived human growth hormone. In the 1980s, purified forms were developed and in the 1990s highly purified urine derivatives of FSH became available, and, finally, recombinant FSH was developed (Figure II.6). The characteristics of the different human gonadotrophin preparations (Table II.4) have been summarized by Loumaye and Howles (1999).

Pregnant Mare Serum Gonadotrophins

The evolution of gonadotrophins started in the 1930s when equine serum gonadotrophin was extracted from pregnant mare serum (Cole and Hart, 1930). The results from using pregnant mare serum gonadotrophins (PMSG) were inconsistent and disappointing because of the formation of antibodies to heterologous gonadotrophin (Schenker and Weinstein, 1978). Until 1961,

Table II.4 Characteristics of different human gonadotrophin preparations
Reproduced with permission from Loumaye and Howles. In (Brinsden P, Ed.), A Textbook of In-Vitro Fertilization and Assisted Reproduction, 1999. Carnforth, UK: Parthenon Publishing, Chapter 7, p. 104

Preparation	Year of first registration	Source of FSH	Protein concentration (IU/mg)	FSH bioassay (IU)	LH bioassay (IU)	Physico-chemical QC	FSH mass content control	Route of administration
Menotropin 1/1	1964	urine	>80	75	75	none	no	im
Menotropin 2/1	1989	urine ·	>80	75	37.5	none	no	im
Urofollitropin	1982	urine	>150	75	<0.1	none	no	im
Urofollitropin HP	1992	urine	= 9000	75	<0.001	++	no	sc
Follotropin	1995	CHO cells	= 12 000	75	–	+++	yes	sc

FSH, follicle stimulating hormone; LH, luteinizing hormone; QC, quality control; HP, highly purified; CHO, Chinese hamster ovary; im, intramuscular; sc, subcutaneous

60 cases of hyperstimulation, including two deaths, were reported when using PMSG (Figueroa-Casas, 1958; Muller, 1963; Schenker and Weinstein, 1978).

Human Pituitary Gonadotrophins

Gemzell et al. (1958) were the first to describe the first successful pregnancy after ovulation induction and pregnancy in humans utilizing follicle stimulating hormone (FSH) derived from human pituitary glands removed at autopsy. Gemzell et al. (1963) reported OHSS in 4 out of 22 cycles, but in 1970 only one case of OHSS was observed by monitoring estradiol levels. Human pituitary gonadotrophins are no longer used. There have been very few reported cases of CJD in Australia in patients treated with pituitary gonadotrophin preparations (Cochius et al., 1990; Brown et al., 1992).

Human Menopausal Gonadotrophin

Human menopausal gonadotrophin (hMG) was developed by extraction of urine based on a process developed in 1947 by Pietro Donini of Serono in Rome (Loumaye and Howles, 1999). This was first successfully used in hypogonatropic hypogonadal women for inducing pregnancy by Bruno Lunenfeld (Lunenfeld et al., 1962; Lunenfeld, 1963).

In 1967, Rabau et al. in their classic article (Rabau et al., 1967), found no relationship between the incidence of OHSS and the dose of gonadotrophin administered. Schenker and Weinstein (1978) found a difference between experimental animal and human studies regarding the impact of hMG dosage and the occurrence of OHSS. In experimental animals, a direct relationship was observed between the hMG dose and the development of OHSS. The change in ovarian size, the degree of capillary permeability, and severity of ascites and

Table II.5 Comparison of the stimulation characteristics of OHSS cycles to normo-ovulatory women who became pregnant after treatment with the same GnRH-a/hMG protocol
Reproduced with permission from Smitz et al. (1990). Hum Reprod 5:933–7

	OHSS	Normal cycles	
	(n = 10)	(n = 40)	Significance
Number of days before desensitization	30.2 ± 6.0	21.0 ± 7.0	p < 0.01
Days of hMG stimulation	9.6 ± 1.7	12.3 ± 2.5	p < 0.01
Number of ampoules of hMG used	21.9 ± 6.9	39.2 ± 14.2	p < 0.001
Preovulatory estradiol concentration (ng/l)	3735.0 ± 1603	1634 ± 492	p < 0.001
Number of oocytes retrieved	19.1 ± 10.3	7.5 ± 4.2	p < 0.001

pleural effusion were all related to the dose of gonadotrophin. In humans, OHSS in the individual patient could be a consequence of overdose of gonadotrophin, whereas, in groups of patients, no correlation between the dose of hMG and the occurrence of OHSS was observed (Schenker and Weinstein, 1978).

OHSS occurred in 0.008–23% of hMG/hCG cycles (Table II.2), compared with 0.6–14% in GnRH-a/hMG/hCG cycles (Table II.1). Comparison of the endocrine patterns (Table II.5) in patients who developed OHSS, and in normo-ovulatory patients who became pregnant after treatment with the same ovarian stimulation protocol, showed that the former required less hMG to achieve a higher preovulatory serum estradiol concentration and a higher number of mature oocytes (Smitz et al., 1990). Rizk and Smitz (1992) found that, in the groups reporting the lowest frequency of severe OHSS, ovarian stimulation was started with 2 × 75 IU hMG, whereas most other groups used 3 × 75 IU hMG. The amount of FSH injected at the start could possibly induce the growth of a larger number of follicles, which could develop sufficiently to acquire receptors for luteinizing hormone (LH), and, as a result, luteinize massively.

Purified Urinary Follicle Stimulating Hormone

Urofollitropin (FSH) has been available since the 1980s. It is devoid of LH but is still contaminated with urinary proteins. Highly purified urofollitropin (FSH-hp) has been available since the 1990s and contains very small amounts of urinary proteins. Lack of urinary proteins diminishes adverse reactions such as local sensitivity (Albano, 1996) while the absence of LH has no negative effects on the stimulation of PCOS patients (Hayden, 1999). Raj et al. (1977) have suggested that the use of FSH in anovulatory patients with PCOS offers a safe treatment compared with hMG, resulting in higher pregnancy rates and lower hyperstimulation rates. These authors suggested that endogenous LH levels in patients with polycystic ovaries are quite adequate for follicular development, and that the administration of exogenous LH is therefore unwarranted. However, it was quickly apparent that the pFSH did not suppress the risks of hyperstimulalation and multiple births when used in the conventional protocol (Check et al., 1985; Garcea et al., 1985, Buvat and Buvat-Herbaut, 1986; Buvat et al., 1989). Check et al. (1985) found a 23.7% incidence of OHSS in 18 women treated with 38 FSH cycles. Severe OHSS occurred in 5.3%, indicating that purified FSH is no safer than hMG.

Seibel et al. (1984) reported a new protocol consisting of chronic, low-dose pFSH administration, starting with 40 IU/day, without any hCG injection. The rate of hyperstimulation was significantly decreased by using a very low dose, and further refinements in the regimen resulted in a significant improvement in the pregnancy rate without a concomitant increase in the OHSS rate.

Recombinant Follicle Stimulating Hormone

Recombinant FSH is made from Chinese hamster ovarian cells, which are the host cells in the production of glycoproteins. The Chinese hamster ovary cells express FSH activity biologically in amounts that are sufficient to make the production process viable. A genomic clone that contains the complete sequence of the FSH β-subunit alone, or together with the gene of the α-subunit, is transferred to the Chinese hamster ovary cells (Figure II.6). The polypeptide chain of the recombinant FSH is identical to the natural one. However, the carbohydrated structures can be identical or closely related. The computer model of the FSH glycoprotein hormone (Gonal-F) is presented in Figure II.7. Furthermore, chimeric molecules have been synthesized with a longer half-life by modifying the carboxy peptide end (Risquez, 2003). The specific bioactivity of bioFSH is ≥ 10 000 IU FSH/mg of proteins (Loumaye and Howles, 1999). The advantages of recombinant FSH compared to urinary products are the consistency of the final product, high biological purity (which allows its subcutaneous injection) as well as chemical characterization for better quality control (Recombinant Human FSH Product Development Group, 1998). The complete lack of LH allows precise studies on ovarian folliculogenesis and, finally, the production of new molecules with short or long activity (Devroey et al., 1994; Tarlatzis and Billi, 1998; Risquez, 2003). The first pregnancies after the use of recombinant FSH for ovulation induction in anovulatory infertility (Donderwinkel et al., 1992) and for ovarian stimulation in IVF (Devroey et al., 1992) were reported more than a decade ago. Today, more than a million babies have been born worldwide. More recently, similar efficacy, tolerability and safety was observed in a randomized comparative IVF/ICSI trial of highly purified menotropin (MENOPUR, Ferring, Copenhagen, Denmark) vs. recombinant follicle stimulating hormone (Gonal-F, Serono, Switzerland) (European Israeli Study Group on highly purified menotropin vs. recombinant FSH, 2002). The OHSS rates were 7% vs. 5.1% respectively and,

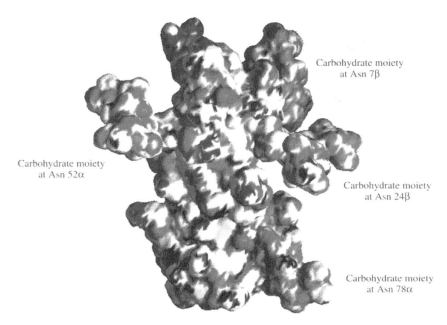

Carbohydrate moiety
at Asn 7β

Carbohydrate moiety
at Asn 52α

Carbohydrate moiety
at Asn 24β

Carbohydrate moiety
at Asn 78α

Fig. II.7: Computer model of the glycoprotein hormone Gonal-F (r-hFSH)
Reproduced with permission from Howles (1996). Hum Reprod Update 2:172–91

interestingly, an advantage of exogenous LH in IVF but not ICSI cycles was observed (Platteau et al., 2004).

What about Recombinant FSH and OHSS?

In a prospective randomized study of low-dose step-up protocols in PCOS patients resistant to clomiphene citrate, Rizk and Thorneycroft (1996) found that the use of recombinant FSH did not abolish the risk of OHSS. In fact, the incidence was comparable to that of purified urinary FSH in a similar low-dose protocol. Aboulghar et al. (1998b) found no difference between recombinant FSH and hMG. In a Cochrane database systematic review, Bayram et al. (2001) studied the safety and effectiveness of recombinant and urinary FSH in terms of ovulation, pregnancy, miscarriage, multiple pregnancy rate and OHSS. Only four randomized clinical trials of rFSH vs. uFSH have been identified. Gonadotrophins used in these studies were Follitropin-beta (Puregon) vs. urofollitropin (Metrodin), Follitropin-alpha (Gonal-F) vs. urofollitropin (Metrodin). No significant differences were demonstrated for the relevant outcomes. The odds ratio (OR) for ovulation was OR = 1.19 (95% CI, 0.78–1.80), pregnancy rate = 0.95 (95% confidence interval (CI), 0.64–1.41); multiple pregnancy rate, OR = 0.44 (95% CI, 0.16–1.21); miscarriage rate, OR = 1.26 (95% CI, 0.59–2.70) and OHSS, OR = 1.55 (95% CI, 0.50–4.84); ovulation rate. A systematic review and meta-analysis of 18 randomized controlled trials comparing recombinant and urinary FSH confirmed that there was no difference in the incidence of OHSS (Daya, 2002).

Long-acting Recombinant Follicle Stimulating Hormone

The relatively short half-life of FSH preparations $(32 \pm 12$ h)(Mannaerts et al., 1993) requires daily injections, which cause considerable discomfort to the patient. In an attempt to create a long-acting FSH preparation, chimeric genes containing the sequence encoding the carboxy terminal peptide (CTP) of beta-hCG fused with beta-FSH were constructed (Fares et al., 1992). The first human trials showed that recombinant FSH—CTP could be administered in hypogonadal males (Bouloux et al., 2001) and showed an extended half-life of 95 h (Duijkers et al., 2002). The pharmacodynamics of a single low dose of long-acting recombinant FSH (Corifollitropin-alpha) has been studied in women in WHO Group II anovulatory infertility (Balen et al., 2004). Following a single dose of long-acting remcombinant FSH, serum FSH—CTP initially rises to peak levels at one to two days and thereafter, serum FSH—CTP slowly decreases. This overall profile mimics the FSH flare-up induced by clomiphene citrate treatment and a step-down approach in classical ovulation induction. The objective of the study was to determine whether a single low dose could replace first- and second-line treatment of anovulatory women, assuming that both clomiphene citrate responders and clomiphene citrate resistors could be treated by this long-acting FSH. At this point, having a single starting dose for all patients is not feasible and additional research is required to achieve monofollicular ovulation. Beckers et al. (2003) reported the first live birth after ovarian stimulation using a chimeric, long-acting human recombinant follicle stimulating hormone agonist (rFSH—CTP) for IVF (Figure II.8).

Fixed-dose Gonadotrophins

A fixed gonadotropin regimen to increase the efficiency of IVF cycles was first used in France without a concomitant increase in the incidence of OHSS (Rainhorn et al., 1987).

Fig. II.8: First live birth after long-acting recombinant FSH
*Reproduced with permission from Beckers et al. (2003). Fertil Steril **79**:621−3*

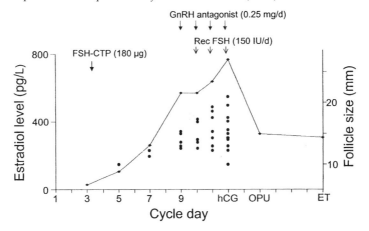

Table II.6 GnRH agonists available worldwide
Reproduced with permission from Edwards RG, Rizquez F (Eds) (2003). Modern Assisted Conception. Cambridge, UK: Reproductive Biomedicine Online: Reproductive Healthcare, Ltd, p. 64

Agonist	Structure
Leuprolide (Lupron®)	pGlu-His-Trp-Ser-Tyr-**DLeu**-Leu-Arg-Pro-**EtNH**$_2$
Triptorelin (Decapeptyl®)	pGlu-His-Trp-Ser-Tyr-**DTrp**-Leu-Arg-Pro-Gly-**NH**$_2$
Buserelin (Suprefact®)	pGlu-His-Trp-Ser-Tyr-**DSer (O^{t}BU)**-Leu-Arg-Pro-**EtNH**$_2$
Histrelin (Supprelin®)	pGlu-His-Trp-Ser-Tyr-**DHis (Bzl)**-Leu-Arg-Pro-**AzaglyNH**$_2$
Nafarelin (Synarel®)	pGlu-His-Trp-Ser-Tyr-**DNal(2)**-Leu-Arg-Pro-Gly-**NH**$_2$
Goserelin (Zoladez®)	pGlu-His-Trp-Ser-Tyr-**DSer (O^{t}Bu)**-Leu-Arg-Pro-**AzaglyNH**$_2$

Interestingly, Rizk et al. (1991b) found that a fixed-regimen protocol with a predetermined date of retrieval has a similar incidence of OHSS of approximately 1%. This study was performed at Norwich in the United Kingdom between 1988 and 1991, where the National Health Service would allocate a fixed operative session to perform Gamete Intrafallopian Transfer (GIFT). There was no observed difference between short and long protocols (Rizk et al., 1991c).

CLOMIPHENE CITRATE

Greenblatt and Barfield (1961) introduced clomiphene citrate for ovulation induction. Severe OHSS with clomiphene citrate (CC) is rare. Southan and Janovsky (1962) reported a patient with polycystic ovaries who developed massive ovarian enlargement, ascites and hydrothorax after the administration of 100 mg of CC for 14 days. Scommegna and Lash (1969) reported a case of ovarian hyperstimulation associated with conception after treatment with CC.

GONADOTROPHIN-RELEASING HORMONE AGONIST

The development of gonadotrophin-releasing hormone agonist has had a tremendous impact on the practice of reproductive endocrinology. Several GnRH agonists are used worldwide (Table II.6) and a wide variety of protocols have been implemented in clinical practice (Figure II.9).

Gonadotrophin-releasing Hormone Agonist without Gonadotrophins

OHSS has rarely been reported following the administration of GnRH agonist without gonadotrophins (Campo et al., 2000; Weissman et al., 1998).

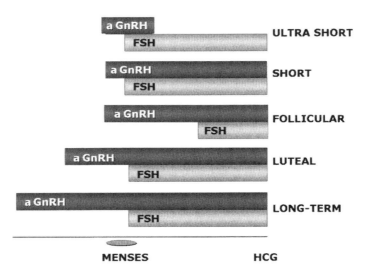

Fig. II.9: GnRH agonists and gonadotrophins: short and ultra-short and long and ultra-long protocols
Reproduced with permission from Edwards RG, Risquez F (Eds) (2003). Modern Assisted Conception. Cambridge, UK: Reprod Biomed Online, Reproductive Health Care Ltd, p. 107

Gonadotrophin-releasing Hormone Agonist Long Protocol

It had been hoped that the use of GnRH-a/hMG protocols would decrease the incidence of OHSS. With the use of GnRH-a, the practice of IVF has been simplified, the blocking of the LH surge permits further stimulation of the ovaries, increasing the number of oocytes (Belaish-Allart et al., 1989; Rizk, 1992, 1993a). Rizk and Smitz (1992) have summarized the major reports of OHSS after the use of GnRH and gonadotrophins for IVF (Table II.1).

Golan et al. (1988) observed a high incidence of OHSS, 8.4%, after combined GnRH-a and hMG for superovulation. The French report of IVF results (Bilan FIVNAT, 1989) showed that the use of GnRH-a led to significantly higher preovulatory estradiol concentrations, and to more frequent severe hyperstimulation (4.6% versus 0.6% for non-GnRH-a/hMG cycles). In a Cochrane database review, Hughes et al. (2000) reported an odds ratio of 1.4 (0.5–3.92) for moderate and severe OHSS in cycles using GnRH agonist as an adjunct to gonadotrophins compared with gonadotrophins alone.

OHSS IN GnRH ANTAGONIST PROTOCOLS

Third generation GnRH antagonists became available for assisted reproductive technology (ART) in the 1990s (Table II.7). They suppress gonadotrophin release by competitive receptor binding, resulting in immediate suppression and blockage of gonadotrophin secretion (Rizk and Nawar, 2004). Several protocols for GnRH antagonists in ART have been used

Table II.7 GnRH antagonists available worldwide
Reproduced with permission from Edwards RG, Rizquez F (Eds) (2003). Modern
Assisted Conception. Cambridge, UK: Reproductive Biomedicine Online:
Reproductive Healthcare, Ltd, p. 64

Name	Structure
Nal-Glu	[N-Ac-DNAL^1, DpCl-Phe^2, **DPal^3, Arg^5, DGlu^6, (AA),** DAla^{10}]GnRH
Detirelix	N-Ac-DNAL^1, DpCl-Phe^2, **DTrp^3, DhArg(ET$_2$)^6,** DAla^{10}]GnRH
Cetrorelix	N-Ac-DNAL^1, DpCl-Phe^2, DPal^3, **DCit^6,** DAla^{10}]GnRH
Ganirelix	N-Ac-DNAL^1, DpCl-Phe^2, DPal^3, **DhArg(ET$_2$)^6, DhArg(ET$_2$)^8,** DAla^{10}]GnRH
Antide	[N-Ac-DNAL^1, DpCl-Phe^2, DPal^3, **Lys(Nic)^5, DLys(Nic)^6, Lys(iPr)^8,** DAla^{10}]GnRH
Antarelix	[N-Ac-DNAL^1, DpCl-Phe^2, DPal^3, **D(HcI)^6, Lys(iPr)^8,** DAla^{10}]GnRH
Azaline B	-Ac-DNAL^1, DpCl-Phe^2, DPal^3, **Daph(at$_z$)^6, D-Aph(at$_z$)^6, Lys(iPr)^8,** DAla^{10}]GnRH

Ganirelix
regimen

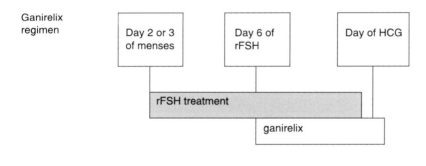

Triptorelin
regimen

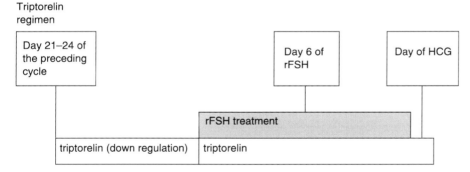

Fig. II.10: GnRH antagonist protocol for assisted reproduction technology
Reproduced with permission from European Middle East Orgalutron Study Group (2001).
Hum Reprod. 16:644—51

(Figure II.10). The efficacy and safety of GnRH antagonists in IVF and ICSI
cycles were reported to be similar to those of the GnRH agonists (Albano et
al., 2000; Ludwig et al., 2000; Olivennes et al., 2000; European Orgalutran
Study Group, 2000; European-Middle East Orgalutran Study Group, 2001;

Fluker et al., 2001). No difference was observed in a Cochrane review between the agonist and antagonist protocols and the incidence of OHSS (Al-Inany and Aboulghar, 2002). As more studies are published, this conclusion could change in favor of the GnRH antagonist, as will be discussed in detail in Chapter VII.

LUTEAL PHASE SUPPORT AND THE ROLE OF LUTEAL hCG IN THE GENESIS OF OHSS

Edwards et al. (1980), in the first extended report on IVF, stated that the luteal phase of virtually all patients was shortened considerably after treatment with gonadotrophins, and it was suggested that high follicular phase estrogen levels due to ovarian hyperstimulation might be involved. In the United States, initial studies in 1983 concerning hMG-stimulated IVF cycles also confirmed the occurrence of an abnormal luteal phase in IVF cycle, with characteristic features of elevated progesterone levels and significantly reduced luteal phase length (Jones, 1996). Seppala (1985) compiled The World Collaborative Report on IVF, which pointed out the non-uniform approach to luteal phase support. Many centers used progesterone and its derivatives, others used hCG and some avoided any luteal support. The introduction of GnRH-a offers advantages in terms of pituitary desensitization and prevention of a premature LH surge, thereby resulting in lower cancellation rates, and increased numbers of preovulatory follicles. However, because of its effect on corpus luteum function, treatment is required if a satisfactory luteal phase endometrium is to be maintained (Rizk, 1992, 1993a, b; Rizk et al., 1997). Smitz et al. (1988) were the first to document luteal phase insufficiency in 23 IVF cycles using GnRH-a when luteal phase support with progesterone was omitted. Golan et al. (1988) observed a high incidence of OHSS (8.4%) after the use of hCG for luteal support. Herman et al. (1990) in a prospective randomized trial, compared the pregnancy rate and incidence of OHSS after luteal hCG in IVF cycles stimulated with GnRH-a and hMG. Nine of the 18 patients who received hCG conceived, compared with 3 out of 18 patients in the placebo group. OHSS occurred in 5 out of 18 patients treated with hCG. None of the 18 patients without luteal hCG support developed OHSS, including those patients who became pregnant. Because the number of patients who conceived in the placebo group was small (3 out of 18), the authors concluded that the question of whether repeated early luteal hCG injections are more important in the pathogenesis of OHSS than endogenous hCG secreted later by the developing conceptus, remains unresolved. A meta-analysis of 18 studies reported a significant reduction in the occurrence of OHSS when progesterone is used for luteal phase support instead of hCG (Soliman et al., 1994) as will be discussed in the section, 'Prevention of OHSS'. Therefore, it is recommended not to use hCG for luteal phase support for all patients (Penzias, 2002; Guibert and Olivennes, 2004; Rizk and Aboulghar, 2005).

Table II.8 Incidence of pregnancy in patients with OHSS
Reproduced with permission from Rizk, B (1993). Progress in Obstetrics and Gynecology. Churchill-Livingstone, Edinburgh, Volume 11, Chapter 18, pp. 311–49

Author	*Year*	*Incidence (%)*	*Number of patients*	*Multiple pregnancies*
Rabau	1967	42	6/14	2/6
Schenker and Weinstein	1978	40	10/25	5/10
Tulandi	1984	34.6	10/29	4/10
Golan	1988	91	10/11	1/10
Borenstein et al.	1989	35	14/39	3/14
Herman	1990	80	4/5	1/4
Forman	1990	88	7/8	2/7
Smitz	1990	70	7/10	3/7
Rizk	1991	57	12/21	5/12

OHSS AND CONCEPTION CYCLES

Frequency of OHSS and Conception Cycles

Rizk (1993a) found OHSS to be much more frequent in conception cycles (Table II.8). In the early 1980s, Haning et al. (1983) found that OHSS was four times more frequent when pregnancy occurs. The pregnancy rate in the reported series of hyperstimulation varied from 34.6% to 91% (Rizk, 1993a). A high incidence of multiple pregnancy (10–42%) was also observed. A statistically significantly higher incidence of multiple pregnancies occurs specifically in the late OHSS patients compared with the non-OHSS patients (Mathur et al., 2000; Papanikolaou et al., 2005). However, OHSS is very rarely reported in association with multiple extrauterine pregnancy as bilateral ectopic or heterotopic pregnancy (Rizk et al., 1990b, 1991d; Reyad et al., 1998; Shiao et al., 2004).

Papanikolaou et al. (2005) designed an observational study to determine whether the onset pattern of OHSS is associated with the occurrence of pregnancy and early pregnancy outcome. In their study, early OHSS occurred in 53 patients, and late OHSS occurred in 60 patients. A total of 96.7% of the late OHSS cases occurred in a pregnancy cycle and were more likely to be severe than the early cases. The authors concluded that the early-onset pattern is associated with exogenously administered hCG and a higher risk of pre-clinical miscarriage, whereas late OHSS may be associated with the conception cycles, especially multiple pregnancy cycles, and will most likely be severe (Papanikolaou et al., 2005).

Duration of OHSS and Conception Cycles

The duration of OHSS is longer and its expression is more severe when pregnancy ensues (Rizk 2001, 2002). Bider et al. (1989) found the average hospitalization stay for pregnant patients with OHSS to be longer, compared to non-pregnant patients. Koike et al. (2004) found that the severity of OHSS is related to the number of conceptions, and this is reflected in the increased number of days in the hospital. Papanikolaou et al. (2005) also observed that late OHSS cases were more likely to be severe, and in fact accounted for 68% of the total cases of severe OHSS.

SPONTANEOUS OHSS

Spontaneous OHSS is a rare event. Rizk (1993a, b) found rare reports of OHSS in spontaneous cycles. However, over the last decade a large number of case reports of spontaneous OHSS have been published, sometimes reoccurring repeatedly in the same patients (Zalel et al., 1995; Lipitz et al., 1996; Regi et al., 1996; Ayhan et al., 1996; Abu-Louz et al., 1997; DiCarlo et al., 1997; Nappi et al., 1998; Todros et al., 1999; Pentz-Vidovic et al., 2000; Hee-Dong et al., 2001; Jung and Kim, 2001; Chae et al., 2001). Most cases of spontaneous OHSS have occurred in patients with PCOS, molar pregnancies and hypothyroidism (Zalel et al., 1992; Nappi et al., 1998) and, very rarely, without any other associated pathology (Chae et al., 2001).

The clinical presentation with ascites and pleural effusion is typical of advanced ovarian cancer in the absence of any previous infertility treatment. In the past, in many cases this has resulted in an exploratory laparotomy, as in the case report of Ayhan et al. (1996). Surgery is generally not advised in the treatment of OHSS (Rizk et al., 1990a; Rizk and Aboulgar, 1991, 1999), and yet, in these extremely rare cases, surgery is often performed, based on an incorrect diagnosis.

Jung et al. (2001) described a case of severe spontaneous OHSS with magnetic resonance (MR) findings. MR scans showed bilateral symmetric enlargement of the ovaries with multiple cystic changes, giving the classic "wheel-spoke" appearance. There was no definite abnormally thickened or enhanced wall, but there was internal hemorrhage in some chambers. The authors emphasized the importance of careful diagnosis to differentiate spontaneous OHSS from ovarian cystic neoplasms.

TIME COURSE DEVELOPMENT OF SPONTANEOUS OHSS

Spontaneous forms of OHSS have been generally reported to develop after between 8 and 14 weeks amenorrhea, differing from iatrogenic OHSS, which usually starts after between 3 and 5 weeks amenorrhea (Delbaere et al., 2004).

SPONTANEOUS OHSS AND hCG LEVELS

Most, if not all, cases of spontaneous OHSS are reported during pregnancy. Endogenous hCG secreted by the trophoblast 7−8 days post-conception is an additional factor in sustaining and exacerbating OHSS (Zalel et al., 1992). Spontaneous OHSS and elevated hCG levels have been described in multiple pregnancies (Leis et al., 1978; Check et al., 2000) as well as in molar pregnancies (Hooper et al., 1966; Moneta et al., 1974; Cappa et al., 1976; Ludwig et al., 1998) and even singleton pregnancy (Rosen and Lew, 1991). On the other hand, spontaneous OHSS and normal hCG levels have been reported by Zalel et al. (1992) and Abu-Louz et al. (1997), and finally, spontaneous OHSS and low hCG has been reported by Todros et al. (1999).

RECURRENT OHSS

A series of cases of recurrent OHSS have been reported, with the development of the syndrome in 2−6 consecutive pregnancies (Zalel et al., 1995; Olatunbosun et al., 1996; Di Carlo et al., 1997; Edi-Osagie and Hopkins, 1997). Zalel et al. (1992) reported a case of OHSS in a spontaneous cycle in a patient with PCOS. The same authors reported a recurrence of OHSS in a spontaneous pregnancy in the same patient with PCOS (Zalel et al., 1995).

FAMILIAL OHSS

Di Carlo et al. (1997) reported the first case of spontaneous, familial, recurrent OHSS, associated with high concentrations of renin and aldosterone. Both the patient and her only sister had suffered from a similar condition in their previous pregnancies. The authors suggested that similar cases of spontaneous OHSS, when admitted to a surgical emergency department, may undergo unnecessary surgical treatment by medical staff with no experience in reproductive medicine. With the increasing awareness of these conditions, more and more cases should be detected and reported. More recently, mutations of the FSH receptor have been reported as the cause of recurrent familial OHSS (Vasseur et al., 2003; Smits et al., 2003; Montanelli et al., 2004a, b). These elegant cases explain not only the occurrence of familial OHSS but also the occurrence of spontaneous cases without exogenous gonado-trophins. The clinical presentation of four pregnancies associated with spontaneous OHSS in a patient with a mutant FSH receptor has been described by Smits et al. (2003) (Table II.9).

HYPOTHYROIDISM AND OHSS

OHSS has been reported in association with hypothyroidism (Rotmensch and Scommegna, 1989; Nappi et al., 1998). Rotmensch and Scommegna (1989) reported the first case of OHSS in a hypothyroid, non-pregnant patient with Down's syndrome. This case deserves a special mention because it antedates the recent studies, where mutation of the FSH receptor was found to be the cause of

Table II.9 Clinical data of the four pregnancies associated with spontaneous ovarian hyperstimulation syndrome in a patient with mutant FSH
Reproduced with permission from Smits et al. (2003). N Eng J Med **349**:760–6

Week of gestation at first ultrasound	Ovaries		Symptoms	HCG level IU/l	Diagnosis	Management	Fetal outcome	Follow-up ultrasound
	Aspect	Size						
First pregnancy, 13	enlarged, multicystic	NA	NA	NA	theca lutein cysts	untreated	term delivery, healthy girl, 2655 g	complete regression at 8 weeks postpartum
Second pregnancy, 14	enlarged, multicystic	13×14 cm each	fluid visible in pelvis and right hypochondrium on ultrasonography	NA	spontaneous OHSS, Grade IV	untreated	in utero fetal death, 41.5 weeks. 2800 g	complete regression at 12 weeks postpartum
Third pregnancy, 9	enlarged, multicystic	14.5×12.5 cm each	hydrothorax, abdominal distension with ascitic fluid visible in abdomen and pelvis on ultrasonography	36, 200 (9 weeks); 21, 350 (10 weeks 3 days); 7430 (10 weeks 5 days)	spontaneous OHSS, Grade IV	paracentesis	nonviable fetus at 10 weeks 3 days gestation; curettage at 10 weeks 6 days	complete regression at 8 weeks after miscarriage
Before pregnancy	multiple subcapsular follicles, 5–8 mm in diameter	4.2×3.2, 4.5×3.5 cm						
Fourth pregnancy, 8	enlarged, multicystic thin hyperechogenic follicles	14×16 cm each	hydrothorax, abdominal distension with ascites; fluid visible in abdomen and pelvis on ultrasonography	101, 190 (8 weeks)	spontaneous OHSS, Grade IV	paracentesis	term delivery, healthy boy, 2860 g	complete regression at 8 weeks postpartum

OHSS, and in at least two cases the mutant FSH receptors were sensitive to TSH (Vasseur et al., 2003; Smits et al., 2003). A 21-year-old black, nulligravid woman with Down's syndrome presented with a two-week history of increasing lower abdominal extension and pain. She denied nausea, vomiting, fever and chills, vaginal bleeding and sexual activity. A pelvic ultrasonogram showed multilateral ovarian cysts with a solid component on the right ovary measuring 10×13.8 mm in diameter. Ascites was noted and a chest X-ray was within normal limits. The urine pregnancy test was negative and the patient was treated with levothyroxin and managed conservatively, and after 16 days her symptoms markedly improved. The authors proceeded to do an exploratory laparotomy because of the presence of the solid components on the ovary and the previous reports of ovarian malignancies masquerading as OHSS. The pathology showed benign follicular cysts. This case is interesting because the patient did not receive exogenous ovarian stimulation and her endogenous gonadotrophin levels were within normal limits. The authors suggested a causal link between the patient's profound hypothyroidism and the development of OHSS because of the temporal relationship between the two and the marked response to thyroid hormone replacement therapy. More recently, a case of familial gestational hyperthyroidism, caused by a mutant thyrotropin receptor hypersensitive to human chorionic gonadotrophin, has been reported (Rodien et al., 1998).

SPONTANEOUS OHSS AND DVT

Todros et al. (1999) have reported a case of DVT associated with spontaneous OHSS, which means that many of the thromboembolic cases seen with OHSS are not related to exogenous gonadotrophins.

THE ROLE OF AN OHSS REGISTRY

The establishment of a reliable OHSS registry is of prime importance. It will serve multiple purposes and have potential advantages for the care of all IVF patients. It will be an accurate method for comparing the incidence of OHSS if the demography of the patients is in the database. It will also identify complications that could not be avoided, and in my opinion that is an important aspect of patient care. Finally, guidelines for treatment could be based on outcomes rather than impressions, particularly in critical cases.

So far, the collection of data on severe and critical OHSS cases has been an informal task for many of us over the last two decades. The European Society for Human Reproduction and Embryology (ESHRE) and the American Society for Reproductive Medicine (ASRM) should take the lead in this important task. A large group of international investigators have taken a lead in the last decade in the study of pathophysiology and prevention of OHSS, and certainly would be more than capable of expanding their role.

REFERENCES

Aboulghar MA, Mansour RT, Serour GI et al. (1992). Follicular aspiration does not protect against the development of ovarian hyperstimulation syndrome after GNRH-agonist/HMG superovulation for in-vitro fertilization. *J Assist Reprod Genet* **9**:238−43.

Aboulghar MA, Rizk B & Mansour RT (1998a). Robert Edwards: a legend of the twentieth century. *Middle East Feril Soc J* **3**:2−3.

Aboulghar MA, Mansour RT, Serour GI et al. (1998b). Recombinant follicle stimulating hormone in the treatment of patients with history of severe ovarian hyperstimulation syndrome. *Ferti Steril* **69**(3 suppl. 2):72S−75S.

Abramov Y, El-chalal U & Schenker JG (1998). Febrile morbidity in severe and critical ovarian hyperstimulation syndrome: a multicenter study. *Hum Reprod* **13**:3128−31.

Abramov Y, Elchalal U & Schenker JG (1999). An 'epidemic' of severe OHSS: a price we have to pay? *Hum Reprod* **14**:2181−3.

Abu-Louz SK, Ahmed AA & Swan RW (1997). Spontaneous ovarian hyperstimulation syndrome with pregnancy. *Am J Obstet Gynecol* **177**:476−7.

Albano C, Smitz J, Camus M et al. (1996). Pregnancy and birth in an in-vitro fertilization cycle after controlled ovarian stimulation in a woman with a history of allergic reactin to human menopausal gonadotrophin. *Hum Reprod* **11**:1632−4.

Albano C, Felberbaum RE, Smitz J et al. (2000). Ovarian stimulation with hMG: results of a prospective randomized phase III European study comparing the luteinizing hormone-releasing hormone (LHRH)-antagonist cetrorelix and the LHRH-agonist buserelin. *Hum Reprod* **15**:526−31.

Asch RH, Li HP, Balmeceda JP et al. (1991). Severe ovarian hyperstimulation syndrome in assisted reproductive technology: definition of high risk groups. *Hum Reprod* **6**:1395−9.

Ayhan A, Tuncer ZS & Aksu AT (1996). Ovarian hyperstimulation syndrome associated with spontaneous pregnancy. *Hum Reprod* **11**:1600−1.

Balen AH, Conway GS, Kaltsas G et al. (1995). Polycystic ovary syndrome: the spectrum of the disorder in 1741 patients. *Hum Reprod* **8**:2107−11.

Balen AH, MacDougall J & Jacobs HS (1999). Polycystic ovaries and their relevance to assisted conception. In (Brinsden PR, Ed.), *A Textbook of In-vitro Fertilization and Assisted Reproduction*, Second Edition. Carnforth, UK: The Parthenon Publishing Group, Chapter 8, pp. 109−29.

Balen AH, Mulders AG, Fauser BC et al. (2004). Pharmacodynamics of a single low dose of long-acting recombinant follicle-stimulating hormone (FSH carboxy terminal peptide, corofollitropin alfa) in women with World Health Organization Group II anovulatory infertility. *J Clin Endocrinol Metab* **89**:6297−304.

Bayram N, van Wely M & van der Veen F (2001). Recombinant FSH versus urinary gonadotrophins or recombinant FSH for ovulation induction for subfertility associated with polycystic ovary syndrome. *The Cochrane Database of Systematic Reviews* 2001; Issue 2. Art. No. CD002121. DOI. 10.1002/14651858.CD002121.

Beckers NG, Macklon NS, Devroey P et al. (2003). First live birth after ovarian stimulation using a chimeric long-acting human recombinant follicle-stimulating hormone (FSH) agonist (recFSH-CTP) for in vitro fertilization. *Fertil Steril* **79**:621−3.

Belaisch-Allart J, De Mouzon J (1989). The effect of luteal phase supplementation with hCG after ovulation stimulation using a LHRH/hMG analogue in in vitro fertilization programmes. *Contracept Fertil Sex* **17**:747−8.

Belaisch-Allart J, Testart J & Frydman R (1989). Utilization of GnRH agonists for poor responders in an IVF programme. *Hum Reprod* **4**:33−4.

Bider D, Menashe Y, Oelsner G et al. (1989). Ovarian hyperstimulation due to exogenous gonadotrophin administration. *Acta Obstet Gynecol Scand* **69**:511−14.

Bilan FIVNAT (1989). Responses aux stimulations de l'ovulation dans les proceations medicalement assistes (PMA). *Contracep Fertil Sex* **18**:592−4.

Blankstein J, Shalev J, Saadon T et al. (1987). Ovarian hyperstimulation syndrome prediction by number and size of preovulatory ovarian follicles. *Fertil Steril* **47**:597−602.

Borenstein R, Elfiyalah N, Limonfeld B et al. (1989). Severe ovarian hyperstimulation syndrome as a re-evaluated approach. *Fertil Steril* **51**:791−5.

Borenstein R, Elhalah U, Lunenfeld B et al. (1989). Severe ovarian hyperstimulation syndrome as a re-evaluated approach. *Fertil Steril* **51**:791−5.

Bouloux PM, Handelsman DJ, Jockenhovel F et al. (2001). First human exposure to FSH-CTP in hypogonadotrophic hypogonadal males. *Hum Reprod* **16**:1592−7.

Brown P, Preece MA & Will RG (1992). Friendly fire in medicine: hormones, homografts, and Creutzfeldt−Jakob disease. *Lancet* **340**:24−7.

Buvat J & Buvat-Herbaut M (1986). Stratégie de l'induction de l'ovulationen cas d'anovulation normoprolactinémique. In (Buvat J & Bringer J, Ed.), *Induction et Stimulation de L'Ovulation*. Paris: Doin Publishers, p. 173.

Buvat J, Buvat-Herbaut M, Marcolin G et al. (1989). Purified follicle stimulating hormone in polycystic ovary syndrome: slow administration is safer and more effective. *Fertil Steril* **5**:553−59.

Campo S, Bezzi I & Garcea N (2000). Ovarian hyperstimulation after administration of triptorelin therapy to a patient with polycystic ovary syndrome. *Fertil Steril* **73**:1256−8.

Cappa F, Pasqua C, Tobia M et al. (1976). Ascites and hydrothorax due to endogenous hyperstimulation of hCG in a case of hydatiform mole destruens with secondary irreversible kidney insufficiency due to disseminated intravascular coagulation. *Riv Ital Ginecol* **56**:363−8.

Carmina E & Lobo RA (1999). Polycystic ovary syndrome (PCOS): arguably the most common endocrinopathy associated with significant morbidity in women. *J Clin Endocrinol Metab* **84**:1897−9.

Caspi E, Levom S, Bukovsky I et al. (1974). Induction of pregnancy with human gonadotrophin after clomiphene failure in menstruating ovulatory infertility patients. *Israeli J Med Sci* **10**:249−58.

Chae HD, Park EJ, Kim SH et al. (2001). Ovarian hyperstimulation syndrome complicating a spontaneous singleton pregnancy: a case report. *J Assist Reprod Genet* **18**:120−3.

Chang RJ (2004). Polycystic ovary syndrome and hyperandrogenic states. In (Strauss, Barbieri, Eds), *Yen and Jaffe's Reproductive Endocrinology: Physiology, Pathophysiology and Clinical Management*, 5th edition. Philadelphia: Elsevier & Saunders, Chapter 19, p. 600.

Charbonnel B, Krempf M, Blanchard P et al. (1987). Induction of ovulation in polycystic ovary syndrome with a combination of luteinizing hormone releasing hormone analogue and exogenous gonadotropins. *Fertil Steril* **47**:920−4.

Check JH, Wu CH, Gocial B et al. (1985). Severe ovarian hyper-stimulation syndrome from treatment with urinary follicle stimulating hormone: two cases. *Fertil Steril* **43**:317−20.

Check JH, Choe JK, Nazari A et al. (2000). Ovarian hyperstimulation can reduce uterine receptivity. A case report. *Clin Exp Obstet Gynecol* **27**:89−91.

Cochius JI, Burns RJ, Blumbergs PC et al. (1990). Creutzfeldt−Jakob disease in a recipient of human pituitary-derived gonadotrophin. *Aust NZ J Med* **20**:592−3.

Daya S (2002). Updated meta-analysis of recombinant follicle-stimulating hormone (FSH) versus urinary FSH for ovarian stimulation in assisted reproduction. *Fertil Steril* **77**:711−14.

Delvigne A (2004). Epidemiology and pathophysiology of ovarian hyperstimulation syndrome. In (Gerris J, Olivennes F, de Sutter P, Eds), *Assisted Reproductive*

Technologies: Quality and Safety. New York: Parthenon Publishing, Chapter 12, pp. 149–62.

Delvigne A & Rozenberg S (2002). Epidemiology and prevention of ovarian hyperstimulation syndrome (OHSS): a review. *Hum Reprod Update* **8**:1353–60.

Delvigne A, Demoulin A, Smitz J et al. (1993a). The ovarian hyperstimulation syndrome in in-vitro fertilization: a Belgian multicenter study. I. Clinical and biological features. *Hum Reprod* **8**:1353–60.

Delvigne A, Dubois M, Battheu B et al. (1993b). The ovarian hyperstimulation syndrome in in-vitro fertilization: a Belgian multicenter study. II. Multiple discriminant analysis for risk prediction. *Hum Reprod* **8**:1361–6.

Delvigne A, Kostyla K, DeLeener A et al. (2002). Metabolic characteristics of OHSS patients who developed ovarian hyperstimulation syndrome. *Hum Reprod* **17**:1994–6.

Devroey P, Van Steirteghem A, Mannaerts B et al. (1992). First singleton term birth after ovarian superovulation with rhFSH. *Lancet* **340**:1108–9.

Devroey P, Mannaerts B, Smitz OJ et al. (1994). Clinical outcome of a pilot efficacy study on recombinant human follicle-stimulating hormone (Org.32489) combined with various gonadotrophin-releasing hormone agonist regimens. *Hum Reprod* **9**:1064–9.

Di Carlo C, Bruno PA, Cirillo D et al. (1997). Increased concentrations of renin, aldosterone and Ca125 in a case of spontaneous, recurrent, familial, severe ovarian hyper-stimulation syndrome. *Hum Reprod* **12**:2115–17.

Donderwinkel PF, Schoot DC, Coelingh Bennink HJ et al. (1992). Pregnancy after induction of ovulation with recombinant human FSH in polycystic ovary syndrome. *Lancet* **340**:943–5.

Duijkers JM, Klipping C, Boerrigter PJ et al. (2002). Single dose pharmacokinetics and effect on follicular growth and serum hormones of a long-acting recombinant FSH preparation (FSH-CtP) in healthy pituitary suppressed females. *Hum Reprod* **17**:1987–93.

Dunaif A, Segal KR, Futterweit W et al. (1989). Profound peripheral insulin resistance, independent of obesity, in polycystic ovary syndrome. *Diabetes* **38**:1165–74.

Edi-Osagie ECO & Hopkins RE (1997). Recurrent idiopathic ovarian hyperstimulation syndrome in pregnancy. *Br J Obstet Gynaecol* **104**:952–4.

Edwards RG, Steptoe PC & Purdy JM (1980). Establishing full-term human pregnancies using cleaving embryos grown in vitro. *Br J Obstet Gynaecol* **87**:737–56.

Edwards RG, Lobo R & Bouchard P (1996). Time to revolutionize ovarian stimulation. *Hum Reprod* **11**:917–19.

Enskog A, Henriksson M, Unander M et al. (1999). Prospective study of the clinical and laboratory parameters of patients in whom ovarian hyperstimulation syndrome developed during controlled ovarian hyperstimulation for in vitro fertilization. *Fertil Steril* **71**:808–14.

European and Israeli Study Group on Highly Purified Menotropin versus Recombinant Follicle-Stimulating Hormone (2002). Efficacy and safety of highly purified menotropin versus recombinant follicle-stimulating hormone in in vitro fertilization/intracytoplasmic sperm injection cycles: a randomized, comparative trial. *Fertil Steril* **78**:520–8.

European Orgalutran Study Group (2000). Treatment with the gonadotrophin-releasing hormone antagonist ganirelix in women undergoing ovarian stimulation with recombinant follicle stimulation hormone is effective, safe and convenient: results of a controlled, randomized, multicenter trial. *Hum Reprod* **15**:1490–8.

European-Middle East Orgalutran Study Group (2001). Comparable clinical outcome using the GnRH antagonist ganirelix or a long protocol of the GnRH agonist triptorelin for the prevention of premature LH surges in women undergoing ovarian stimulation. *Hum Reprod* **16**:644–51.

Fares FA, Suganuma N, Nishimori K et al. (1992). Design of a long-acting follitropin agonist by fusing the C-terminal sequence of the chorionic gonadotrophin beta subunit to the follitropin beta subunit. *Proc Natl Acad Sci USA* **89**:4304−8.

Fauser BC, Devroey P, Yen SS et al. (1999). Minimal ovarian stimulation for IVF: Appraisal of potential benefits and drawbacks. *Hum Reprod* **14**:2681−6.

Fedorcsak P, Dale PO, Stroeng R et al. (2001). The impact of obesity and insulin resistance on the outcome of IVF or ICSI in women with polycystic ovarian syndrome. *Hum Reprod* **16**:1086−91.

Figueroa-Casas P (1958). Reaccion ovariaa monstruosa a las gonadotrophines a proposito de un caso fatal. *Ann Cirug* **23**:116−18.

Fluker M, Grifo J, Leader A et al. (2001). Efficacy and safety of ganirelix acetate versus leuprolide acetate in women undergoing controlled ovarian hyperstimulation. *Fertil Steril* **75**:38−45.

Forman RG, Frydman R, Egan D et al. (1990). Severe ovarian hyperstimulation syndrome using agonists of gonadotrophin-releasing hormone for in-vitro fertilization: a European series and a proposal for prevention. *Fertil Steril* **53**:502−9.

Fulghesu AM, Villa P, Pavone V et al. (1997). The impact of insulin secretion on the ovarian response to exogenous gonadotrophins in polycystic ovary syndrome. *J Clin Endocrinol Metab* **82**:644−8.

Garcea N, Campo S, Panetta V et al. (1985). Induction of ovulation with purified urinary follicle-stimulating hormone in patients with polycystic ovarian syndrome. *Am J Obstet Gynecol* **151**:635−8.

Gemzell CA, Diczfalusy E & Tillinger G (1958). Clinical effect of human pituitary follicle stimulating hormone (FSH). *J Clin Endocrinol Metab* **18**:1333.

Gemzell CA (1963). The use of human gonadotrophins in gynecological disorders. In (Keller, Ed.), *Modern Trends in Gynecology*. London: Butterworth, p. 133.

Golan A, Ron-El R, Herman A et al. (1988). Ovarian hyperstimulation syndrome following D-Trp-6 luteinizing hormone-releasing hormone microcapsules and menotropin for in-vitro fertilization. *Fertil Steril* **50**:912−16.

Goldfarb AF & Rakoff AE (1973). Experience with hyperstimulation syndrome during menotropin therapy. In (Rosenberg E, Ed.), *Gonadotrophin Therapy in Female Infertility*. Amsterdam: Excerpta Medica, p. 225.

Greenblatt RB & Barfield WE (1961). Induction of ovulation with MRL/41. *JAMA* **178**:101−10.

Hammond CB & Marshall JR (1973). Ovulation induction with human gonadotrophins. In (Rosemberg E, Ed.), *Gonadotrophin Therapy in Female Infertility*. Amsterdam: Excerpta Medica, p. 117.

Haning RV Jr, Austin CW, Carison IH et al. (1983). Plasma estradiol is superior to ultrasound and urinary estriol glucuronide as a predictor of ovarian hyperstimulation during induction of ovulation with menotropins. *Fertil Steril* **40**:31−6.

Hayden CJ, Balen AH & Rutherford AJ (1999). Recombinant gonadotrophins. *Br J Obstet Gynecol* **5**:793−9.

Hee-Dong C, Eun-Joo P, Sung-Hoon K et al. (2001). Ovarian hyperstimulation complicating a spontaneous singleton pregnancy: case report. *J Assist Reprod Genet* **18**:120−3.

Herman A, Ron-El R, Golan A et al. (1990). Pregnancy rate and ovarian hyperstimulation after luteal human chorionic gonadotrophin in vitro fertilization stimulated with gonadotrophin-releasing hormone analog and menotropins. *Fertil Steril* **53**:92−6.

Hooper AA, Mascarenhas AM & O'Sullivan JV (1966). Gross ascites complicating hydatiform mole. *J Obstet Gynecol Br Commonw* **73**:854−5.

Howles CM (1996). Genetic engineering of human FSH. *Human Reprod Update* **2**:172−91.

Hughes E, Collins J & Vandekerckhove P (2002). Gonadotrophin-releasing hormone analogue as an adjunct to gonadtropin therapy for clomiphene-resistant polycystic ovarian syndrome. *Cochrane Database Syst Rev*. CD000097.

Jewelewicz R, Dyrenfurth I, Warren MP et al. (1973). Ovarian overstimulation syndrome. In (Rosenberg E, Ed.), *Gonadotrophin Therapy in Female Infertility*. Amsterdam: Excerpta Medica, p. 235.

Jones HWJ (1996). What happened? Where are we? *Hum Reprod* **11**(Suppl. 1):7–21.

Jung BG & Kim H (2001). Severe spontaneous ovarian hyperstimulation syndrome with MR findings. *J Comput Assist Tomogr* **25**:215–17.

Leis D, Richter K & Schmid K (1978). Spontaneous hyperstimulation of the ovaries with luteal cysts and ascites during a twin pregnancy – extreme case of the syndrome of painful early pregnancy. *Geburtshilfe Frauenheilkd* **38**:1085–7.

Lewis C, Warnes G, Wang X & Matthews C (1990). Failure of body mass index or body weight to influence markedly the response to ovaian hyperstimulation in normal cycling women. *Fertil Steril* **53**:1097–9.

Lipitz SM, Grisaru D, Achiron R et al. (1996). Spontaneous ovarian hyperstimulation mimicking ovarian tumor. *Hum Reprod* **11**:720–1.

Loumaye E & Howles C (1999). Superovulation for assisted conception: the new gonadotrophins. In (Brinsden P, Ed.), *A Textbook of In-vitro Fertilization and Assisted Reproduction*, Second Edition. Carnforth, UK: The Parthenon Publishing Group, Chapter 7, pp. 103–8.

Ludwig M, Gembruch U, Bauer O et al. (1998). Ovarian hyperstimulation syndrome (OHSS) in a spontaneous pregnancy with fetal and placental triploidy: information about the general pathophysiology of OHSS. *Hum Reprod* **13**:2082–7.

Ludwig M, Felberbaum RE, Devroey P et al. (2000). Significant reduction of the incidence of ovarian hyperstimulation syndrome (OHSS) by using the LHRH antagonists Cetrorelix (Cetrotide) in controlled ovarian stimulation for assisted reproduction. *Arch Gynecol Obstet* **264**:29–32.

Lunenfeld B, Sulimovici S, Rabau E et al. (1962). L'induction de l'ovulation dans les amenorrhees hypophysaires par un traitement combine de gonadotrophins urinaires menopausiques et de gonadotropins chorioniques. *Comptes Rendis Soc Francaise Gynecol* **5**:30–4.

Lunenfeld B (1963). Treatment of anovulation by human gonadotrophins. *J Int Fed Gynecol Obstet* **1**:153–8.

Lunenfeld B & Insler V (1974). Classification of amenorrheic states and their treatment by ovulation induction. *Clin Endocrinol* **3**:223.

MacDougall MJ, Tan SL, Jacobs HS (1992). In-vitro fertilization and the ovarian hyperstimulation syndrome. *Hum Reprod* **7**:597–600.

MacDougall JM, Tan SL, Balen AH et al. (1993). A controlled study comparing patients with and without polycystic ovaries undergoing in-vitro fertilization and the ovarian hyperstimulation syndrome. *Hum Reprod* **8**:233–7.

Mannaerts B, Shoham Z, Schoot D et al. (1993). Single-dose pharmokinetics and pharmacodynamics of recombinant human follicle-stimulating hormone (Org 32489∗) in gonadotropin-deficient volunteers. *Fertil Steril* **59**:108–14.

Mathur RS, Akande AV, Keay SD et al. (2000). Distinction between early and late ovarian hyperstimulation syndrome. *Fertil Steril* **73**:901–7.

Moneta E, Menini E, Scirpa P et al. (1974). Urinary excretion of steroids in a case of hydatiform mole with ascites. *Obstet Gynecol* **44**:47–52.

Montanelli L, Delbaere A, Di Carlo C et al. (2004a). A mutation in the follicle-stimulating hormone receptor as a cause of familial spontaneous ovarian hyperstimulation syndrome. *J Clin Endocrinol Metab* **89**:1255–8.

Montanelli L, Van Durme JJ, Smits G et al. (2004b). Modulation of ligand selectivity associated with activation of the transmembrane region of the human follitropin receptor. *Mol Endocrinol* **18**:2061–73.

Muller P (1963). Gonadotrophines en Gynecologie. In (Beclere C, Ed.), *Ovulation Induction*. Paris, Masson, p. 137.

Nappi RG, Di Nero E, D'Aries AP & Nappi I (1998). Natural pregnancy in hypothyroid woman complicated by spontaneous ovarian hyperstimulation syndrome. *Am J Obstet Gynecol* **178**:610−11.

Navot D, Relou A, Birkenfeld A et al. (1988). Risk factors and prognostic variables in the ovarian hyperstimulation syndrome. *Am J Obstet Gynecol* **159**:210−15.

Olatunbosun OA, Gilliland B, Brydon LA et al. (1996). Spontaneous ovarian hyperstimulation syndrome in four consecutive pregnancies. *Clin Exp Obstet Gynecol* **23**:127−32.

Olivennes F, Belaisch-Allart J, Emperaire JC et al. (2000). Prospective, randomized, controlled study of in vitro fertilization-embryo transfer with a single dose of a luteininzing hormone-releasing hormone (LH-RH) antagonist (Cetrorelix) or a depot foumula of an LH-RH agonist (triptorelin). *Fertil Steril* **73**:314−20.

Papanikolaou EG, Tournaye H, Verpoest W et al. (2005). Early and late ovarian hyperstimulation syndrome: early pregnancy outcome and profile. *Hum Reprod* **20**:636−41.

Penzias AS (2002). Luteal phase support. *Fertil Steril* **77**:318−23.

Pentz-Vidovic I, Skoric T, Grubisic G et al. (2000). Evolution of clinical symptoms in young women with a recurrent gonsdotrophadenoma causing ovarian hyperstimulation. *Eur J Endocrinol* **143**:607−14.

Platteau P, Smitz J, Albano C et al. (2004). Exogenous luteinizing hormone activity may influence the treatment outcome in in vitro fertilization but not in intracytoplasmic sperm injection cycles. *Fertil Steril* **81**:1401−4.

Rabau E, Serr DM, David A et al. (1967). Human menopausal gonadotrophin foranovulation and sterility. *Am J Obstet Gynecol* **98**:92−8.

Rainhorn JD, Forman RG, Belaisch-Allart J et al. (1987). One year's experience with programmed oocyte retrieval. *Hum Reprod* **2**:491−4.

Raj SG, Berger MJ, Grimes EM & Taymor ML (1977). The use of gonadotrophin for the induction of ovulation in women with polycystic ovarian disease. *Fertil Steril* **28**:1280−4.

Recombinant Human FSH Product Development Group (1998). Recombinant follicle stimulation hormone: development of the first biotechnology product for the treatment of infertility. *Hum Reprod Update* **4**:862−81.

Regi A, Mathai M, Jasper P et al. (1996). Ovarian hyperstimulation syndrome (OHSS) in pregnancy not associated with ovulation induction. *Acta Obstet Gynecal Scand* **75**:599−600.

Reyad RM, Aboulghar MA, Serour GI et al. (1988). Bilateral ectopic pregnancy with an intact intrauterine pregnancy following an ICSI procedure. *Middle East Fertil Soc J* **3**:91−4.

Risquez F (2003). Induction of follicular growth and ovulation with urinary and recombinant gonadotrophins. In (Edwards R, Risquez F, Eds), *Modern Assisted Conception Reproductive Biomedicine Online*. Cambridge, UK: Reproductive Healthcare, Ltd, Chapter 9, pp. 92−110.

Rizk B (1992). Ovarian hyperstimulation syndrome. In (Brinsden PR, Rainsbury PA, Eds), *A Textbook of In-Vitro Fertilization and Assisted Reproduction*. Cambridge, UK: Parthenon Publishing Group, Chapter 23, pp. 369−84.

Rizk B (1993a). Ovarian hyperstimulation syndrome. In (Studd J, Ed.), *Progress in Obstetrics and Gynecology*. Edinburgh: Churchill Livingstone, Volume 11, Chapter 18, pp. 311−49.

Rizk B (1993b). *Prevention of ovarian hyperstimulation syndrome: the Ten Commandments*. Presented at the European Society of Human Reproduction and Embryology Symposium, Tel Aviv, Israel, pp. 1−2.

Rizk B (2001). Ovarian hyperstimulation syndrome: prediction, prevention and management. In (Rizk B, Meldrum DR, Devroey P, Eds), *Advances and Controversies in Ovulation Induction*. Proceedings of the 34th ASRM Annual Postgraduate Program,

Middle East Fertility Society Pre-Congress Course, ASRM, 57th Annual Meeting, Orlando, FL, pp. 23–46.

Rizk B (2002). Can OHSS in ART be eliminated? In (Rizk B, Meldrum DR, Schoolcraft W, Eds), *A Clinical Step-by-Step Course for Assisted Reproductive Technologies.* Proceedings of the 35th ASRM Annual Postgraduate Program, Middle East Fertility Society Pre-Congress Course, ASRM, 58th Annual Meeting, Seattle, WA , pp. 65–102.

Rizk B & Aboulghar M (1991). Modern management of ovarian hyperstimulation syndrome. *Hum Reprod* **6**:1082–7.

Rizk B & Smitz J (1992). Ovarian hyperstimulation syndrome after superovulation for IVF and related procedures. *Hum Reprod* **7**:320–7.

Rizk B & Thorneycroft IH (1996). Does recombinant follicle stimulating hormone abolish the risk of severe ovarian hyperstimulation syndrome? Abstracts of the 52nd Annual Meeting of the American Society for Reproductive Medicine. *Fertil Steril* S151–2.

Rizk B & Nawar MG (2004). Ovarian hyperstimulation syndrome. In (Serhal P, Overton C, Eds), *Good Clinical Practice in Assisted Reproduction.* Cambridge, UK: Cambridge University Press, Chapter 8, pp. 146–66.

Rizk B & Aboulghar MA (2005). Classification, pathophysiology and management of ovarian hyperstimulation syndrome. In (Brinsden P, Ed.), *A Textbook of In-vitro Fertilization and Assisted Reproduction.* New York and London: Parthenon Publishing, Chapter 12, pp. 217–58.

Rizk B & Abdalla H (2006). *Infertility and Assisted Reproductive Technology.* Oxford, UK: Health Press, Chapter I.4, pp. 54–8.

Rizk B, Meagher S & Fisher AM (1990a). Ovarian hyperstimulation syndrome and cerebrovascular accidents. *Hum Reprod* **5**:697–8.

Rizk B, Morcos S, Avery S et al. (1990b). Rare ectopic pregnancies after in-vitro fertilization: One unilateral twin and four bilateral tubal pregnancies. *Hum Reprod* **5**:1025–8.

Rizk B, Aboulghar MA, Mansour RT et al. (1991a). Severe ovarian hyperstimulation syndrome: analytical study of twenty-one cases. Proceedings of the VII World Congress on In-vitro Fertilization and Assisted Procreations, Paris. *Hum Reprod* S368–9.

Rizk B, Lenton W, Vere M et al. (1991b). The use of gonadotrophin releasing hormone agonist in programmed oocyte retrieval for GIFT. Proceedings of the VII World Congress on In-vitro Fertilization and Assisted Reproduction, Paris. *Hum Reprod* S368–9.

Rizk B, Vere MF, Martin R & Lenton W (1991c). *Short and long GnRH-hMG protocols of ovarian stimulation for fixed oocyte retrieval for assisted conception.* ESHRE Symposium, Cairo, Egypt.

Rizk B, Tan SL, Morcos S & Edwards RG (1991d). Heterotopic pregnancies after in-vitro fertilization and embryo transfer. *Am J Obstet Gynecol* **164**:161–4.

Rizk B, Manners CV, Davies MC et al. (1992). Immunohistochemical expression of endometrial proteins and pregnancy outcomes in frozen embryo replacement cycles. *Hum Reprod* **7**:413–17.

Rizk B, Aboulghar MA, Smitz J & Ron-El R (1997). The role of vascular endothelial growth factor and interleukins in the pathogenesis of severe ovarian hyperstimulation syndrome. *Hum Reprod Update* **3**:255–66.

Rodien P, Bremont C, Sanson ML et al. (1998). Familial gestational hyperthyroidism caused by a mutant thyrotropin receptor hypersensitive to human chorionic gonadotrophin. *N Eng J Med* **339**:1823–6.

Rosen GF & Lew MW (1991). Severe ovarian hyperstimulation in a spontaneous singleton pregnancy. *Am J Obstet Gynecol* **165**:1312–13.

Rotmensch S & Scommegna A (1989). Spontaneous ovarian hyperstimulation syndrome associated with hypothyroidism. *Am J Obstet Gynecol* **160**:1220–2.

Rotterdam ESHRE/ASRM Sponsored PCOS Consensus Workshop Group (2004). Revised 2003 consensus on diagnostic criteria and long-term health risks related to polycystic ovary syndrome (PCOS). *Hum Reprod* **19**:41−7.

Schenker JG & Weinstein D (1978). Ovarian hyperstimulation syndrome: a current survey. *Fertil Steril* **30**:255−68.

Schwartz M, Jewelwicz R & Dyrenfurth I (1980). The use of human menopausal and chorionic gonadotrophins for induction of ovulation. Sixteen years' experience at Sloane Hospital for Women. *Am J Obstet Gunecol* **138**:801−7.

Scommegna A & Lash SR (1969). Ovarian overstimulation with massive ascites and singleton pregnancy after clomiphene. *J Am Med Assoc* **207**:753.

Seibel MM, Kamrava MM, McArdle C et al. (1984). Treatment of polycystic ovarian disease with chronic low dose follicle stimulating hormone: biochemical changes and ultrasound correlation. *Int J Fertil* **29**:39−43.

Seppala M (1985). The world collaborative report on in-vitro fertilization and embryos replacement: current state of art in January 1984. *Ann NY Acad Sci* **442**:558−63.

Serour GI, Aboulghar M, Mansour R et al. (1998). Complications of medically assisted conception in 3,500 cycles. *Fertil Steril* **70**:638−42.

Shiau CS, Chang MY, Chiang CH et al. (2004). Severe ovarian hyperstimulation syndrome coexisting with a bilateral ectopic pregnancy. *Chang Gung Med J.* **27**:143−7.

Smits G, Olatunbosun O, Delbaere A et al. (2003). Ovarian hyperstimulation syndrome due to a mutation in the follicle-stimulating hormone receptor. *N Eng J Med* **349**:760−6.

Smitz J, Devroey P, Camus M et al. (1988). The luteal phase and early pregnancy after combined GnRH-agonist/HG treatment for superovulation in IVF and GIFT. *Hum Reprod* **3**:585−90.

Smitz J, Camus M, Devroey P et al. (1990). Incidence of severe ovarian hyperstimulation syndrome after GnRH-agonist/HMG superovulation for in-vitro fertilization. *Hum Reprod* **5**:933−7.

Soliman S, Daya S, Collins J et al. (1994). The role of luteal phase support in infertility treatment: a meta-analysis of randomized trials. *Fertil Steril* **61**:1068−76.

Southan AL & Janovsky NA (1962). Massive ovarian hyper-stimulation with clomiphene citrate. *J Am Med Assoc* **200**:443−5.

Steptoe P & Edwards RG (1978). Birth after the reimplantation of a human embryo (letter). *Lancet* **2**:366.

Tarlatzis BC & Billi H (1998). Impact of the use of recombinant follicle stimulation hormone. In (Kempers RD, Cohen J, Haney AF, Younger JB, Eds), *Fertility and Reproductive Medicine*. Amsterdam: Elsevier Science, pp. 103−112.

Taymor ML (1968). Gonadotrophin therapy. *J Am Med Assoc* **203**:362.

Thompson C & Hansen M (1970). Pergonal: summary of clinical experience in induction of ovulation and pregnancy. *Fertil Steril* **21**:844−9.

Todros T, Carmazzi CM, Bontempo S et al. (1999). Spontaneous ovarian hyperstimulation syndrome and deep vein thrombosis in pregnancy: case report. *Hum Reprod* **14**:2245−8.

Tulandi T, McInnes RA & Arronet GH (1984). Ovarian hyperstimulation syndrome following ovulation induction with hMG. *Int J Fertil* **29**:113−17.

Tyler E (1968). Treatment of anovulation with menotropins. *JAMA* **205**:16−18.

Van de Wiele RL & Turksoy RN (1965). Treatment of amenorrhea and anovulation with human menopausal and chorionic gonadotrophins. *J Clin Endocrinol Metab* **25**:369−74.

Vasseur C, Rodien P, Beau I et al. (2003). A chorionic gonadotrophin-sensitive mutation in the follicle-stimulating hormone receptor as a cause of familial gestational spontaneous ovarian hyperstimulation syndrome. *N Engl J Med* **349**:753−9.

Weissman A, Barash A, Shapiro H et al. (1998). Ovarian hyperstimulation following the sole administration of agonistic analogues of gonadotrophin releasing hormone. *Hum Reprod* **13**:3421–4.

WHO Scientific Group (1973). Agents stimulating gonadal functions in the human. Technical Report Series no. 514, World Health Organization, Geneva.

Zalel Y, Katz Z, Caspi B et al. (1992). Spontaneous ovarian hyperstimulation syndrome concomitant with spontaneous pregnancy in a woman with polycystic ovary disease. *Am J Obstet Gynecol* **167**:122–4.

Zalel Y, Orvieto R, Ben-Rafael Z et al. (1995). Recurrent spontaneous ovarian hyperstimulation syndrome associated with polycystic ovary syndrome. *Gynecol Endocrinol* **9**:313–15.

III

PATHOPHYSIOLOGY OF OVARIAN HYPERSTIMULATION SYNDROME

Rizk et al. (1997) have extensively reviewed the pathophysiology of OHSS. OHSS is marked by massive bilateral cystic ovarian enlargement (Figure I.1). The ovaries are noted to have a significant degree of stromal edema, interspersed with multiple hemorrhagic follicular and theca-lutein cysts, areas of cortical necrosis and neovascularization. The second pathological phenomenon is that of acute body fluid shifts, resulting in ascites (Figure I.2) and pleural effusion. Most investigators believe that these fluid shifts are the result of enhanced capillary permeability (Rizk and Aboulghar, 1991, 1999; El-Chalal and Schenker, 1997; Kaiser, 2003). This has been demonstrated in several animal models including hyperstimulated rats (Gomez et al., 2002), and rabbits (Schenker and Weinstein, 1978). More recently, Tollan et al. (1990) showed that, during ovarian stimulation for IVF, there is infiltration of fluid from the vascular space to the interstitial compartment one day before oocyte aspiration. Significant advances have been made in our understanding of the nature of the vasoactive agents involved (Figure III.1).

ROLE OF PERIPHERAL ARTERIOLAR DILATATION

In contrast to our classic concept of increased capillary permeability (Rizk, 1993a, b; Aboulghar et al., 1996; Rizk et al., 1997). Balasch et al. (1991) adopted a very different and interesting view. They studied the hemodynamic changes in severe OHSS and suggested that the circulatory disturbances are not secondary to reduction in circulating blood volume, but are a consequence of an intense peripheral arteriolar vasodilatation that leads to underfilling of the arterial vascular component, arterial hypotension and a compensatory increase in heart rate and cardiac output (Balasch et al., 1991). During the syndrome, all five patients studied showed arterial hypotension, tachycardia, increased cardiac output and low peripheral vascular resistance. They observed high plasma levels of renin, norepinephrine and antidiuretic hormone and increased urinary excretion of PGE_2 and 6-keto-$PGF_{1\alpha}$. However, it must be mentioned that none of their patients in this study had hemo-concentration − a common finding among patients with severe OHSS. Balasch et al. (1994) evaluated endogenous vasoactive neurohormonal factors and renal function in 31 patients with severe OHSS. These patients were evaluated at the appearance of the syndrome and four to five weeks later after the condition resolved. They recorded increased hematocrit and cardiac output, and decreased mean arterial pressure and

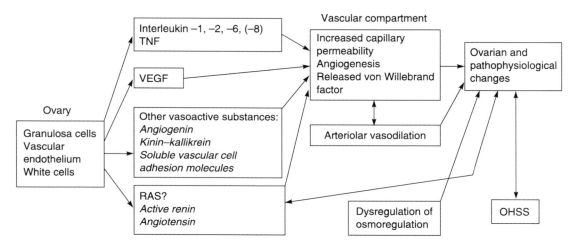

Fig. III.1: Pathophysiology of OHSS. TNF, tumor necrosis factor; VEGF, vascular endothelial growth factor; RAS, renin–angiotensin system

peripheral vascular resistance. This was accompanied by marked increases in plasma renin, norepinephrine, antidiuretic hormone, and atrial natriuetic peptide. Hemoconcentration was observed in 50% of the patients. Balasch et al. (1994) analyzed these results with and without hemoconcentration. They observed similar values for cardiac output, arterial pressure and peripheral vascular resistance. However, higher levels of renin, norepinephrine and antidiuretic hormone were observed in patients with hemoconcentration. The authors suggested that, in addition to increased capillary permeability, severe OHSS is associated with arterial vasodilatation. The argument is that if circulatory dysfunction occurred solely as a result of extravascular fluid shift, then we would expect that the contraction of the circulating blood volume would result in a reduction in the cardiac output, as well as an increase in peripheral vascular resistance as well as atrial natriuretic peptide. The actual findings were increased cardiac output and atrial natriuretic, and markedly reduced peripheral vascular resistance. The authors concluded that these findings indicate a marked peripheral arteriolar vasodilataion.

OSMOREGULATION IN PATIENTS WITH OHSS

The hemodynamic relationship between hematocrit and plasma volume was nicely illustrated by Van Beaumont in 1872. It is accepted that, in the face of a constant red cell volume, a rising hematocrit signifies a fall in plasma volume. It appears that, when the red cell volume remains constant, the change in hematocrit can never be numerically commensurate with the change in plasma volume. The change in plasma volume must always be larger than the change reflected by the hematocrit. Thus a change of two percentage points in the hematocrit from 45% to 47% is four times smaller than the actual 8% drop in plasma volume. It is extremely important to keep this in mind when treating patients with OHSS. Any increase in the hematocrit as it approaches 45% does not accurately reflect the magnitude of plasma volume depletion, and thus the seriousness of the patient's condition. Likewise, in the face of hemoconcentration, small drops in the hematocrit may represent significant improvements in plasma volume (Rizk, 2001, 2002).

Evbuomwan et al. (2000) performed a prospective longitudinal study on women undergoing ovulation induction to analyze the osmolality and hematocrit prior to the onset of clinical symptoms of OHSS. In OHSS patients, a 20% decrease of blood volume occurred between days two and four after administration of hCG. This was followed by a sustained 30% increase above baseline from day 8 to day 12 after administration of hCG. These blood volume alterations were not seen in patients without OHSS ($p < 0.006$). In OHSS patients an unexpected increase of 6 mOsm/kg in osmolality was observed during the later stages of follicular growth two days before hCG administration. Thereafter, the osmolality decreased from day 2 to day 12 after hCG administration. Decreased osmolality in severe OHSS is maintained despite significant increases and decreases in blood volume. In control patients, the osmolality decreased gradually from the beginning of gonadotropin injections until two days after injecting hCG and started to recover from the fourth day after hCG. This prospective longitudinal study is the first to track changes in osmolality and blood volume during spuperovulation, and in severe OHSS from onset to resolution. Previous studies have investigated women who already had the fully developed syndrome (Balasch et al., 1994) or who were pregnant (Haning et al., 1985). Evbuomwan et al. (2000) demonstrated that blood volume does not change significantly with superovulation alone, and that alterations in osmolality are observed in women even if they do not develop OHSS. The paradox of hypoosmolality with hypovolemia demonstrated during severe OHSS is suggestive of osmoregulatory adjustments. Furthermore, the unexpected but significant decrease in osmolality between two days before and the day of hCG administration in patients who developed severe OHSS demonstrates that significant changes are apparent even before hCG administration.

Evbuomwan et al. (2000) therefore postulated that the significant decrease in serum osmolality by day two after hCG may be achieved by a resetting of the threshold for arginine vasopressin secretion to lower serum osmolality values, as they have demonstrated in their second study (Evbuomwan et al., 2001). There is a precedent for the resetting of the threshold for arginine vasopressin secretion in pregnant women (Davison et al., 1981, 1984). The authors investigated the hypothesis that the decrease in and the maintenance of a new steady state in plasma osmolality and sodium level in OHSS are due to the altered osmoregulation of arginine vasopressin secretion and thirst. They found that the osmotic thresholds for arginine vasopressin secretion and thirst are reset to lower plasma osmolality during superovulation for IVF-ET. This new lower body tonicity is maintained until at least day 10 after hCG in OHSS. The decrease in plasma osmolality and plasma sodium levels in OHSS are due to altered osmoregulation rather than electrolyte losses; correction of apparent "electrolyte imbalance" in OHSS is therefore inappropriate.

INCREASED ERYTHROCYTE AGGREGATION IN OHSS

Levin et al. (2004) conducted a study to evaluate the erythrocyte aggregation in OHSS. The degree of erythrocyte aggregation is enhanced in the peripheral venous blood of patients with both COH and OHSS. This finding, known to cause capillary leak, may contribute to the pathophysiology of the OHSS.

IMMUNOGLOBULINS IN OHSS

The major event in the pathophysiology appears to be an increase in capillary permeability. Hypoalbuminemia occurs because of leakage of albumin into the third space, which is a well-established feature of OHSS (Schenker and Weinstein, 1978; Polishuk and Schenker, 1969). The status of other plasma proteins and specific immunoglobulins has been studied by Abramov et al. (1999) in 10 patients with severe OHSS after induction of ovulation for IVF. Significantly lower levels of gamma-globulins, specifically IgG and IgA, were detected in the plasma of patients with severe OHSS, whereas alpha-and beta-globulin levels, as well as IgM levels, were not significantly different from those in controls (Abramov et al., 1999). Both IgG and IgA levels increased as the patients improved. Ascitic fluid contained high IgG, moderate IgA and negligible IgM levels. Severe OHSS is therefore characterized by hypogamma-globulinemia attributable to leakage of medium-molecular-weight immuno-globulins, such as IgG and IgA, into the peritoneal cavity.

SOURCE OF THE PERITONEAL FLUID

In the absence of ovarian stimulation, the volume of normally present peritoneal fluid was found to be directly related to cyclical ovarian activity; it was consistently low in postmenopausal women and women on oral contraceptives. In normal ovulatory women, the volume of peritoneal fluid was diminished in the early proliferative phase and increased until the time of ovulation (Donnez et al., 1982). Following ovulation, there was a sudden increase in the volume of peritoneal fluid, which lingered throughout the luteal phase and diminished at the commencement of menses (Maathuis et al., 1978). Since this peritoneal fluid production was not dependent on the patency or presence of the fallopian tubes or uterus, its origin was felt to be ovarian or peritoneal.

Yarali et al. (1993) assessed the direct ovarian contribution to ascites formation in OHSS in the rabbit by the microsurgical isolation of the ovaries from the peritoneal cavity. Despite extraperitonealization of both ovaries, ascites occurred in all animals. This was considered to be evidence against a direct ovarian contribution to ascites formation. They postulated that the development of ascites was caused by a substance that increased capillary permeability of the peritoneum and the omentum, and possibly the pleura.

MEDIATORS OF INCREASED CAPILLARY PERMEABILITY

Extensive research has focused on the pathogenesis of increased capillary permeability in OHSS (Rizk, 1992, 1993a, b; El-Chalal and Schenker, 1997; Kaiser, 2003).

Estrogens

The association between severe OHSS and high estradiol levels is well established (Rizk et al., 1991). Asch et al. (1991) reported an overall incidence of 1% for severe OHSS, but when the estradiol concentration on the day of hCG administration was more than 22 000 pmol/1, the incidence of severe OHSS rose to 38%. Estrogens were shown to induce increased capillary permeability of the uterine and ovarian circulation. Because levels of estrogen are greatly increased in OHSS patients, it was postulated that the increase in its production and levels causes the increase in capillary permeability.

On the other hand, large doses of estrogens could not reproduce OHSS in the rabbit model. Furthermore, Pellicer et al. (1991) reported moderate to severe OHSS during pregnancy in a woman with partial 17, 20-desmolase deficiency and very low serum estradiol concentration. Levy et al. (1996) presented a case report of a woman with hypogonadotropic hypogonadism who developed severe OHSS during ovulation induction, with urinary FSH and hCG in the presence of low circulating estradiol concentrations. Therefore, the role of estrogen as a mediator of increased capillary permeability is seriously questioned.

Progesterone

It is well established that the use of progesterone rather than hCG in the luteal phase decreases the occurrence of late-onset OHSS (Rizk and Nawar, 2004; Rizk and Aboulghar, 2005). However, the role of progesterone in OHSS has been unclear, because of evidence of its ability to induce Vascular Endothelial Growth Factor (VEGF) and hence, vascular permeability (Novella-Maestre et al., 2005). Ohba et al. (2003) demonstrated that, in the rat model, hCG elicits VEGF production, whereas the potent progesterone synthetic antagonist decreases VEGF production in a dose-dependent fashion. The VEGF gene expression was stable. Their studies suggested that progesterone is implicated in part in the development of OHSS to enhance ovarian VEGF production by post-transcriptional and organ-specific control.

Novella-Maestre et al. (2005) have recently studied the role of progesterone on the VEGF expression in the ovary and vascular permeability in OHSS, using the rat model with dopamine agonists with or without progesterone. To induce clinical manifestations of OHSS, mature female Wistar rats (22 days old), were injected with 10 IU Pregnant Mare Serum Gonadotrophin (PMSG) on days 22 to 25 and with hCG 30 IU on day 26. This ovarian stimulation protocol has been shown by the authors to result in significant ovarian enlargement (ten-fold), ascites and increased vascular permeability, with maximum levels 48 h after the hCG administration (day 28). In the first set of investigations, Novella-Maestre et al. (2005) blocked progesterone synthesis by administering dopamine agonist on the day of hCG injection. The rats were treated with:

(1) Dopamine agonist, bromocriptine 100 or 600 µg
(2) Cabergoline, 3 or 10 µg
(3) Untreated (placebo group).

In the second set of investigations the previous study was repeated but the dopamine agonist treated rats were supplemented with progesterone pellets at a dose of 400 mg 24 h after hCG administration. In the first set of experiments, significant inhibition of vascular permeability, prolactin and progesterone synthesis was observed in the dopamine-agonist groups compared to the untreated rats. However, VEGF levels were unchanged. In the second set of experiments, progesterone administration recovered progesterone levels in the dopamine-agonist treated rats but was unable to recover vascular permeability or VEGF expression. Novella-Maestre et al. (2005) concluded that progesterone neither affects ovarian VEGF expression nor vascular permeability. It is postulated that the inhibitory effects of vascular permeability is due to apoptosis, or the post-transcriptional mechanism, and, furthermore, exogenous progesterone supplementation was unable to recover ovarian function once prolactin was deprived in this animal model.

The Ovarian Renin–Angiotensin System

The role of the ovarian renin–angiotensin system (RAS) in OHSS has been extensively investigated (Rizk, 1993a; Rizk and Abdalla, 2006). In humans, 90% of circulating renin is prorenin. The major source of plasma renin and prorenin is the kidney (Peach, 1977; Hsueh et al., 1983). However, the ovary is also a source of circulating prorenin, as has been reported in a bilaterally nephrectomized woman (Blankestijn et al., 1990). Prorenin is synthesized without conversion to renin in the monkey and the human ovarian theca cells and corpus luteum (Paulson et al., 1989). Luteinizing hormone (LH) and hCG switch on the renin gene expression (Itskovits et al., 1992; Lightman et al., 1987). In a spontaneous menstrual cycle, the peak of plasma renin expression occurs in response to the LH surge. In early pregnancy, there is an increase in plasma renin that correlates with the rise of hCG (Derkx et al., 1986).

Does the Ovarian Renin–Angiotensin System Play a Role in OHSS?

The role of the ovarian renin–angiotensin system in the pathogenesis of OHSS has been investigated (Navot et al., 1987; Pepperell et al., 1993; Morris et al., 1995; Aboulghar et al., 1996; Delbaere et al., 1997; Rizk et al., 1997). The angiogenic properties of human follicular fluid demonstrated by Frederick et al. (1984) in addition to the high levels of prorenin (Glorioso et al., 1986; Itskovitz and Sealey, 1987) renin-like activity (Itskovitz and Sealey, 1987; Fernandez et al., 1985a), angiotensin II (Culler et al., 1986) in the follicular fluid, as compared with the plasma, is the cornerstone of the hypothesis that the ovarian renin–angiotensin system is central to the pathogenesis of OHSS.

Fernandez et al. (1985a) demonstrated preovulatory follicular fluid levels of prorenin up to 12 times higher than those of plasma prorenin after gonadotrophin stimulation. The magnitude of the mid-cycle rise of prorenin in response to hCG is related to the number of ovarian follicles. Fernandez et al. (1985b), in a study investigating the development of new vessel formation in the New Zealand white rabbit cornea, concluded that angiotensin II not only facilitates the activation of pre-existing collateral vascular pathways but also has angiogenic properties, and could therefore play an active role not only in the fast but also in the slow phase of collateral revascularization characterized by formation of new vessels. Navot et al. (1987) studied plasma renin activity and aldosterone in patients with ovarian hyperstimulation. A direct correlation between plasma renin activity and the severity of OHSS was established. Elevated plasma aldosterone levels were observed in OHSS cycles, especially in conceptual cycles with OHSS. Pronounced elevations in plasma renin activity and plasma aldosterone concentrations were reported in patients with OHSS by Ong et al. (1991) despite significant therapeutic plasma volume expansion.

The investigations performed on the ascites collected from patients that developed OHSS rekindled interest in the concept of a significant stimulation of the ovarian renin–angiotensin system in OHSS (Pride et al., 1990; Rizk, 1992, 1993a). Rosenberg et al. (1994) observed a very high renin concentration in the ascites of severe OHSS compared to control ascites. Prorenin was the measured form identified. Delbaere et al. (1994) demonstrated levels of angiotensin II-immunoreactive 100 times higher in the ascites of severe OHSS patients compared with control ascites, and 6.9 times higher than in the plasma during OHSS. An ovarian origin of angiotensin II in the ascites was therefore suggested by Delbaere et al. (1994). The absence of a parallel concentration gradient between plasma and ascites for renin activity and angiotensin II-immunoreactive during severe OHSS prompted these investigators to evaluate more accurately the active as well as inactive levels of renin, together with their respective plasma-to-ascites ratio in the syndrome. Delbaere et al. (1997) measured total renin, active renin, prorenin, and aldosterone in the plasma and ascites of nine patients who developed severe OHSS. Total renin and prorenin concentrations were significantly higher in the ascites than in the plasma. The concentration gradient between the plasma and the ascites supports the hypothesis of an ovarian origin in the ascites, and to a large extent in the plasma also.

It is, however, likely that the high plasma renin and active renin activity reflect a peripheral activation of the renin—angiotensin system. Delbaere et al. (1997) concluded that their findings are consistent with a marked stimulation of both the ovarian and the renal renin—angiotensin system during OHSS.

Studies of Angiotensin-converting Enzyme Inhibitors and Angiotensin Receptor Blockers

Data on the effect of angiotensin-converting enzyme (ACE) inhibitors on OHSS in a rabbit model are conflicting (Rizk, 2001, 2002). Sahin et al. (1997) investigated the possible effects of the ACE inhibitor, cilazapril and the angiotensin II antagonist, saralasin on ovulation, ovarian steroidogenesis and ascites formation in OHSS in a rabbit model. They concluded that the ACE inhibitor cilazapril and the angiotensin II antagonist saralasin did *not* prevent ascites formation in OHSS. The ovarian renin—angiotensin system may not be the only factor acting in ascites formation in OHSS. Morris et al. (1995) conducted an experiment to determine whether the use of the ACE inhibitor enalapril would prevent the occurrence of OHSS in a rabbit model. In contrast to the work done by Sahin et al. (1997) ACE inhibition resulted in a 40% decrease in the occurrence of OHSS in the rabbit model (Morris et al., 1995).

Teruel et al. (2002) studied the hemodynamic state in 16 hyperstimulated New Zealand rabbits, and investigated the role of angiotensin II in the pathophysiology of OHSS. Angiotensin-converting enzyme inhibition decreases the incidence of OHSS in a rabbit model by 30%, suggesting that angiotensin II may plan a role in the formation of ascites. These authors also studied the effect of an angiotensin-converting enzyme inhibitor on renal function in OHSS in rabbits. They found that angiotensin II may play a significant role in this phenomenon, since angiotensin-converting enzyme inhibition normalized the pressure—natriuresis relationship (Teruel et al., 2001).

Ando et al. (2003) studied the efficacy of combined oral administration of angiotensin-converting enzyme inhibitor and angiotensin II receptor blocker in the prevention of early OHSS in IVF patients at very high risk of this syndrome. Four women who had estradiol concentrations of ≥ 8000 pg/ml were treated with a combination of the ACE inhibitor alacepril and the angiotensin II receptor blocker candesartan cilexetil for eight days, starting the day after oocyte retrieval. All embryos were cryopreserved and transfer postponed. Despite the extremely large ovaries, no ascites accumulated, and hematocrit and serum albumin remained normal. The authors concluded that dual renin—angiotensin blockage therapy may be useful in prevention of early OHSS. Further prospective randomized studies should be encouraged. It is tempting to speculate that ACE inhibitors may be useful in the treatment of OHSS in humans. Since severe OHSS commonly occurs with pregnancy, possible fetal effects are important (Rizk 1993a). ACE inhibitors may alter steroid synthesis within the ovary and inhibit ovulation (Pellicer et al., 1988), resulting in retention of oocytes and follicular fluid, leading to larger ovaries.

Prostaglandins

Prostaglandins have been investigated as possible mediators by Schenker and Polishuk (1976) and prostaglandin synthetase inhibitors have been used to prevent the fluid shift responsible for the manifestations of OHSS. However, Pride et al. (1986) found that indomethacin, in pharmacological doses, did not influence the clinical features of OHSS (ovarian weight and ascites formation). Katz et al. (1984) found indomethacin to be useful in the prevention of ascites associated with OHSS. However, the same group later demonstrated that that was not the case (Borenstein et al., 1989).

Therefore, the rationale for treatment of OHSS with nonsteroidal anti-inflammatory drugs should be seriously questioned (Rizk, 1992, 1993a; Rizk and Aboulghar, 1999; Rizk and Nawar, 2004). Furthermore, Balasch et al. (1990) suggested that renal prostaglandin PGE_2 and PGI_2, by antagonizing the renal vasoconstrictor effect of angiotensin II and norepinephrine (noradrenaline), play a major role in the maintenance of renal function in severe OHSS. They reported a case of prerenal failure in a patient treated with prostaglandin synthetase inhibitors.

von Willebrand Factor

The von Willebrand factor (vWF) is a large adhesive plasma glycoprotein produced mainly by vascular endothelial cells and released mainly as multimers (Handin and Wagner, 1989). The largest vWF multimers are stored in the endothelial cells in the organelles called weibel-palad bodies. The endothelium deposits vWF into the basement membrane of blood vessels (Meyer et al., 1991). von Willebrand factor is a marker of activation of endothelial cells. Its levels are diminished in von Willebrand syndrome and increased in clinical conditions characterized by endothelial cell dysfunction, such as pre-eclampsia in pregnancy and thrombocytopenic purpura. Plasma levels of vWF are raised by desmopressin due to a selective effect on endothelial permeability. This effect is used in the treatment of patients with von Willebrand syndrome (Mannucci et al., 1981).

Todorow et al. (1993) were the first to demonstrate elevated vWF in patients with severe OHSS, which subsided when the clinical syndrome improved. In a retrospective study, Ogawa et al. (2001) found that a rise of the serum level of vWF occurs before clinical manifestation of the severe form of OHSS, but not in patients with mild OHSS.

Endothelin-1

Endothelin-1 is a vasoconstrictor that increases vascular permeability that was observed to be 100- to 300-fold higher in follicular fluid than in plasma. In OHSS patients, serum endothelin-1 is elevated, but in parallel with other neurohormonal vasoactive substances and without correlation with the severity of OHSS, suggesting a homeostatic response rather than an initiating role in the development of the syndrome (Balasch et al., 1994).

VASCULAR ENDOTHELIAL GROWTH FACTOR

Discovery and Cloning

Rizk et al. (1997) extensively reviewed the role of vascular endothelial growth factor (VEGF) in the pathogenesis of OHSS. VEGF is a member of a family of heparin-binding proteins that act directly on endothelial cells to induce proliferation and angiogenesis (Gospodarowicz et al., 1989; Ferrara and Henzel, 1989; Millauer et al., 1993; Rizk and Nawar, 2004). Vascular permeability factor (VPF) was characterized as a protein that promotes extravasation of proteins from tumor-associated blood vessels (Senger et al., 1983). It was subsequently realized that the permeability inducing factor and the endothelial cell growth factor are encoded by a single VEGF gene. Several VEGF isoforms are produced from this gene by alternate slicing to form active disulfide-linked homodimers (Keck et al., 1989; Leung et al., 1989; Tischer et al., 1989).

The first human VEGF were cDNAs cloned from a phorbol ester-activated HL60 promyelocytic leukemia cell library (Leung et al., 1989) and histiocytic lymphoma cell line U937 (Connolly et al., 1989). Both the cDNAs were screened with oligonucleotides designed on the basis of the amino-acid sequence of the previously purified protein. The VEGF family (Figure III.2) includes four different dimeric forms (A–D) and placental growth factors, which all bind differently to the three receptors (VEGF-R 1–3) that are expressed on endothelial cells (Neufeld et al., 1999).

VEGF RECEPTORS

Tyrosine Kinase Receptors

Two VEGF receptors belonging to the tyrosine kinase receptor family have been identified and cloned: the VEGFR-1 and the VEGFR-2 receptors. The third VEGF receptor, VEGFR-3 receptor, is expressed in lymph vessels and binds VEGF-C and VEGF-D. These three receptors form a subfamily characterized by the presence of seven immunoglobulin-like loops in their extracellur part and a split tyrosine–kinase domain in their intracellular part. The homologous tyrosine kinase receptors, fms-like tyrosine kinase receptor VEGFR-1 (flt), and kinase insert domain-containing receptor VEGFR-2 (KDR), function as high affinity VEGF receptors (Millauer et al., 1993). KDR and flt are selectively expressed by vascular endothelial cells (Kendall and Thomas, 1993). VEGFR-1 is also expressed in the trophoblast cells, monocytes and mesangial renal cells. VEGFR-2 is also expressed in the hematopoietic stem cells, megakaryocytes and retinal progenital cells (Neufeld et al., 1999). The expression of VEGFR-1 and

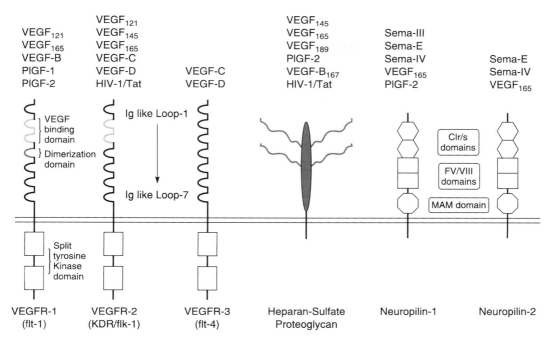

Fig. III.2: Growth factors and receptors of the VEGF family
Reproduced with permission from Neufeld et al. (1999). FASEB Journal 13:9–22

VEGFR-2 is affected by hypoxia, but to a lesser degree than for VEGF (Neufeld et al., 1999).

VEGF$_{165}$ Specific Receptor Neuropilin-1

Endothelial cells also contain VEGF receptors with a lower mass than VEGFR-1 or VEGFR-2 (Gitay-Goren et al., 1992). It was subsequently discovered that these smaller receptors of the endothelial cells are isoform-specific, and bind to VEGV$_{165}$ and not to VEGF$_{121}$. The binding of VEGF$_{165}$ to these receptors is mediated by amino acids residing at the carboxy terminal part of the exon 7 encoded peptide of VEGF$_{165}$. Two such receptors have been identified: neuropilin-1 and neuropilin-2. Neuropilin-1 also functions as a receptor for the heparin-binding form of placental growth factor. The neuropilins have a short intracellular domain and therefore cannot function as independent receptors (Figure III.2). No responses to VEGF$_{165}$ were observed when cells were expressing neuropilin-1 but no other VEGF receptors were stimulated with VEGF$_{165}$ (Soker et al., 1998).

VEGF GENE EXPRESSION

The human VEGF gene has been mapped to chromosome 6p12 and is made up of eight exons. Exons 1–5 and 8 are always present in VEGF mRNA, whereas the expression of exon 6 and 7 is regulated by alternative splicing. The phenomenon produces various VEGF isoforms which differ in length but have a common region.

REGULATION OF VEGF PRODUCTION

VEGF production is upregulated by hypoxia, cytokines and prostaglandins (Ferrara et al., 1992; Rizk et al., 1997). Cytokines and growth factors that do not stimulate angiogenesis directly can still modulate angiogenesis by impacting VEGF expression in certain cell types (Neufeld et al., 1999). In other words, cytokines may have an indirect angiogenic or anti-angiogenic effect. Growth factors that potentiate VEGF production include transforming growth factor β, fibroblast growth factor-4, platelet derived growth factor, insulin-like growth factor-1, interleukin-1β and interleukin-6 (Goad et al., 1996; Li et al., 1995; Cohen et al., 1996; Neufeld et al., 1999). VEGF production is downregulated by thrombospondin, hyperoxia and interleukin-10 (Enskog et al., 2001a, b). VEGF is produced and stored in granules in T-lymphocytes, mast cells, neutrophils and megakaryocytes.

VEGF Isoforms

VEGF-A, commonly known as just VEGF, exists in at least five isoforms of different molecular weights. Five human VEGF mRNA species encoding VEGF isoforms of 121, 145, 165, 189 and 206 amino acids ($VEGF_{121-206}$) are produced by alternative splicing of the VEGF mRNA. The major difference between the different VEGF isoforms is their heparin and heparin-sulfate binding ability. The most potent and well-characterized isoform is $VEGF_{165}$. It is made up of two subunits of 165 amino acids. The three secreted VEGF splice forms, $VEGF_{121}$, $VEGF_{145}$ and $VEGF_{165}$, induce proliferation of endothelial cells and in vivo angiogenesis.

Role of VEGF in Physiological and Pathological States

In vivo, VEGF is a powerful mediator of vessel permeability. It is also strongly implicated in the initiation and development of angiogenesis in thedeveloping embryo and in adult tissue undergoing profound angiogenesis, such as cycling endometrium and the leutinizing follicle (Charnok-Jones et al., 1993). In addition to its physiological role, VEGF is implicated as a critical angiogenic factor in the development of tumor vascularization (Kim et al., 1993) and the excessive neovascularization seen in conditions such as rheumatoid arthritis (Koch et al., 1994). Its levels are also increased in the peritoneal fluid of women with endometriosis compared with normal controls (Rizk and Abdalla, 2003; McLaren et al., 1996).

Role of VEGF in Reproductive Function and Ovarian Cyst Formation

VEGF may also play a role in the regulation of cyclic ovarian angiogenesis, and its ability to increase vascular permeability may be an important factor in the production of Fallopian tube effluent and fluid formation in ovarian cysts. Gordon et al. (1996) demonstrated that, in normal ovaries, VEGF within healthy follicles was localized to the theca cell layer with minimal VEGF peptide detected in the granulosa cell layer. VEGF was not expressed in atretic follicles or degenerating corpus luteum. However, intense VEGF immunostaining was observed within the highly vascularized corpora luteum. In normal ovaries from postmenopausal women, VEGF was detected only in epithelial inclusion cysts and serous cystadenoma. The authors concluded that, during reproductive life, VEGF plays an important role in growth and maintenance of ovarian follicles and corpus luteum by mediating angiogenesis. In addition, VEGF within the fallopian tube luminal epithelium increased the vascular permeability and modulated the tubal luminal secretions. Similarly, VEGF in the epithelial lining of benign ovarian neoplasms may contribute to fluid formation in ovarian cysts.

WHAT IS THE LINK BETWEEN VEGF AND OHSS?

The role of VEGF in OHSS has been extensively evaluated (Aboulghar et al., 1996; Rizk et al., 1997; Pellicer et al., 1999). The association will be discussed in this section but it has been very well summarized by Albert et al. (2002), who suggested three important reasons affirming the role of VEGF as a potential mediator in the development of OHSS. First, VEGF and its isoforms have vasoactive properties (Senger et al., 1983; Motro et al., 1990); second, VEGF has been identified in follicular fluid; and third, mRNA transcripts and proteins have been detected in granulosa luteal cells (Yan et al., 1993; Neulen et al., 1995a, b; Gordon et al., 1996). Finally, VEGF is increased in serum and peritoneal fluid of women who develop OHSS compared with control patients (Abramov et al., 1997; Agrawal et al., 1998, 1999; Artini et al., 1998; Ludwig et al., 1999; Aboulghar et al., 1999).

VEGF AS A CAPILLARY PERMEABILITY AGENT IN OHSS

McClure et al. (1994) pioneered investigation of the role of VEGF as the capillary permeability agent in OHSS. Two similar peaks of permeability activity were observed in OHSS ascites and liver ascites spiked with human VEGF (rhVEGF). No activity was observed in control liver ascites. Incubation with rhVEGF antiserum decreased activity in the two OHSS peaks by 79% and 65%, and in the two spiked liver peaks by 49% and 50%. In contrast, control serum produced 24% and 27%, and 17% and 0% reductions, respectively.

These results have led investigators to conclude that VEGF is the major capillary permeability agent in ascites fluid (McClure et al., 1994).

VEGF mRNA Expression in the Rat and Primate Ovary

Molecular biology studies suggest a strong link between VEGF and hCG, which is important in the development of VEGF (Rizk and Nawar, 2004). First, hybridization studies demonstrated VEGF mRNA expression in the rat (Phillips et al., 1990) and primate ovary (Ravindranath et al., 1992) predominantly after the LH surge. This surge is also essential for OHSS. Second, luteal phase treatment with GnRH antagonist to suppress LH secretion decreased VEGF mRNA expression, implying such expression is dependent on LH (Ravindranath et al., 1992). Similarly, luteal phase supplementation with progesterone rather than hCG decreases the likelihood of OHSS (Smitz et al., 1990; Rizk and Smitz, 1992; Novella-Maestra et al., 2005).

Low-dose LH Decreases VEGF Expression in Superovulated Rats

The administration of a combination of pregnant mare serum gonadotrophins (PMSG) and hCG in high doses induces OHSS, which is characterized by increased vascular permeability and overexpression of VEGF in the ovarian cells. It is established that hCG has a longer half-life than LH and a greater biologic activity expressed in a higher incidence of OHSS. FSH may also be related to the ovulatory changes within the follicle, based on the fact that there are cases of spontaneous LH surges without the administration of hCG or LH. Gomez et al. (2004) compared the capacity of hCG, LH and FSH to induce ovulation and simultaneously prevent OHSS in the animal model. Immature female rats were given PMSG (10 IU) for four days. Ovulation was triggered by using 10 IU of hCG, 10 IU FSH, 10 IU LH, 60 IU LH or saline. The number of oocytes ovulated into the tubes, vascular permeability and mRNA VEGF expression were evaluated and compared. All the hormones utilized in this investigation were equally effective in triggering ovulation, with similar significant p values when compared with saline controls. The administration of 10 IU of LH resulted in significantly lower vascular permeability and VEGF expression than that observed in the groups treated with 10 IU of hCG, 10 IU of FSH or 60 IU of LH. The authors concluded that FSH and hCG, as well as a six-fold increase in LH, demonstrated similar biologic acitivities, including increased vascular permeability, such as VEGF expression (Gomez et al., 2004). In fact, the lower doses of LH produced similar ovulation rates but, at the same time, prevented the undesired permeability changes and perhaps the risk of OHSS.

VEGF m-RNA Expression in Human Luteinized Granulosa Cells

Yan et al. (1993) were the first to demonstrate the presence of VEGF mRNA in human luteinized granulosa cells. Neulen et al. (1995a, b), from the same group, later demonstrated that the expression of VEGF mRNA is enhanced by hCG in a dose- and time-dependent fashion. VEGF mRNA expression in granulosa cells was enhanced by increasing amounts of hCG, with maximum enhancement at 1 IU of hCG/ml of medium. Further dosage increments revealed no additional augmentation of VEGF expression. VEGF mRNA expression also reached maximum values at 3 h. Kamat et al. (1995) used immunohistochemistry to demonstrate the increased activity of VEGF with Graafian follicle development, which reaches strong cytoplasmic staining for VEGF with the formation of the corpus luteum.

Is hCG-induced OHSS Associated with Upregulation of VEGFG?

Wang et al. (2002) investigated whether the effects of hCG on the pathogenesis of OHSS were mediated through the VEGF produced by luteinized granulosa cells. They measured estradiol, VEGF, and insulin-like growth factor II (IGF-II) in serum and follicular fluid, and analyzed mRNA expression in luteinized granulosa cells obtained from 101 women (58 with OHSS and 43 controls) who underwent IVF/ET. HCG upregulated VEGF expression of granulosa cells in the OHSS and not in the control group. Follicular VEGF worked through an autocrine mechanism using its kinase insert domain-containing receptor. The authors calculated total follicular production of VEGF by multiplying follicular concentrations by volumes. They verified that an increase in total follicular production of VEGF accounted for elevated serum levels of VEGF, which was associated with the development of OHSS.

VEGF Dynamic Studies and OHSS

A large series of investigations have been completed between 1995 and 2005 that address the relation between VEGF and OHSS (Delvigne, 2004; Rizk and Nawar, 2004; Rizk and Aboulghar, 2005). While many studies have reported the correlation between OHSS and serum/plasma, peritoneal fluid/follicular fluid VEGF levels, others have reported contradictory results with no difference between the OHSS and the control groups (Geva et al., 1999; D'Ambrogio et al., 1999; Enskog et al., 2001a). Delvigne (2004) explained several potential mechanisms for the contradictory results in the large number of VEGF investigations.

(1) VEGF can be measured in plasma or in serum but the clotting process increases VEGF 8- to 10-fold in serum.
(2) Degranulation or hemoconcentration in OHSS may cause misinterpretation of the real level of free, active VEGF.
(3) VEGF could be trapped in the ascites fluid and the large corpora luteal cysts of the ovary.
(4) The biologically active isoform of VEGF could vary from one patient to another.

(5) Immunoassays may not be able to differentiate between the four or more isoforms of VEGF.

(6) Soluble VEGF receptors may influence the biologic activity of VEGF.

Krasnow et al. (1996) measured VEGF in serum, peritoneal fluid and follicular fluid of eight patients considered at risk of OHSS. Serum VEGF was significantly higher in the group who developed severe OHSS compared with those who did not. The detection of high serum VEGF levels in the circulation of patients with OHSS suggests that this factor may play a role in the pathogenesis of OHSS. The large amount of VEGF in follicular fluid relative to serum or peritoneal fluid suggests that the ovary is a significant source of VEGF. In an unstimulated menstrual cycle, the development of a single corpus luteum does not result in OHSS. In patients with severe OHSS in whom VEGF was significantly higher in the serum, a mean of 21 follicles were present before hCG administration. It is possible that the hCG that rescues the corpus luteum results in an increase in ovarian VEGF secretion, which in turn causes an exacerbation of OHSS, confirming the work of Neulen et al. (1995a, b). The effect of follicular aspiration on the incidence of OHSS has been debated in clinical studies (Rizk, 2001, 2002).

Abramov et al. (1996) followed the kinetics of VEGF in the plasma of seven patients with severe OHSS from the time of admission to the hospital until clinical resolution. High levels of VEGF were detected in the plasma of all patients admitted for severe OHSS compared with controls, who received similar ovulation-induction regimens but did not develop OHSS after IVF and embryo transfer. Levels dropped significantly, accompanied by clinical improvement, reaching minimum values after complete resolution. A statistically significant correlation was found between plasma VEGF levels and certain biological characteristics of OHSS, and of capillary leakage such as leukocytosis with increasing VEGF levels. Ascitic fluid obtained from the study patients also confirmed high VEGF levels. These findings suggest the involvement of VEGF in the pathogenesis of capillary leakage in OHSS.

Lee et al. (1997) studied the relationship between serum and follicular fluid levels of VEGF, estradiol and progesterone in patients undergoing IVF, to quantify the effects of hCG on serum levels of VEGF during early pregnancy and to report serial measurements of serum and ascitic fluid levels of VEGF in a patient with severe OHSS. They found a significant ovarian contribution to the circulating VEGF levels in early pregnancy. They concluded that elevated serum VEGF levels may be a factor in the etiology of OHSS symptoms.

D'Ambrogio et al. (1999) found that serum VEGF levels before starting gonadotrophin treatment in women who have developed moderate forms of OHSS showed no significant difference with a control group.

Aboulghar et al. (1999) observed higher VEGF plasma levels in patients hospitalized for OHSS than in controls. The VEGF value dropped significantly with clinical improvement, reaching minimal values after resolution. There was a significant correlation between VEGF values and hematocrit as well as white blood cell count.

Agrawal et al. (1999) suggest that serum VEGF concentrations in IVF cycles predict the risk of OHSS, and that VEGF increases may predict risk better than the estradiol concentration, the number of follicles, and the number of oocytes, which individually predict only 15%−25% of cases.

In a prospective cohort study Enskog et al. (2001a) evaluated whether differences in plasma $VEGF_{165}$ concentrations exist during gonadotrophin stimulation in IVF patients developing severe OHSS compared to matched controls. They found that patients developing OHSS do not have raised plasma $VEGF_{165}$ levels during gonadotrophin stimulation. The lack of positive correlation between $VEGF_{165}$ levels and follicle numbers/progesterone in the OHSS group suggests a disruption of the normal controlled follicular VEGF expression in patients with OHSS.

The prognostic importance of serial cytokine changes in ascites and pleural effusion in women with severe OHSS was evaluated and compared with ascitic fluid in IVF cycles before oocyte retrieval. The results suggest that local cytokines may be involved in the evolution of severe OHSS and possibly serve as prognostic marker for this syndrome. Geva et al. (1999) concluded that pre-ovulatory FF levels are not useful predictors for the development of OHSS. The increased capillary permeability found in OHSS may be due to its systemic effect.

McElhinney et al. (2002) studied the variations in serum vascular endothelial growth-factor-binding profiles and the development of OHSS, and observed than patients who do not develop OHSS appear to have a high-molecular-weight protein (α-2 macroglobulin) that binds VEGF to a greater degree than occurs in patients who develop OHSS.

Gomez et al. (2002) reported that vascular endothelial growth-factor receptor-2 activation induces vascular permeability in hyperstimulated rats (Figures III.3 and III.4), and this effect is prevented by receptor blockade.

Fig. III.3: Time course of permeability among OHSS, control and PMSG groups, at different time points after hCG
*Reproduced with permission from Gomez et al. (2002). Endocrinology **143**:4339−48*

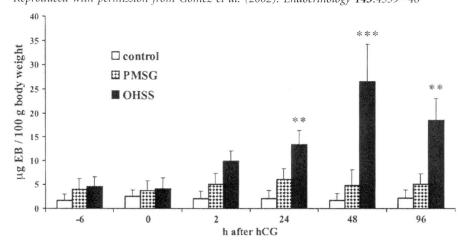

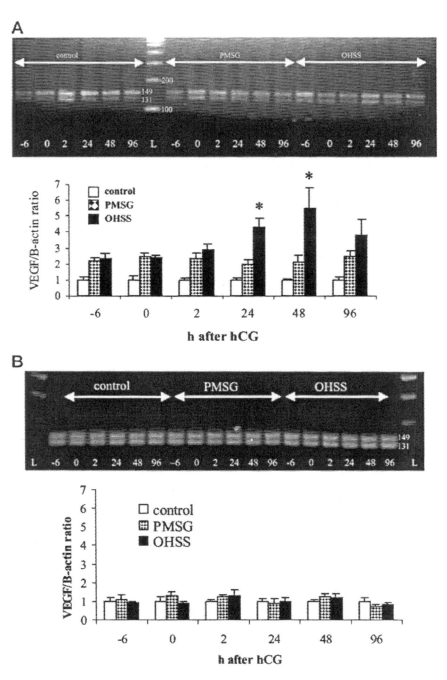

Fig. III.4: Reverse transcriptase polymerase chain reaction detection of β-actin and whole VEGF in the ovary and mesentery from OHSS, PMSG and control groups at different time points after hCG

*Reproduced with permission from Gomez et al. (2002). Endocrinology **143**:4338—49*

Mathur et al. (1967) studied whether serum VEGF levels can distinguish highly responsive women who subsequently developed OHSS from women with a similar ovarian response who do not. They found out that serum VEGF levels are poorly predictive of subsequent OHSS in highly responsive women undergoing assisted conception.

Artini et al. (1998) studied VEGF, interleukin-6 (lL-6) and interleukin-2 (lL-2) in serum and follicular fluid of patients with OHSS. Patients presented with follicular fluid IL-6 levels higher than both the patients at risk and control ($p<0.05$). On the day of the oocyte retrieval the patients developing OHSS showed serum and follicular VEGF values higher than those of the patients at risk ($p<0.05$). Serum and follicular fluid IL-2 levels showed no differences between the examined groups. IL-2, IL-6 and VEGF values were not correlated with each other. The authors concluded that angiogenesis and inflammation processes are both present in severe OHSS.

Gomez et al. (2003) observed that administration of moderate and high doses of gonadotrophins to female rats increases ovarian vascular endothelial growth factor (VEGF) and VEGF receptor-2 expression that is associated with vascular hyperpermeability.

Kitajima et al. (2004) observed that gonadotrophin-releasing hormone agonist administration reduced VEGF, VEGF receptors, and vascular permeability of the ovaries of hyperstimulated rats. They speculated that GnRH-a treatment may prevent early OHSS by reducing vascular permeability through the decrease in VEGF and its receptors.

VEGF in Follicular Fluid and GnRH Antagonist

Recent investigation of the impact of GnRH antagonist on IVF on the follicular fluid VEGF content demonstrated no change. VEGF follicular fluid content is associated with embryo maturation, gonadotrophins dose and those of follicular hypoxia. Some investigators reported an increase in follicular fluid VEGF concentration in poor responders, which is most likely a compensatory mechanism (Friedman et al., 1998).

VEGF Soluble Receptor

VEGF functions through a distinct membrane-spanning tyrosine kinase receptor. The c-DNA encoding a soluble truncated form of one such receptor, fms-like tyrosine kinase receptor, has been cloned from a human vascular endothelial cell library (Kendall and Thomas, 1993). The m-RNA coding region distinctive to this c-DNA has been confirmed to be present in vascular endothelial cells. The recombinant soluble human receptor binds VEGF with high affinity and inhibits its mitogenic activity for vascular endothelial cells. This soluble receptor could potentially act as an efficient specific antagonist of VEGF in vivo (Kendall and Thomas, 1993).

Free VEGF or Total VEGF

Alonso-Muriel et al. (2005) recently investigated the role of systemic total VEGF and free VEGF as well as its physiologic inhibitors, such as soluble receptor (sVEGFR-1) and α2-macroglobulin in the pathogenesis of OHSS. Alonso-Muriel et al. (2005) concluded that free VEGF and not total VEGF is related to the development of OHSS. The ratios of free VEGF to total VEGF and free VEGF to α2-macroglobulin could be useful predictors of the development of the syndrome.

Interleukins

Rizk et al. (1997) recently reviewed the role of interleukins (IL) in the pathogenesis of OHSS. There is growing evidence for a role of the immune system and, in particular, cytokines as mediators of pathophysiologic changes in OHSS (Mathur et al., 1997). Cytokines are a family of low-molecular-weight proteins that play important roles in the regulation of immunological and non-immunological homeostatic responses (Mathur et al., 1997). They exert their effects on cellular differentiation and activation.

Interleukins are a subset of cytokines originally thought to be lymphocyte products involved in interactions between leukocytes. Interleukins have a variety of actions on endothelium, fibroblasts and granulosa and luteal cells (Wang et al., 1991; Wang and Norman, 1992; Mathur et al., 1997).

Interleukin-2

Interleukin-2 is a glycoprotein with a molecular weight of 15 400 kDa. It is released from activated T-lymphocytes and is rapidly cleared from circulation with a half life of 3–22 minutes (Oppenheim et al., 1991). Interleukin-2 is not central in the cascade of events leading to OHSS (Aboulghar et al., 1999; Rizk and Aboulghar, 2005). Barak et al. (1992) studied the correlation between IL-2 and estradiol, progesterone and testosterone levels in periovulatory follicles of IVF patients. There was no correlation between follicular fluid IL-2 concentration and follicular fluid estradiol and progesterone concentrations. Furthermore, no correlation between follicular fluid IL-2 and serum estradiol concentrations was observed. Orvieto et al. (1995) elected to use pooled aspirated follicular fluid from each patient rather than to evaluate each follicle separately. They demonstrated a significantly higher IL-2 concentration in follicular fluid obtained at the time of oocyte recovery from patients who developed OHSS as compared with the control group. A possible role for follicular fluid IL-2 concentrations in the prediction of OHSS was suggested. In a multicenter study, Revel et al. (1996) found undetectable IL-2 levels in all samples of peritoneal fluid from patients with severe OHSS. Aboulghar et al. (1999) found these conflicting data for IL-2 levels in the peritoneal fluid difficult to explain. One possible explanation is the very short half-life of IL-2. Based on these studies and their own data, Aboulghar et al. (1999) concluded that there is no solid evidence for the involvement of interleukin-2 as the major mediator of vascular permeability in OHSS.

Interleukin-6

Circulating levels of IL-6 increase in a variety of acute illnesses including septic shock (Damas et al., 1992). IL-6 mediates the acute phase response to injury, a systemic reaction characterized by leukocytosis, increased vascular permeability and increased levels of acute phase proteins synthesized by the liver (Kishimoto, 1989). Interleukin-6 has been described in the follicular fluid in women undergoing stimulation. A role for IL-6 in normal ovarian function has been suggested by the observation that IL-6 mRNA is produced during the neovascularization or angiogenesis that occurs in the development of ovarian follicles. The rapid growth and luteinization of the stimulated ovary require extensive angiogenesis.

Friedlander et al. (1993) examined the role of IL-6 and other cytokines in four patients with OHSS. Five healthy women at the time of elective laparoscopic tubal ligation served as controls. Control serum was also obtained from healthy volunteers, and control peritoneal fluid was obtained from patients on peritoneal dialysis. Both serum and ascitic fluid from women with OHSS contained significantly greater levels of IL-6 than control serum and peritoneal fluid. No significant differences in tumor necrosis factor (TNF) levels in serum, ascitic fluid or peritoneal fluid could be found by enzyme-linked immunosorbent assay (ELISA) or bioassay. The mechanism by which IL-6 might mediate the pathogenesis of this syndrome is not clear. However, elevated levels of plasma IL-6 have been recorded in both acute pancreatitis and acute alcoholic hepatitis, conditions in which ascites and hypotension are common complications of severe disease. It was also found that the albumin level was markedly lower than would be expected in two of the patients with severe OHSS. This observation provides further clinical support for the hypothesis that IL-6 plays a key pathophysiological role in OHSS, because IL-6 is a potent inhibitor of hepatic albumin production, switching the liver to synthesis of acute-phase reactants.

Loret de Mola et al. (1996a) examined the production and immunolocalization of IL-6 in patients with OHSS. Significantly higher serum and ascites IL-6 levels were found in OHSS, compared with post-ovulatory serum and peritoneal fluid from normal controls or serum after menotropin stimulation. The same authors, having found a significant increase in cytokines in OHSS, addressed the possibility of whether preovulatory cytokine levels could predict the occurrence of OHSS. Preovulatory cytokine values were similar in OHSS compared to controlled ovarian hyperstimulation. They therefore concluded that cytokine measurement cannot be used to predict the occurrence of OHSS prior to the administration of hCG (Loret de Mola et al., 1996b).

Abramov et al. (1996) studied the kinetics of four inflammatory cytokines in the plasma of patients who developed severe OHSS after IVF. Higher concentrations of IL-1, IL-6 and TNF were detected in all individuals upon admission for severe OHSS. Concentrations dropped significantly along with clinical improvements, with normal values recorded after complete resolution. A statistically significant correlation was found between plasma cytokine concentration and certain biological characteristics of the syndrome, such as leukocytosis, increased hematocrit and elevated plasma estradiol concentrations.

Interleukin-8

IL-8 is a chemoattractant and an activating cytokine to neutrophils and a potent angiogenic agent (Rizk and Aboulghar, 1999, 2005). IL-8 is produced by a number of cell types including monocytes, endothelial cells, fibroblasts, mesothelial cells and endometrial stromal cells. Significantly higher peritoneal fluid levels of IL-8 were found in 12 patients with severe OHSS compared with 20 controls. However, no statistical significance was observed in the serum levels of patients and controls. This may imply a direct spill of IL-8 from the ovaries to the peritoneal fluid. Chen et al. (2000) suggest that follicular fluid IL-6 concentrations at the time of oocyte retrieval and serum IL-8 concentrations on the day of embryo transfer may serve as early predictors for this syndrome.

Interleukin-10

Manolopoulos et al. (2001) found high concentrations of IL-10 in peritoneal fluid and suggested a role for this anti-inflammatory cytokine during OHSS. 17 beta-estradiol and progesterone were elevated in peritoneal fluid and serum during OHSS but no correlation with IL-10 concentrations was found. Therefore, they assumed that IL-10 has a role in OHSS as a local mediator of inflammation; however, it presents different aspects of the OHSS than the sex steroids 17 β-estradiol and progesterone (Enskog et al., 2001b) (Figure III.5).

Interleukin-18

Barak et al. (2004) investigated the role of interleukin-18 (IL-18) in the pathophysiology of severe OHSS, its potential use as a marker of OHSS and correlation to capillary permeability. They studied 24 patients with severe OHSS in a prospective controlled study. Two control groups were used. The first consisted of 40 age-matched women without ovulation induction treatment, and the second group consisted of 19 women receiving the same medication as a group of 19 women who did not develop OHSS. Significantly higher levels of interleukin-18 were detected in the peritoneal and pleural fluids as well as the serum of the women who developed severe OHSS in comparison with the two control groups. Serum IL-18 dropped significantly when the patient progressed to the diuretic phase and resolution of OHSS. A statistically significant correlation was observed between serum IL-18 and capillary permeability, as judged by the hematocrit and white blood cell count as well as serum estradiol and IL-6 levels.

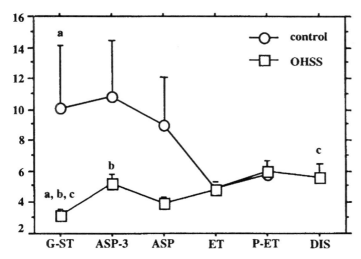

Fig. III.5: Interleukin-10 concentrations in plasma of OHSS and control patients
*Reproduced with permission from Enskog et al. (2001b). J Reprod Immunol **49**:71−82*

Angiogenin

Aboulghar et al. (1998) investigated the possible role of angiogenin in the pathogenesis of OHSS. The study group consisted of ten healthy women who developed severe OHSS, following ovarian stimulation by the long GnRH-a/hMG protocols for IVF. A control group of ten patients underwent stimulation according to the same protocol and did not develop OHSS. Blood samples were taken from the OHSS group on the day of admission to hospital for treatment and in the control group one week after oocyte retrieval. Ascitic fluid samples were aspirated during the routine aspiration of ascitic fluid as treatment for severe OHSS, and peritoneal fluid samples were aspirated transvaginally before oocyte retrieval in the control group.

In the OHSS group, the mean serum level of angiogenin, mean ascitic fluid level of hCG administration and the mean hematocrit were 8390 ± 6836 ng/ml, 2794 ± 1024 ng/ml, 6300 ± 2450 pg/ml and 46.6 ± 4.4; as compared with 234 ± 91 ng/ml, 254 ± 105 ng/ml, 1850 ± 1100 pg/ml and 36.8 ± 4.6 in the control group, respectively. The difference was highly significant between all parameters. Angiogenin seems to play an important role in the formation of neovascularization responsible for the development of OHSS.

THE ROLE OF SELECTINS AND ICAM IN THE PATHOPHYSIOLOGY OF OHSS

The selectins, a group of cell adhesion molecules, are major mediators of inflammatory, immunologic and angiogenic reactions (Rizk and Abdalla, 2006). Daniel et al. (1999) performed a prospective case-control study to determine whether plasma and peritoneal fluid levels of vascular cell adhesion molecule-1 (sVCAM-1) and soluble intercellular adhesion molecule (sICAM-1) are altered in women with OHSS. The study group consisted of 16 women with severe OHSS and the control group consisted of ten women treated with controlled ovarian hyperstimulation and eight women with normal findings at diagnostic laparoscopy. The mean peritoneal fluid levels of sVCAM-1 and sICAM-1 and the mean plasma levels sVCAM-1 were significantly higher in the women with OHSS than the control group. However, the mean plasma levels of sICAM-1 were comparable. The authors observed a positive correlation between the levels of plasma estradiol at the time of hCG and sVCAM-1, and between the number of oocytes retrieved and the levels of sICAM-1. Soluble cell adhesion molecules may therefore have a role in the pathogenesis and progression of OHSS (Daniel et al., 1999).

Daniel et al. (2001) carried out a prospective case-control study involving 16 women with OHSS. Ten matched women treated by ovarian stimulation and eight women with normal diagnostic laparoscopy results served as controls. Peritoneal fluid and serum were assayed for soluble endothelial selectin and soluble platelet selectin by specific enzyme-linked immunoabsorbent assay (ELISA). Significantly higher levels of soluble endothelial selectin and soluble platelet selectin were found in the peritoneal fluid of the women with OHSS compared with the basal levels in unstimulated women. Women with OHSS had significantly lower soluble serum endothelial selectin levels compared with those treated by controlled ovarian stimulation who did not develop OHSS. The serum soluble platelet selectin levels were similar in both groups. Daniel et al. (2001) concluded that ascitic fluid of women with OHSS contains appreciable amounts of soluble selectins, suggesting their ovarian origin and possible involvement in the syndrome.

Abramov et al. (2001) studied the potential involvement of the soluble endothelial cell-leukocyte adhesion molecules E-selectin and intercellular adhesion molecule (ICAM-1) in the pathophysiology of capillary hyper-permeability in the OHSS. Soluble ICAM-1 and soluble E-selectin are potentially involved in the pathophysiology of capillary hyperpermeability in severe OHSS.

ROLE OF THE IMMUNE SYSTEM IN THE PATHOGENESIS OF OHSS

Several cytokines have important functions in reproductive physiology (Adashi, 1990; Ben-Rafael and Orvieto, 1992). Immunochemistry reveals the presence in the ovary of T-lymphocytes that are capable of secreting IL-2. The human corpus luteum cell population has a concentration of macrophages at the junction of the theca, granulosa and lutein cells (Wang et al., 1992). Enskog et al. (2001b) hypothesized that patients developing OHSS may have a disturbed responsiveness or delayed activation of the immunosuppressive cytokine system. They performed a prospective cohort study on 428 patients undergoing IVF. Fifteen patients who developed severe OHSS were compared with matched control patients. Levels of IL-4, IL-10 and IL-13, estradiol and progesterone were measured throughout the stimulation and up to seven days after embryo transfer and during hospitalization for OHSS. Significantly lower levels of IL-10 levels were observed at the initiation of gonadotrophin therapy in OHSS patients with an increase observed after OHSS development. In OHSS patients, a negative correlation was observed between IL-10 levels and the number of follicles at the time of oocyte retrieval. No correlation was observed between IL-10 and steroid levels. Levels of IL-13 and IL-14 were low in both groups and did not change during stimulation. Enskog et al. (2001b) hypothesized that the lower levels of IL-10 at the initiation of stimulation in OHSS patients, as compared with controls, might be of pathophysiological significance by allowing for an enhanced Th-1 type immune response and therefore an increased and generalized inflammation (Figure III.5). The increase in IL-10 after the development of OHSS may suggest that IL-10 is induced in a systemic attempt to suppress the inflammation of OHSS.

ROLE OF ENDOTHELIAL CELLS IN THE PATHOGENESIS OF OHSS

The role of endothelial cells in the pathogenesis of OHSS was elegantly investigated by Albert et al. (2002). The hypothesis of involvement of the endolthelial cell was based upon their observation of high levels of VEGF in serum and lower levels of VEGF in the follicular fluid in women at risk of developing OHSS (Pellicer et al., 1999). This interesting observation suggested that cells other than ovarian follicles could be a potential cellular source and target of VEGF. To test this hypothesis, Albert et al. (2002) developed an in-vitro model using high estradiol and hCG concentrations in human microvascular endothelial cells. They investigated the ability of the micro-vascular endothelial cells to express and secrete the mediators that could be involved in the development of the syndrome.

The endothelium is a source of both VEGF (Banerje et al., 1997) and IL-6 (Van der Meeren et al., 1991). Once VEGF and IL-6 are produced, they may act at the paracrine and autocrine level, inducing the vascular changes leading to the syndrome. Receptors for both VEGF (Shweiki et al., 1993) and IL-6 (Mantovani et al., 1997) have been identified in luteal cells and have been shown to increase capillary permeability in human (Goldsman et al., 1995) and animal models (Rizk et al., 1997; Schenker, 1999).

Albert et al. (2002), in their study of the response of the endothelium, observed that hCG induced an upregulation of the VEGF receptor KDR in human endothelial cells. This receptor, the most functional receptor for human VEGF, transduces signals for mitogenicity, angiogenesis and cytoskeletal organization. On the basis of these findings, Albert et al. (2002) postulated that hCG induces the secretion and reception of VEGF in the endothelial cells, generating an acute response manifested by vascular permeability. The lack of a role of estradiol in the pathogenesis of OHSS was demonstrated when the presence of regulation of VEGF and hCG receptors was investigated. Estradiol alone was unable to upregulate either type of receptor at the messenger RNA or protein levels. Again, that it was the addition of hCG that induced a cascade of events that resulted in a significant increase of the VEFG KDR receptor.

The integrity of the endothelial cytoskeleton is important for the functional competence of an endothelial barrier. Permeability to water and solutes depend on the shape and configuration of the endothelial cells. Albert et al. (2002) used confocal microscopy to analyze the monolayers. They observed an irregular alignment and arrangement of the active filaments and morphological changes of cell shape and gap formation of adjacent cells and in HUMEC-L treated with estradiol and hCG, but not in endothelial cells treated with estradiol only. This effect was reversed by anti-VEGF. The authors deduced three important messages:

(1) that estradiol alone does not increase vascular permeability
(2) hCG acts through VEGF
(3) blocking VEGF action is a valid alternative to overcome the changes induced in the endothelium by hCG.

Albert et al. (2002) concluded that the endothelium along with the ovary is a primary target for hCG (Figure III.6). As a result, VEGF and its KDR receptor are stimulated, resulting in an acute biological response in the capillaries causing increased permeability. Blocking VEGF action with specific antibodies prevents the changes induced by hCG, providing the rationale for new therapeutic approaches to prevent or treat OHSS.

Fig. III.6: The role of endothelial function in the pathophysiology of OHSS
Reproduced with permission from Albert et al. (2002). Mol Hum Reprod 8:409–18

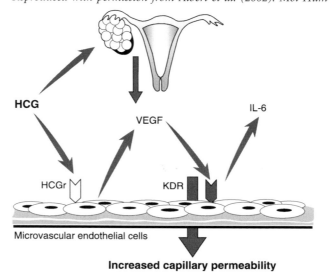

SPONTANEOUS OHSS AND GONADOTROPH ADENOMAS

Gonadotroph adenomas are benign tumors that arise from the gonado-troph cells of the anterior pituitary gland. They comprise approximately 10% of all pituitary adenomas (Snyder, 1987). Unlike most pituitary adenomas, such as corticotrope adenomas associated with Cushing's syndrome and somatotrope adenomas causing acromegaly, gonadotroph adenomas often do not cause a recognizable clinical syndrome (Snyder, 1985). The majority of patients will present with symptoms of intracranial masses (Kwekkboom et al., 1989).

Some of the clinical presentations in patients with gonadotroph adenomas resemble those with PCOS in several ways, such as infertility, amenorrhea and oligorrhea, and enlarged ovaries with multiple cysts. However, women with gonadotroph adenomas differ from those with PCOS in several ways (Castelbaum et al., 2002). Several cases of spontaneous OHSS associated with FSH secretion of pituitary adenomas have been reported recently (Djerassi et al., 1995; Christin-Maitre et al., 1998; Catargi et al., 1999; Valimaki et al., 1999; Pentz-Vidovic et al., 2000; Shimon et al., 2001; Castelbaum et al., 2002; Roberts et al., 2005). Roberts et al. (2005) recently reported a case of spontaneous OHSS caused by an FSH-secreting pituitary adenoma (Figure III.7). No ascites or hematological abnormalities were observed as in some of the reported cases, so, by definition, the patient could not be classified as having OHSS (Roberts et al., 2005). However, the ovaries were hyperstimulated and it is interesting to hypothesize the reasons for the absence of ascites in this case (Figure III.7), despite supraphysiologic serum estradiol levels.

Fig. III.7: MRI of gonadotroph adenoma
Reproduced with permission from Roberts et al. (2005). Fertil Steril 83:208–10

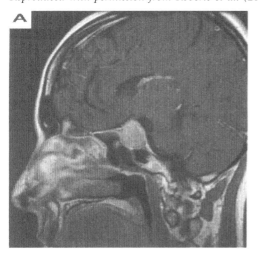
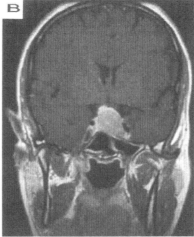

REFERENCES

Aboulghar MA, Mansour RT, Serour GI & Rizk B (1996). Ovarian hyperstimulation syndrome: modern concepts in pathophysiology and management. *Middle East Fertil Soc J* **1**:3–16.

Aboulghar MA, Mansour RT, Serour GI et al. (1998). Elevated levels of angiogenin in serum and ascitic fluid from patients with severe ovarian hyperstimulation syndrome. *Hum Reprod* **13**:2068–71.

Aboulghar MA, Mansour RT, Serour GI et al. (1999). Elevated levels of interleukin-2, soluble interleukin-2 receptor alpha, interleukin-6, soluble interleukin-6 receptor and vascular endothelial growth factor in serum and ascitic fluid of patients with severe ovarian hyperstimulation syndrome. *Eur J Obstet Gynecol Reprod Biol* **87**:81–5.

Abramov Y, Schenker JG, Lewin A et al. (1996). Plasma inflammatory cytokines correlate to the ovarian hyperstimulation syndrome. *Hum Reprod* **11**:1381–6.

Abramov Y, Barak V, Nisman B et al. (1997). Vascular endothelial growth factor plasma levels correlate to the clinical picture in severe ovarian hyperstimulation syndrome. *Fertil Steril* **67**:261–5.

Abramov Y, Naparstek Y, Elchalal U et al. (1999). Plasma immunoglobulins in patients with severe ovarian hyperstimulation syndrome *Fertil Steril* **71**:102–5.

Abramov Y, Schenker JG, Lewin A et al. (2001). Soluble ICAM-1 and E-selection levels correlate with clinical and biological aspects of severe ovarian hyperstimulation syndrome. *Fertil Steril* **76**:51–7.

Adashi EY (1990). The potential relevance of cytokines to ovarian physiology: the emerging role of resident ovarian cells of the white blood cell series. *Endocr Rev* **11**:454–64.

Agrawal R, Conway G, Sladkevicius P et al. (1998). Serum vascular endothelial growth factor and Doppler blood flow velocities in in vitro fertilization: relevance to ovarian hyperstimulation syndrome and polycystic ovaries. *Fertil Steril* **79**:651–8.

Agrawal R, Tan SL, Wild S et al. (1999). Serum vascular endothelial growth factor concentrations in in vitro fertilization cycles predict the risk of ovarian hyperstimulation syndrome. *Fertil Steril* **71**:278–93.

Albert C, Garrido N, Mercader A et al. (2002). The role of endothelial cells in the pathogenesis of ovarian hyperstimulation syndrome. *Mol Hum Reprod* **8**:409–18.

Alonso-Muriel I, Gomez-Gallego R, Pau E et al. (2005). Free VEGF but not total VEGF is responsible for ovarian hyperstimulation syndrome (OHSS) onset. *J Soc Gyn Invest* **12** (Suppl 6):87A.

Ando H, Furugori K, Shibata K et al. (2003). Dual renin-angiotensin blockade therapy in patients at high risk of early ovarian hyperstimulation syndrome recieving IVF and elective embryo cryopreservation: a case series. *Hum Reprod* **18**:1219–22.

Artini PG, Fasciani A, Monti M et al. (1998) Changes in vascular endothelial growth factor concentrations and the risk of ovarian hyperstimulation syndrome in women enrolled in an in vitro fertilization program. *Fertil Steril* **70**:560–4.

Asch RH, Li HP, Balmeceda JP et al. (1991). Severe ovarian hyperstimulation syndrome in assisted reproductive technology; definition of high risk groups. *Hum Reprod* **6**:1395–9.

Balasch J, Carmona F, Llach J et al. (1990). Acute prerenal failure and liver dysfunction in a patient with severe ovarian hyperstimulation syndrome. *Hum Reprod* **5**:348–51.

Balasch J, Arroyo V, Carmona F et al. (1991). Severe ovarian hyperstimulation syndrome: role of peripheral vasodilation. *Fertil Steril* **56**:1077–83.

Balasch J, Arroyo V, Fabregues F et al. (1994). Neurohormonal and hemodynamic changes in severe cases of ovarian hyperstimulation syndrome. *Ann Intern Med* **121**:27–33.

Barak V, Mordel N, Zakicek G et al. (1992). The correlation between interleukin 2 and interleukin 2 receptors to oestradiol, progesterone and testosterone levels in preovulatory follicles of in vitro fertilization patients. *Hum Reprod* **7**:926−9.

Barak V, Elchalal U, Edelstein M et al. (2004). Interleukin-18 levels correlate with severe ovarian hyperstimulation syndrome. *Fertil Steril* **82**:415−20.

Banarjee SK, Sarkar DK, Weston AP et al. (1997). Over expression of vascular endothelial growth factor and its receptors during the development of estrogen induced rat pituitary tumors may mediate estrogen-initiated tumor angiogenesis. *Carcinogenesis* **18**:1155−61.

Ben-Rafael Z & Orvieto R (1992). Cytokines-involvement in reproduction. *Fertil Steril* **58**:1093−9.

Blankestijn PF, Derkx FHM, Van Geelen JA et al. (1990). Increase in plasma prorenin during the mesntrual cycle of a bilaterally nephrectomized woman. *Br J Obstet Gynaecol* **97**:1038−42.

Borenstein R, Elhalah U, Lunenfeld B & Schwartz ZS (1989). Severe ovarian hyperstimulation syndrome: a reevaluated therapeutic approach. *Fertil Steril* **51**:791−5.

Buyalos RP, Watson JM, Martinez Maza O et al. (1992). Detection of IL-6 in human follicular fluid. *Fertil Steril* **57**:1230−40.

Castelbaum AJ, Bigdeli H, Post KD et al. (2002). Exacerbation of ovarian hyperstimulation by leuporlide reveals a gonadotroph adenoma. *Fertil Steril* **78**:1311−3.

Catargi B, Felicie-Dellan E & Tabarin A (1999). Comment on gonadotrophin adenoma causing ovarian hyperstimulation. *J Clin Endocrinol Metab* **84**:3404−6.

Chae HD, Park EJ, Kim SH et al. (2001). Ovarian hyperstimulation syndrome complicating a spontaneous singleton pregnancy: a case report. *J Assist Reprod Genet* **18**:120−3.

Charnock-Jones DS, Sharkey AM, Rajput-Williams J et al. (1993). Identification and localization of alternately spliced mRNAs for vascular endothelial growth factor in human uterus and estrogen regulation in endometrial carcinoma cell line. *Biol Reprod* **48**:1120−60.

Chen CD, Wu MY, Chen HF et al. (2000). Relationships of serum pro-inflammatory cytokines and vascular endothelial growth factor with liver dysfunction in severe ovarian hyperstimulation syndrome. *Hum Reprod* **15**:66−71.

Christin-Maitre S, Rongieres-Bertrand C, Kottler ML et al. (1998). A spontaneous and severe hyperstimulation of the ovaries revealing a gonadotroph adenoma. *J Clin Endocrinol Metab* **83**:3450−3.

Cohen T, Hahari D, Cerem-Weiss L et al. (1996). Interleukin-6 induces the expression of vascular endothelial growth factor. *J Biol Chem* **271**:736−41.

Connolly DT, Olander JV, Heuvelman D et al. (1989). Human vascular permeability factor. Isolation from U937 cells. *J Biol Chem* **264**:20017−24.

Culler MD, Tarlatzis BC, Rzasa PJ et al. (1986). Renin-like activity in ovarian follicular fluid. *J Clin Endocrinol Metab* **62**:613−5.

Cunha-Filho JS, Lemos N, Stein N et al. (2005). Vascular endothelial growth factor and inhibin A in follicular fluid of infertile patients who underwent in vitro fertilization with a gonadotropin-releasing hormone antagonist. *Fertil Steril* **83**:902−7.

D'Ambrogio G, Fasciani A, Monti M et al. (1999). Serum vascular endothelial growth factor levels before starting gonadotrophin treatment in women who have developed moderate forms of ovarian hyperstimulation syndrome. *Gynecol Endocrinol* **13**:311−15.

Damas P, Ledoux D, Nys M et al. (1992). Cytokine serum level during severe sepsis in humans IL-6 as a marker of severity. *Ann Surg* **215**:356−62.

Daniel Y, Geva E, Amit A et al. (1999). Levels of soluble vascular cell adhesion molecule-1 and soluble intercellular adhesion molecule-1 are increased in women with ovarian hyperstimulation syndrome. *Fertil Steril* **71**:896−901.

Daniel Y, Geva E, Amit A et al. (2001). Soluble endothelial and platelet selectins in serum and ascitic fluid of women with ovarian hyperstimulation syndrome. *Am J Reprod Immunol* **45**:154–60.

Davison JM, Vallotton MV & Lindheimer MD (1981). Plasma osmolality and urinary concentration and dilution during and after pregnancy: evidence that lateral recombency inhibits maximal urinary concentrating ability. *Br J Obstet Gynaecol* **88**:472–9.

Davison JM, Gilmore EA, Durr J et al. (1984). Altered osmotic threshold for vasopressin secretion and thirst in human pregnancy. *Am J Physiol* **246**:F105–109.

Delbaere A, Bergmann PJM & Gervy-Decoster C (1994). Angiotensin II immunoreactivity is elevated in ascites during severe ovarian hyperstimulation syndrome: implications for pathophysiology and clinical management. *Fertil Steril* **62**:731–7.

Delbaere A, Bergmann PJM, Gervy-Decoster C et al. (1997). Prorenin and active renin concentrations in plasma and ascites during severe ovarian hyperstimulation syndrome. *Hum Reprod* **12**:236–40.

Delvigne A (2004). Epidemiology and pathophysiology of ovarian hyperstimulation syndrome. In (Gerris G, Olivennes F & De Sutter P, Eds), *Assisted Reproductive Technologies: Quality and Safety*. New York: Parthenon Publishing, Chapter 12, pp. 149–62.

Derkx FHM, Stuenkel C, Schalekamp MPA et al. (1986). Immunoreactive renin, prorenin, and enzymatically active renin in plasma during pregnancy and in women taking oral contraceptives. *J Clin Endocrinol Metab* **63**:1008–15.

Djerassi A, Coutifaris C, West VA et al. (1995). Gonadotroph adenoma in a premenopausal woman secreting follicle-stimulating hormone and causing ovarian hyperstimulation. *J Clin Endocrinol Metab* **80**:591–4.

Do YS, Sherrod A, Lobo RA et al. (1988). Human ovarian theca cells are a source of renin. *Proc Natl Acad Sci USA* **85**:1957–8.

Donnez J, Langerock S & Thomas K (1982). Peritoneal fluid volume and 17β-estradiol and progesterone concentrations in ovulatory, anovulatory, and postmenopausal women. *Obstet Gynecol* **59**:687–92.

El-Chalal U & Schenker JG (1997). The pathophysiology of ovarian hyperstimulation syndrome – views and ideas. *Hum Reprod* **12**:1129–37.

Enskog A, Nilsson L & Bränström M (2001a). Plasma levels of free vascular endothelial growth factor165 (VEGF165) are not elevated during gonadotropin stimulation in in vitro fertilization (IVF) patients developing ovarian hyperstimulation syndrome (OHSS): results of a prospective cohort study. *Eur J Obstet Gynecol Reprod Biol* **96**:196–201.

Enskog A, Nilsson L & Bränström M (2001b). Low peripheral blood levels of the immunosuppressive cytokine interleukin-10 (IL-10) at the start of gonadotrophin stimulation indicates increased risk for development of ovarian hyperstimulation syndrome (OHSS). *J Reprod Immunol* **49**:71–85.

Evbuomwan IO, Davison JM & Murdoch AP (2000). Coexistent hemoconcentration and hypoosmolality during superovulation and in severe ovarian hyperstimulation syndrome: volume homeostasis paradox. *Fertil Steril* **74**:67–72.

Evbuomwan IO, Davison JM, Baylis PM et al. (2001). Altered osmotic thresholds for arginine vasopressin secretion and thirst during superovulation and in the ovarian hyperstimulation syndrome (OHSS): relevance to the pathophysiology of OHSS. *Fertil Steril* **75**:933–41.

Fernandez LA, Tarlatzis BC, Rzasa QJ et al. (1985a). Renin like activity in ovarian follicular fluid. *Fertil Steril* **44**:219–23.

Fernandez LA, Twickler J & Mead A (1985b). Neovascularization produced by angiotensin II. *J Lab Clin Med* **105**:141–2.

Ferrara N & Henzel WJ (1989). Pituitary follicular cells secrete a novel heparin-binding growth factor specific for vascular endothelial cells. *Biochem Biophys Res Commun* **161**:851–8.

Ferrara N, Houck K, Jakeman L et al. (1992). Molecular and biological properties of the vascular endothelial growth factor family of proteins. *Endocr Rev* **13**:18—32.

Frederick JL, Shimanuki T & DiZerega GS (1984). Initiation of angiogenesis by human follicular fluid. *Science* **224**:389—92.

Friedlander MA, de Mola JR & Goldfarb JM (1993). Elevated levels of interleukin-6 in ascites and serum from women with ovarian hyperstimulation syndrome. *Fertil Steril* **60**:826—32.

Friedman CI, Seifer DB, Kennard EA et al. (1998). Elevated level of follicular fluid vascular endothelial growth factor is a marker of diminished pregnancy potential. *Fertil Steril* **64**:268—72.

Geva E, Amit A, Lessing JB et al. (1999). Follicular fluid levels of vascular endothelial growth factor. Are the premarkers for ovarian hyperstimulation syndrome? *J Reprod Med* **44**:91—6.

Gitay-Goren H, Soker S, Vlodavsky I et al. (1992). The binding of vascular endothelial growth factor to its receptors is dependent on cell surface-associated heparin-like molecules. *J Biol Chem* **267**:6093—8.

Glorioso N, Atlas SA, Laragh JH et al. (1986). Prorenin in high concentrations in human ovarian follicular fluid. *Science* **233**:1422—4.

Goad DL, Rubin J, Wang H et al. (1996). Enhanced expression of vascular endothelial growth factor in human SaOS-2 osteoblast-like cells and murine osteoblasts induced by insulin-like growth factor I. *Endocrinology* **137**:2262—8.

Goldsman MP, Pedram A, Dominguez CE et al. (1995). Increased capillary permeability induced by human follicular fluid: a hypothesis for an ovarian origin of the hyperstimulation syndrome. *Fertil Steril* **63**:268—72.

Gomez R, Simon C, Remohi J et al. (2002). Vascular endothelial growth factor receptor-2 activation induces vascular permability in hyperstimulated rats, and this effect is prevented by receptor blockade. *Endocrinology* **143**:4338—49.

Gomez R, Simon C, Remohi J et al. (2003). Administration of moderate and high doses of gonadotropins to female rats increases ovarian vascular endothelial growth factor (VEGF) and VEGF receptor-2 expression that is associated to vascular hyperpermeability. *Biol Reprod* **299**:2164—71.

Gomez R, Lima I, Simon C & Pellicer A (2004). Administration of low-dose LH induces ovulation and prevents vascular hyperpermeability and vascular endothelial growth factor expression in superovulated rats. *Reproduction* **127**:483—9.

Gordon JD, Mesiano S, Zaloudek CJ et al. (1996). Vascular endothelial growth factor localization in human ovary and fallopian tubes: possible role in reproductive function and ovarian cyst formation. *J Clin Endocrinol Metab* **81**:353—9.

Gospodarowicz D, Abraham JA & Schilling J (1989). Isolation and characterization of a vascular endothelial cell mitogen produced by pituitary-derived folliculo stellate cells. *Proc Natl Acad Sci* **86**:7311—5.

Handin RI & Wagner KK (1989). Molecular and cellular biology of von Willebrand factor. In (Coller BS, Ed.), *Progress in Hemostasis and Thrombosis*. Philadelphia: WB Saunders, Vol. 9, p. 233.

Haning RV, Estil Y & Nolten WE (1985). Pathophysiology of the ovarian hyperstimulation syndrome. *Obstet Gynecol* **66**:220—4.

Hsueh WA, Carlson EJ & Dzau VJ (1983). Characterization of inactive renin from human kidney and plasma: evidence of a renal source of circulating inactive renin. *J Clin Invest* **71**:506—9.

Itskovitz J & Sealey JE (1987). Ovarian prorenin-renin-angiotensin system. *Obstet Gynecol Surv* **42**:545—9.

Itskovitz J, Bruneval P, Soubrier F et al. (1992). Localization of renin gene expression in monkey ovarian theca cells by in situ hybridization. *J Clin Endocrinol Metab* **75**:1374—80.

Kaiser UB (2003). The pathogenesis of the ovarian hyperstimulation syndrome. *New Engl J Med* **349**:729–32.

Kamat BR, Brown LF, Manseau EJ et al. (1995). Expression of vascular permeability factor/vascular endothelial growth factor by human granulosa and theca lutein cells. *Am J Pathol* **146**:157–65.

Katz Z, Lancet M, Borenstein R et al. (1984). Absence of teratogenicity of indomethacin in ovarian hyperstimulation syndrome. *Int J Fertil* **29**:186–8.

Keck PJ, Hauser SD, Krivi G et al. (1989). Vascular permeability factor, an endothelial cell mitogen related to PDGF. *Science* **246**:1309–12.

Kendall RL & Thomas KA (1993). Inhibition of vascular endothelial cell growth factor activity by an endogenously encoded soluble receptor. *Proc Natl Acad Sci USA* **90**:10705–9.

Kim KJ, Li B, Winer J et al. (1993). Inhibition of vascular endothelial growth factor induced angiogenesis suppresses tumor growth in vivo. *Nature* **362**:841–4.

Kishimoto T (1989). The biology of IL-6. *Blood* **74**:1–10.

Kitajima Y, Endo T, Manase K et al. (2004). Gonadotropin-releasing hormone agonist administration reduced vascular endothelial growth factor (VEGF), VEGF receptors, and vascular permeability of the ovaries of hyperstimulated rats. *Fertil Steril* **81**(Suppl 2):842–9.

Koch AE, Harlow LA, Haines GK et al. (1994). Vascular endothelial growth factor: a cytokine modulating endothelial function in rheumatoid arthritis. *J Immunol* **152**:4149–56.

Krasnow JJ, Berga SL, Guzick DS et al. (1996). Vascular permeability factor and vascular endothelial growth factor in ovarian hyperstimulation syndrome. *Fertil Steril* **65**:552–5.

Kwekkeboom DJ, de Jong FH & Lamberts SW (1989). Gonadotrophin release by clinically nonfunctioning and gonadotroph pituitary adenomas in vivo and in-vitro: relation to sex and effects of thryotropin-releasing hormone, gonadotrophin-releasing hormone, and bromocriptine. *J Clin Endocrinol Metab* **68**:1128–35.

Lee A, Christenson LK, Stouffer RL et al. (1997). Vascular endothelial growth factor levels in serum and follicular fluid of patients undergoing in-vitro fertilization. *Fertil Steril* **68**:305–11.

Leung DW, Cachianes G, Kuang WJ et al. (1989). Vascular endothelial growth factor is a secreted angiogenic mitogen. *Science* **246**:1306–9.

Levin I, Gamzu R, Hasson Y et al. (2004). Increased erythrocyte aggregation in ovarian hyperstimulation syndrome: a possible contributing factor in the pathophysiology of this disease. *Hum Reprod* **19**:1076–80.

Levy T, Oriveto R, Homburg R et al. (1996). Severe ovarian hyperstimulation syndrome despite low plasma oestrogen concentrations in a hypogonadotrophic, hypogonadal patient. *Hum Reprod* **11**:1177–9.

Li J, Perrella MA, Tsai JC et al. (1995). Induction of vascular endothelial growth factor gene expression by interleukin-1 beta in rat aotic smooth muscle cells. *J Biol Chem* **270**:308–12.

Lightman A, Tarlatzis BC, Rzasa PJ et al. (1987). The ovarian renin–angiotensin system: renin-like activity and angiotensin II/III immunoreactivity in gonadotropin-stimulated human follicular fluid. *Am J Obstet Gynecol* **156**:808–16.

Loret de Mola JR, Flores JP, Baumgardner GP et al. (1996a). Elevated interleukin-6 levels in the ovarian hyperstimulation syndrome: ovarian imunohistochemical localization of interleukin-6 signal. *Obstet Gynecol* **87**:581–7.

Loret de Mola JR, Baumgardner GP, Goldfarb JM et al. (1996b). Ovarian hyperstimulation syndrome: pre-ovulatory serum concentrations of interleukin-6, interleukin-1 receptor antagonist and tumor necrosis factor cannot predict its occurrence. *Hum Reprod* **11**:1377–80.

Ludwig M, Gembruch U, Bauer O et al. (1998). Ovarian hyperstimulation syndrome (OHSS) in a spontaneous pregnancy with a fetal and placental triploidy: information about the general pathophysiology of OHSS. *Hum Reprod* **13**:2082−7.

Ludwig M, Jekmann W, Bauen O et al. (1999). Prediction of severe ovarian hyperstimulation by free serum vascular endothelial growth factor concentration on the day of human chorionic gonadotropin administration. *Hum Reprod* **14**:2437−41.

Maathuis JB, Van Look PF & Michie EA (1978). Changes in volume, total protein and ovarian steroid concentrations of peritoneal fluid through the human menstrual cycle. *J Endocrinol* **76**:123−4.

Mannucci PM, Canciani MT, Rota L et al. (1981). Response of factor VIII/von Willebrand factor to DDAVP in healthy subjects and patients with haemophilia A and von Willebrand's disease. *Br J Hematal* **47**:283−93.

Manolopoulos K, Lang U, Gips H et al. (2001). Elevated interleukin-10 and sex steroid levels in peritoneal fluid of patients with ovarian hyperstimulation syndrome. *Eur J Obstet Gynecol Reprod Biol* **99**:226−31.

Mantovani A, Bussolino F & Introna M (1997). Cytokine regulation of endothelial cell function: from molecular level to the bedside. *Immunol Today* **18**:231−40.

Mathur RS, Jenkins JM & Bansal AS (1997). The probable role of the immune system in the pathogenesis of ovarian hyperstimulation syndrome. *Hum Reprod* **12**:2629−34.

McClure N, Healy DL, Rogers PA et al. (1994). Vascular endothelial growth factor as capillary permeability agent in ovarian hyperstimulation syndrome. *Lancet* **344**:235−6.

McElhinney B, Ardill J, Caldwell C et al. (2002). Variations in serum vascular endothelial growth factor binding profiles and the development of ovarian hyperstimulation syndrome. *Fertil Steril* **78**:286−90.

McLaren J, Prentice A, Charnock-Jones DS et al. (1996). Vascular endothelial growth factor (VEGF) concentrations are elevated in peritoneal fluid of women with endometriosis. *Hum Reprod* **11**:220−3.

Meyer D, Pietu G, Fressinaud E et al. (1991). Von Willebrand factor: structure and function. *Proc Mayo Clin* **66**:516−23.

Millauer B, Wizigmann-Voos S, Schnurch H et al. (1993). High affinity VEGF binding and developmental expression suggest FLK-1 as a major regulator of vasculogenesis and angiogenesis *Cell* **72**:835−46.

Morris RS, Wong IL, Kirkham E et al. (1995). Inhibition of ovarian-derived prorenin to angiotensin cascade in the treatment of ovarian hyperstimulation syndrome. *Hum Reprod* **10**:1355−8.

Motro B, Itin A, Sacjs L et al. (1990). Pattern of IL-6 gene expression in vivo suggests a role for this cytokine in angiogenesis. *J Cell Biol* **87**:3092−6.

Navot D, Margalioth E & Laufer N (1987). Direct correlation between plasma renin activity and severity of the ovarian hyperstimulation syndrome. *Fertil Steril* **48**:57−61.

Neufeld G, Cohen T, Gengrinovitch S et al. (1999). Vascular endothelial growth factor (VEGF) and its receptors. *The FASEB Journal* **13**:9−22.

Neulen J, Yan Z, Raczek S et al. (1995a). Ovarian hyperstimulation syndrome: vascular endothelial growth factor/vascular permeability factor from luteinized granulosa cells is the patho-physiological principle. In *Abstracts of the 11th Annual Meeting of the ESHRE*, Hamburg.

Neulen J, Yan Z, Raczek S et al. (1995b). Human chorionic gonadotropin-dependent expression of vascular endothelial growth factor/vascular permeability factor in human granulosa cells: importance in ovarian hyperstimulation syndrome. *J Clin Endocrinol Metab* **80**:1967−71.

Novella-Maestre E, Gomez-Gallego R, Alonso-Muriel I et al. (2005). Progesterone has no role in the increased vascular permeability which onsets OHSS. *J Soc Gyn Invest* **12** (Suppl 364):202A.

Ogawa S, Minakami H, Araki S et al. (2001). A rise of the serum level of von Willebrand factor occurs before clinical manifestation of the severe form of ovarian hyperstimulation syndrome. *J Assist Reprod Genet* **18**:114−19.

Ohba T, Ujioka T, Ishikawa K et al. (2003). Ovarian hyperstimulation syndrome-model rats; the manifestation and clinical implication. *Mol Cell Endocrinol* **202**:47−52.

Ong ACM, Eisen V, Rennie DP et al. (1991). The pathogenesis of the ovarian hyperstimulation syndrome (OHS): a possible role for ovarian renin. *Clin Endocrinol* **34**:43−9.

Oppenheim JJ, Ruscetti FW & Faltynek C (1991). Cytokines. In (Stites DP, Terr AI, Eds), *Basic and Clinical Immunology* (7th Edn). East Norwalk, CT: Appleton and Lange, p. 78.

Orvieto R, Voliovitch I, Fishman P et al. (1995). Interleukin-2 and ovarian hyperstimulation syndrome: a pilot study. *Hum Reprod* **10**:24−7.

Paulson RJ, Do YS, Hsueh WA et al. (1989). Ovarian renin production in vitro and in vivo: characterization and clinical correlation. *Fertil Steril* **51**:634−8.

Peach MJ (1977). Renin-angiotensin system: biochemistry and mechanism of action. *Physiol Rev* **57**:313−7.

Pellicer A, Palumbo A, DeCherney AH et al. (1988). Blockage of ovulation by an angiotensin antagonist. *Science* **240**:1660−1.

Pellicer A, Miru F, Sampaia M et al. (1991). In-vitro fertilization as a diagnostic and therapeutic tool in a patient with partial 17, 20 desmolase deficiency. *Fertil Steril* **55**:970−5.

Pellicer A, Albert C, Mercader A et al. (1999). The pathogenesis of ovarian hyperstimulation syndrome: in vivo studies investigating the role of interleukin-1β, interleukin-6, and vascular endothelial growth factor. *Fertil Steril* **71**:482−9.

Penz-Vidovic I, Skori T, Grubisi G et al. (2000). Evolution of clinical symptoms in a young woman with a recurrent gonadotroph adenoma causing ovarian hyperstimulation. *Eur J Endocrinol* **143**:607−14.

Pepperell JR, Nemeth G, Plaumbo A et al. (1993). The intraovarian renin−angiotensin system. In (Adashi EY, Leung PCK, Eds), *The Ovary*. New York: Raven Press, pp. 363−80.

Phillips HS, Hains J, Leung DW et al. (1990). Vascular endothelial cell growth factor is expressed in rat corpus luteum. *Endocrinology* **127**:965−7.

Polishuk WZ & Schenker JG (1969). Ovarian overstimulation syndrome. *Fertil Steril* **20**:443−5.

Pride SM, Ho Yuen B, Moon YS et al. (1986). Relationship of gonadotrophin-releasing hormone, danazol and prostaglandin blockage to ovarian enlargement and ascites formation of the ovarian hyperstimulation syndrome. *Am J Obstet Gynecol* **154**:1155−60.

Pride SM, James C & Ho Yuen B (1990). The ovarian hyperstimulation syndrome. *Semin Reprod Endocrinol* **8**:247−60.

Ravindranath N, Little-Ihrig LL, Phillios HS et al. (1992). Vascular endothelial growth factor messenger ribonucleic acid expression in the primate ovary. *Endocrinol* **131**:254−60.

Revel A, Barak V, Lavy Y et al. (1996). Characterization of intraperitoneal cytokines and nitrites in women with severe ovarian hyperstimulation syndrome. *Fertil Steril* **66**:66−71.

Rizk B (1992). Ovarian hyperstimulation syndrome. In (Brinsden PR, Rainsbury PA, Eds), *A Textbook of In-Vitro Fertilization and Assisted Reproduction*. Carnforth, UK: Parthenon Publishing, Chapter 23, pp. 369−83.

Rizk B (1993a). Ovarian hyperstimulation syndrome. In (Studd J, Ed.), *Progress in Obstetrics and Gynecology*, Volume 11. Edinburgh: Churchill Livingstone, Chapter 18, pp. 311−49.

Rizk B (1993b). Prevention of ovarian hyperstimulation syndrome: the Ten Commandments. *European Society of Human Reproduction and Embryology Symposium*, Tel Aviv, Israel, pp. 1−2.

Rizk B (2001). Ovarian hyperstimulation syndrome: prediction, prevention and management. In (Rizk B, Devroey P, Meldrum DR, Eds), *Advances and Controversies in Ovulation Induction.* Proceedings of the 34th ASRM Annual Postgraduate Program, Middle East Fertility Society Precongress Course. ASRM, 57th Annual Meeting, Orlando, FL, October 2001, pp. 23–46.

Rizk B (2002). Can OHSS in ART be eliminated? In (Rizk B, Meldrum D, Schoolcraft W, Eds), *A Clinical Step-By-Step Course For Assisted Reproductive Technologies.* Proceedings of the 35th ASRM Annual Postgraduate Program, Middle East Fertility Society Precongress Course. ASRM, 58th Annual Meeting, Seattle, WA, October 2002, pp. 65–102.

Rizk B & Abdalla H (2003). Pathogenesis of endometriosis. In (Rizk B, Abdalla H, Eds), *Endometriosis,* 2nd edn. Oxford: Health Press, Chapter 1, pp. 9–23.

Rizk B & Aboulghar M (1991). Modern management of ovarian hyperstimulation syndrome. *Hum Reprod* **6**:1082–7.

Rizk B & Aboulghar MA (1999). Classification, pathophysiology and management of ovarian hyperstimulation syndrome. In (Brinsden P, Ed.), *A Textbook of In-Vitro Fertilization and Assisted Reproduction,* 2nd edn. London: Parthenon Publishing, Chapter 9, pp. 131–55.

Rizk B & Aboulghar MA (2005). Classification, pathophysiology and management of ovarian hyperstimulation syndrome. In (Brinsden P, Ed.), *A Textbook of In-Vitro Fertilization and Assisted Reproduction,* 3rd edn. London: Parthenon Publishing, Chapter 12, pp. 217–58.

Rizk B & Nawar MG (2004). Ovarian hyperstimulation syndrome. In (Serhal P, Overton C, Eds), *Good Clinical Practice in Assisted Reproduction.* Cambridge: Cambridge University Press, Chapter 8, pp. 146–66.

Rizk B & Abdalla H (2006). Ovulatory dysfunction and its management. In (Rizk B & Abdullah M, Eds), *Infertility and Assisted Reproductive Technology.* Oxford: Health Press, Chapter 1, pp. 87–9.

Rizk B & Smitz J (1992). Ovarian hyperstimulation syndrome after superovulation for IVF and related procedures. *Hum Reprod* **7**:320–7.

Rizk B, Meagher S & Fisher AM (1990). Ovarian hyperstimulation syndrome and cerebrovascular accidents. *Hum Reprod* **5**:697–8.

Rizk B, Aboulghar MA, Mansour RT et al. (1991). Severe ovarian hyperstimulation syndrome: analytical study of twenty-one cases. *Proceedings of the VII World Congress on In-Vitro Fertilization and Assisted Procreations, Paris. Hum Reprod* **8**:368–9.

Rizk B, Aboulghar MA, Smitz J & Ron-El R (1997). The role of vascular endothelial growth factor and interleukins in the pathogenesis of severe ovarian hyperstimulation syndrome. *Hum Reprod Update* **3**:255–66.

Roberts JE, Spandorfer S, Fasouliotis SJ et al. (2005). Spontaneous ovarian hyperstimulation caused by a follicle-stimulating hormone-secreting pituitary adenoma. *Fertil Steril* **83**:208–10.

Rosenberg ME, Mckinzie JK, Mckenzie LM et al. (1994). Increased ascitic fluid prorenin in the ovarian hyperstimulation syndrome. *Am J Kidney Dis* **23**:427–9.

Sahin Y, Kontas O, Muderris II et al. (1997). Effects of angiotensin converting enzyme inhibitor cilasaprin and angiotensin II antagonist saralasin in ovarian hyperstimulation syndrome in the rabbit. *Gynecol Endocrinol* **11**:231–6.

Schenker JG (1999). Clinical aspects of ovarian hyperstimulation syndrome. *Eur J Gynecol Reprod Biol* **85**:10–3.

Schenker JG & Polishuk WZ (1976). The role of prostaglandins in ovarian hyperstimulation syndrome. *Obstet Gynecol Surv* **31**:74–8.

Schenker JG & Weinstein D (1978). Ovarian hyperstimulation syndrome: a current survey. *Fertil Steril* **30**:255–68.

Senger DR, Galli SJ, Dvorak AM et al. (1983). Tumor cells secrete a vascular permeability factor that promotes accumulation of ascites fluid. *Science* **219**:983–5.

Shimon J, Rubinek T, Bar-Hava I et al. (2001). Ovarian hyperstimulation without elevated serum estradiol associated with pure follicle-stimulating hormone-secreting pituitary adenoma. *J Clin Endocrinol Metab* **86**:3635—40.

Shweiki D, Itin A, Neufeld G et al. (1993). Patterns of expression on vascular endothelial growth factor (VEGF) receptors in mice suggest a role in hormonally regulated angiogenesis. *J Clin Invest* **91**:2235—43.

Smitz J, Camus M, Devroey P et al. (1990). Incidence of severe ovarian hyperstimulation syndrome after GnRH-agonist—HMG treatment in super ovulation in vitro fertilization. *Hum Repord* **5**:933—7.

Snyder PJ (1985). Gonadotroph cell adenomas of the pituitary. *Endocrinol Rev* **6**:552—63.

Snyder PJ (1987). Gonadotroph cell pituitary adenomas. *Endocrinol Metab Clin North Am* **16**:755—64.

Soker S, Takashima S, Miao H et al. (1998). Neuropilin-1 is expressed by endothelial and tumor cells as an isoforms specific receptor for vascular endothelial growth factor. *Growth Factors* **92**:735—45.

Tischer E, Gospodarowicz D, Mitchell R et al. (1989). Vascular endothelial growth factor: a new member of the platelet-derived growth factor gene family. *Biochem Biophys Res Commun* **165**:1198—206.

Tollan A, Holst N, Forsdahl F et al. (1990). Transcapillary fluid dynamics during ovarian stimulation for in-vitro fertilization. *Am J Obstet Gynecol* **162**:554—6.

Teruel MJ, Carbonell LF, Llanos MC et al. (2002). Hemodynamic state and the role of angiotensin II in ovarian hyperstimulation syndrome in the rabbit. *Fertil Steril* **77**:1256—60.

Teruel MJ, Carbonell LF, Teruel MG et al. (2001). Effect of angiotensin-converting enzyme inhibitor on renal function in ovarian hyperstimulation syndrome in the rabbit. *Fertil Steril* **76**:1232—7.

Todorow S, Schricker ST, Siebzinruebl ER et al. (1993). Von Willebrand factor: an endothelial marker to monitor in vitro fertilization patients with ovarian hyper-stimulation syndrome. *Hum Reprod* **8**:2039—49.

Valimaki MJ, Tiitinen A, Alfthan H et al. (1999). Ovarian hyperstimulation caused by gonadotroph adenoma secreting follicle-stimulating hormone in a 28 year old woman. *J Clin Endocrinol Metab* **84**:4204—8.

Van Beaumont W (1872). Evaluation of hemoconcentration from hematocrit measurements. *J Appl Physiol* **5**:712—3.

Van der Meeren A, Squiban C, Guormelon P et al. (1991). Differential regulation by IL-4 and IL-10 of radiation induced IL-6 and IL-8 production and ICAM-1 expression by human endothelial cells. *Cytokine* **11**:831—8.

Wang LJ & Norman RJ (1992). Concentrations of immunoreactive interleukin-1 and interleukin-2 in human preovulatory follicular fluid. *Hum Reprod* **7**:147—50.

Wang LJ, Robertson S, Seamark RF et al. (1991). Lymphokines, including interleukin-2 alter gonadotrophin-stimulated progesterone production and proliferationof human granulosa-luteal cells in vitro. *J Clin Endocrinol Metab* **72**:824—31.

Wang LJ, Pascoe V, Petrucco OM et al. (1992). Distribution of leukocyte subpopulations in the human corpus luteum. *Hum Reprod* **7**:197—202.

Wang TH, Horng SG, Chang CL et al. (2002). Human chorionic gonadotropin-induced ovarian hyperstimulation syndrome is associated with up-regulation of vascular endothelial growth factor. *J Clin Endocrinol Metab* **87**:3300—8.

Yan Z, Weich HA, Bernart W et al. (1993). Vascular endothelial growth factor (VEGF) messenger ribonucleic acid (mRNA) expression in luteinized human granulosa cells in-vitro. *J Clin Endocrinol Metab* **77**:1723—5.

Yarali H, Fleige-Zahradka BG, Yuen BH et al. (1993). The ascites in the ovarian hyperstimulation syndrome does not originate from the ovary. *Fertil Steril* **59**: 657—61.

IV

GENETICS OF OVARIAN HYPERSTIMULATION SYNDROME

FOLLICLE STIMULATING HORMONE: STRUCTURE, FUNCTION AND RECEPTOR

Follicle stimulating hormone (FSH) is the central hormone of human reproduction necessary for gonadal development and maturation at puberty and for gamete production during the fertile phase of life (Simoni et al., 1997; Rizk and Abdalla, 2006). Together with luteinizing hormone (LH), FSH is produced and secreted by the pituitary gland as a highly heterogenous glycoprotein. FSH, LH and hCG consist of a *common alpha subunit* and a *receptor specific beta subunit* (Figures IV.1, IV.2 and IV.3). FSH acts by binding to specific receptors localized specifically in the gonads.

The FSH receptor is a glycoprotein belonging to the family of G-protein-coupled receptors. Complex transmembrane proteins are characterized by seven hydrophobic helices inserted in the plasmalemma and by intracellular and extracellular domains, depending on the type of the ligand (Figure IV.4). The large extracellular domain of the glycoprotein hormone receptors is a unique feature within the G-protein-coupled receptor family. The intracellular portion of the FSH receptor is coupled to a Gs protein, and upon receptor activation by the hormonal interaction with the extracellular domain, initiates a cascade of events that finally leads to the specific biologic effects of the gonadotrophin (Figure IV.5). The intramolecular mechanisms involved in the transduction of the activation signal from the binding step to the activation of the G protein have been the subject of intense investigations (Montanelli et al., 2004a) whereas in most rhodopsin-like GPCRs, there is evidence for a direct interaction between agonists and serpentine domains. Following receptor activation by the ligand, the activated $G_{\alpha s}$ subunit (GTP-bound) stimulates the effector enzyme adenylyl cyclase, and the generation of the cyclic AMP (cAMP) from ATP. The cAMP then activates protein kinase A (A-kinase), triggering a phosphorylation (P) cascade and activating intracellular proteins (Figure IV.5). The models for the activation of gonadotrophin receptors suggest that binding of the hormones to the receptors would promote a conformational change in their ectodomains, transforming them into full agonist of the serpentine domain (Vlaeminck-Guillem et al., 2002; Montanelli et al., 2004a).

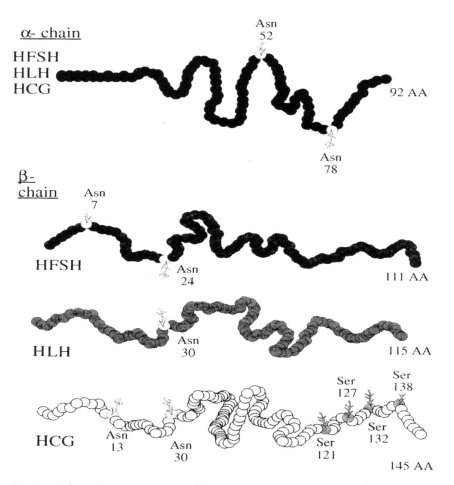

Fig. IV.1: Schematic representation of the primary structure of α- and β-subunits of the gonadotrophin family
Reproduced with permission from Olijve et al. (1996). Mol Hum Reprod **2***:371—82*

FSH RECEPTOR GENE

The chromosomal mapping of the FSH receptor gene has been performed by fluorescence in situ hybridization using cDNA or genomic probes and by linkage analysis (Rousseau-Merck et al., 1993; Gromoll et al., 1994). The FSH receptor gene is located at chromosome 2p21 in the human (Simoni et al., 1997; Themmen and Huhtaniemi, 2000; Simoni et al., 2002). The LH receptor gene can be mapped to the same chromosomal location whereas the human TSH receptor is located on chromosome 14 q31. The FSH receptor gene is a single-copy gene and spans a region of 54 kbp in the human as determined by restriction analysis of genomic clones and size determination of PCR probes. It consists of 10 exons and 9 introns (Simoni et al., 1997).

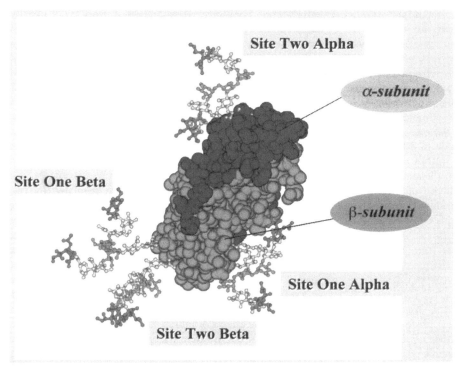

Fig. IV.2: Model of a fully glycosylated and sialylated human FSH molecule
*Reproduced with permission from Edwards RG, Risquez F, Eds (2003). Modern Assisted
Conception. Cambridge, UK. Reproductive Biomedicine Online: Reproductive Health Care
Ltd, p. 66*

Fig. IV.3: The sequence of the common human α-subunit (hFSHα; upper panel and
human FSHβ (lower panel)
*Reproduced with permission from Edwards RG, Risquez F, Eds (2003). Modern Assisted
Conception. Reproductive Biomedicine Online: Reproductive Health Care Ltd, p. 66*

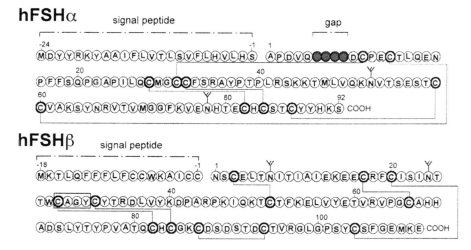

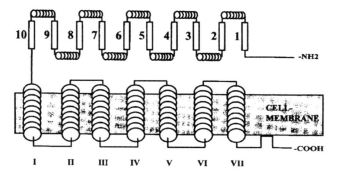

Fig. IV.4: FSH receptor
Reproduced with permission from Simoni et al. (1997). Endocr Rev. 18:739–73

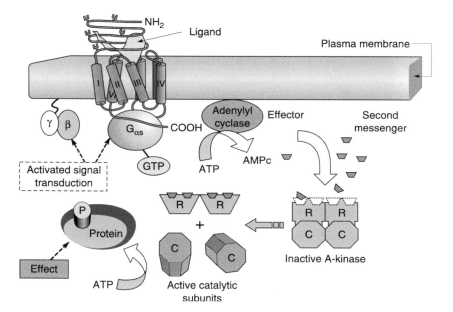

Fig. IV.5: Attachment to FSH receptor and signal transduction mediated by the $G_{\alpha s}$ protein pathway in response to a gonadotrophic stimulus (ligand)
Reproduced with permission from Edwards RG, Risquez F, Eds (2003). Modern Assisted Conception. Cambridge, UK. Reproductive Biomedicine Online: Reproductive Healthcare Ltd, p. 70

OVARIAN RESPONSE AND FSH RECEPTOR

FSH plays a central role in oogenesis. It triggers the maturation of follicles, proliferation of granulosa cells and aromatase enzyme induction (Rizk and Abdalla, 2006). Its role is pivotal in the recruitment of the dominant follicle. FSH action is mediated by the FSH receptor (Figure IV.4) and, therefore, screening for mutations in the FSH receptor has been pursued in the search for causes of infertility (Aittomaki et al., 1995; Whithney et al., 1995; Gromoll et al., 1996).

De Castro et al. (2003) analyzed the clinical outcome of 102 controlled ovarian hyperstimulation cycles and the role of $Ser^{680}Asn$ in recombinant FSH. Although the results suggest Ser/Ser patients have a lower response to recombinant FSH during controlled ovarian stimulation cycles and increased risk of cycle cancellation, the presence of Asn/Asn homozygotes among poor responders and among patients whose cycles were cancelled indicates that the Ser^{680} allele alone is not sufficient to cause a lower response to recombinant FSH. Furthermore, variables of ovulation induction were similar among genotypes, suggesting that other factors such as age, ovarian reserve or other genes may contribute to the oucome (De Castro et al., 2003).

Serum FSH levels are among the best predictors of ovarian response. A significant variability from cycle to cycle in the same patient is observed. The distribution of FSH isoforms and the interference of circulating FSH inhibitors or FSH antibodies also play a role. Ovarian response to FSH stimulation depends on the FSH receptor genotype (Perez Mayorga et al., 2000). Two nonsynonymous polymorphisms have been described in exon 10 of the transmembrane region of the FSH receptor (Simoni et al., 2002). The first one is A919G ($Thr^{307}Ala$), located just before the beginning of the first transmembrane helix and the second polymorphism is A2039G ($Asn^{680}Ser$), located intracellularly at the end of the C permanent tail of the receptor. In Caucasian populations, four haplotypes have been described by Simoni et al. (2002). The common haplotypes are $T^{307}N^{680}$ and $A^{307}S^{680}$ (60% and 40%, respectively). The rare haplotypes are $A307N^{680}$ $T^{307}S^{680}$ (approximately 1% each). The presence of a serine in position 680 is associated with high basal levels of FSH on day 2 to 4 of the menstrual cycle and higher requirements of exogenous FSH for ovarian stimulation (Perez Mayorga et al., 2000; Sudo et al., 2002). This means that an FSH receptor with a serine in position 680 is less efficient than an FSH receptor with an asparagine in position 680 (Perez Mayorga et al., 2000; Sudo et al., 2002). DeCastro et al. (2003) have demonstrated an association between the presence of serine in position 680 to poor responses to gonadotrophin therapy in IVF patients. DeCastro et al. (2003) suggested that the S^{680} allele was associated with a diminished sensitivity to FSH. However, Laven et al. (2003) could not establish altered ovarian sensitivity to exogenous FSH during ovulation induction in clomiphene-resistant normo-gonadotrophic anovulatory patients. The in-vivo association of S^{680} with higher levels of basal FSH on day 2 to 4 of the menstrual cycle has not yet been explained in molecular terms (Perez Mayorga et al., 2000; Sudo et al., 2002; Simoni et al., 2002; Daelemans et al., 2004).

NATURALLY OCCURRING FSH RECEPTOR MUTATIONS

After two decades of investigations, the FSH receptor cDNA was finally cloned in 1990 (Sprengel et al., 1990). The first mutations were described with a major impact on the reproductive phenotype (Aittomaki et al., 1995; Gromoll et al., 1996). The new information emerging from the naturally occurring mutations and the molecular work provides insights into FSH physiology (Gromoll et al., 1996; Simoni et al., 1997).

FSH RECEPTOR MUTATIONS AND OHSS

The association between FSH receptor mutations and OHSS (Figure IV.6) has opened new horizons in our understanding of the pathophysiology of this syndrome (Kaiser, 2003; Rizk and Aboulghar, 2005). Recently, three naturally occurring mutations in the serpentine region of the FSH receptor (FSHr)

Fig. IV.6: Pathogenesis of familial gestational spontaneous OHSS
*Reproduced with permission from Kaiser, B (2003). N Engl J Med **349***:729–32*

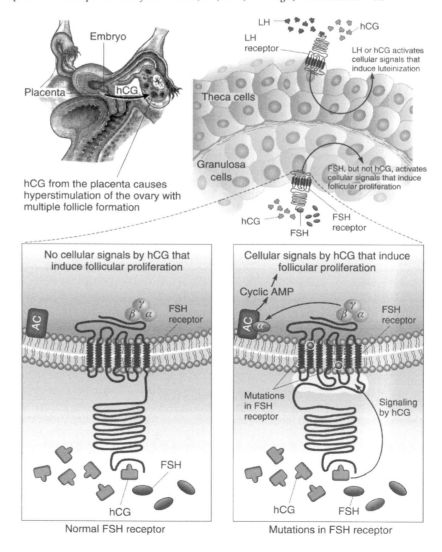

(D567N and T449I/A) have been identified in three families with spontaneous ovarian hyperstimulation syndrome. All mutant receptors displayed abnormally high sensitivity to human chorionic gonadotrophin, and, in addition, D567N and T449A displayed a concomitant increase in sensitivity to TSH and detectable constitutive activity (Vasseur et al., 2003; Smits et al., 2003; Montanelli et al., 2004a, b). Up until that point in time, few mutations in the FSH receptor (Themmen and Huhtaniemi, 2000), and only one resulting in a gain of function (Gromoll et al., 1996), have been reported. These three recently published mutations broaden the specificity of the FSH receptor so that it responds to another ligand, chorionic gonadotrophin (Figure IV.6).

Vasseur et al. (2003) identified a chorionic-gonadotrophin-sensitive mutation in the FSH receptor as a cause of familial gestational spontaneous ovarian hyperstimulation syndrome. The patient developed OHSS during all of her four pregnancies that went beyond 6 weeks of gestation. The patient's sisters, who also had OHSS in their pregnancies, had the same mutation, but another sister who did not develop OHSS did not have the mutation. The mutation consisted of a substitution of thymidine for cytosine in exon 10 of the follitropin receptor gene. This resulted in the replacement of threonine by an isoleucine at position 449 of the follitropin protein (Figure IV.7). In-vitro characterization of the mutated receptor showed an increased sensitivity to hCG.

Smits et al. (2003) identified another mutation in the FSH receptor gene in a patient with spontaneous OHSS during each of her four pregnancies. The mutation consisted of a substitution of an adenine for a guanine at the first base of the codon 567 in exon 10 of the follitropin receptor gene, resulting in the replacement of an aspartic acid with asparagine (Figure IV.8). The functional response of the mutant receptor when tested in-vitro displayed an increased sensitivity to hCG.

Fig. IV.7: FSH receptor mutation and spontaneous OHSS. Sequence of exon 10 of the follicle-stimulating hormone receptor in the proband; the arrow indicates the heterozygous position at 449
*Reproduced from Vasseur et al. (2003). N Engl J Med **349**:753–9*

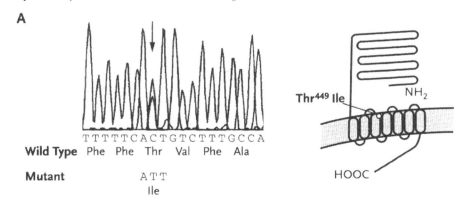

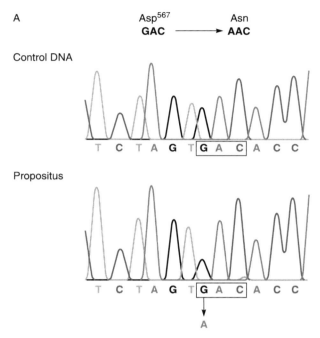

Fig. IV.8: FSH receptor mutation and spontaneous OHSS. Nucleotide sequence traces of follicle-stimulating hormone receptor around codon 567, in a control subject and in a patient with recurrent spontaneous ovarian hyperstimulation syndrome
*Reproduced with permission from Smits et al. (2003). N Engl J Med **349**:760–6*

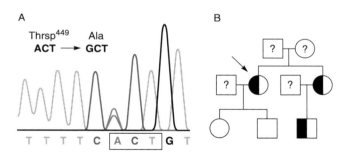

Fig. IV.9: FSH receptor mutation and spontaneous OHSS. Detection of the T449A mutation. Panel A: Nucleotide sequence traces of exon 10 of the FSHr around codon 449 in a patient with spontaneous OHSS. Panel B: Family pedigree
*Reproduced with permission from Montanelli et al. (2004). J Clin Endocrinol Metab **89**:1255–8*

Montanelli et al. (2004b) recently described a new familial case of recurrent spontaneous OHSS associated with a different mutation affecting the residue 449 of the FSH receptor. The affected women were heterozygous for a different mutation involving codon 449, where an alanine was substituted for threonine (Figure IV.9). Similar to D567N, the T449A FSHr mutant shows an increased sensitivity to both hCG and TSH, together with an increase in basal activity.

How do FSH Receptor Mutations Result in OHSS?

Human chorionic gonadotropin activity is normally limited to LH receptors expressed in the corpus luteum and assists in the maintenance of pregnancies. The three mutations of the FSH receptor result in promiscuous stimulation by hCG of the FSH receptors expressed on the granulosa cells of the ovarian follicles, resulting in excessive follicular development. Kaiser (2003) hypothesized that excessive follicular recruitment in association with luteinization of the follicles mediated by LH receptors results in OHSS (Figure IV.6).

Unexpected Location for the FSH Mutations

The mutations in the FSH receptor led to reduction of ligand specificity, permitting activation by hCG. It was very unexpected that the mutaions were not in the hormone-binding ectodomain, but rather in the serpentine domain that is responsible for the activation of signaling (Kaiser, 2003; Montanelli et al., 2004a). The affinity for FSH was not affected and no direct binding of hCG could be detected. These findings argue against changes in ligand binding. Kaiser (2003) suggested that the mutations affect the specificity of ligand recognition by allowing the low-affinity interaction of hCG with the ectodomain of the FSH receptor to be sufficient to "flip the switch". This would result in inducing an active confirmation of the serpentine domain and downstream signaling (Figure IV.6). Furthermore, the mutation in the FSH receptor reported by Smits et al. (2003) was such that the ligand specificity was reduced to an even greater extent, permitting downstream signaling induction by TSH in addition to hCG and FSH and also permitting constitutive activity in the absence of ligand (Kaiser, 2003).

Are There Other Effects of the FSH Receptor Mutations

Kaiser (2003) discussed three interesting possible effects of the FSH receptor mutations identified in association with spontaneous OHSS. The first possibility is that such mutations may lead to increased susceptibility to iatrogenic OHSS in patients undergoing ovulation induction. The second predisposition is multiple pregnancy as a result of increased stimulation of ovarian follicular development. However, in the three reported cases, no multiple pregnancies were observed. Finally, there is an unresolved concern that ovulation induction may increase the risk of cancer of the ovary, breast or uterus. Therefore, patients with activating mutations of the FSH receptor require careful and diligent follow-up, perhaps for a long time (Kaiser, 2003).

SPONTANEOUS AND IATROGENIC OHSS

The recent identification of mutations in the FSH receptor gene which display an increased sensitivity to hCG and are responsible for the development of spontaneous OHSS, provides for the first time the molecular basis for the physiopathology of spontaneous OHSS (Delbaere et al., 2004; Rizk and Aboulghar, 2005). In the three reported cases, the abnormal function of mutant FSH receptors in vitro provides a reasonable explanation for their implication of their role in OHSS development in vivo. During pregnancy there is a significant decrease in the FSH receptor expression in the corpus luteum. However, the expression of FSH receptor in the granulosa cells of the developing follicles remains constant (Simoni et al., 1997). Since the pituitary gonadotrophins fall to very low levels in the serum, these receptors are not usually stimulated during pregnancy (Delbaere et al., 2004). The mutant FSH receptor expressed in the developing follicles could be stimulated by the pregnancy-derived hCG and the follicle would start growing and enlarge. Finally, the granulosa cells acquire LH receptors which may also be stimulated by hCG (Delbaere et al., 2004). This would induce follicular luteinization and secretion of vasoactive substances that is implicated in the pathophysiology of the syndrome.

The interaction between the FSH receptor and hCG is therefore a requirement for the development of spontaneous OHSS. Delbaere et al. (2004) highlighted the differences between spontaneous and iatrogenic OHSS, and proposed a model to account for the different chronology between the two forms of the syndrome (Figure IV.10). In the iatrogenic form, the follicular recruitment and enlargement occur during ovarian stimulation with exogenous FSH (Dahl Lyons et al., 1994), while in the spontaneous form, the follicular recruitment occurs later through the stimulation of the FSH receptor by pregnancy-derived hCG. In both forms, massive luteinization of enlarged stimulated ovaries ensues, inducing the release of vasoactive mediators, leading to the development of the symptoms of OHSS. It is possible that the stimulation of the mutated FSH receptor occurs at the threshold hCG level. That threshold value could vary according to the type of mutation. In the first trimester of pregnancy, hCG peaks between 8 and 10 weeks and declines thereafter. It follows therefore that the initiation of follicular growth by pregnancy-derived hCG could start between 6 and 10 weeks of amenorrhea (Delbaere et al., 2004). If these follicles develop at the same rate as ovarian stimulation, the development of OHSS will occur at the time of massive follicular luteinization, between 8 and 12 weeks amenorrhea (Figure IV.10).

PREDICTION OF SEVERITY OF SYMPTOMS IN IATROGENIC OHSS BY FSH RECEPTOR POLYMORPHISM

The potential association of the S^{680} allele with poor responders to ovarian stimulation for IVF (Perez Mayorga et al., 2000; DeCastro et al., 2003) led to the hypothesis that the N^{680} allele could be associated with hyper-responders, i.e. patients at risk of iatrogenic OHSS. In an elegant study published by Daelemans et al. (2004), no statistically significant differences were found in allelic and genotypic frequencies between the IVF control population and the

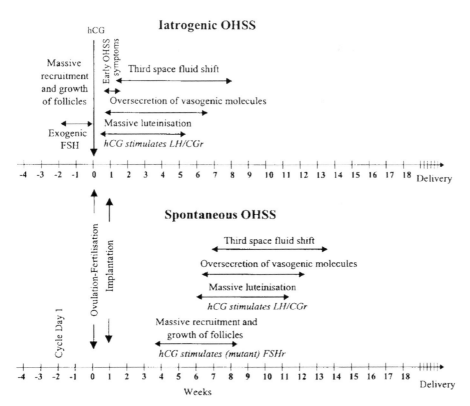

Fig. IV.10: Chronological development of iatrogenic and spontaneous OHSS
*Reproduced with permission from Delbaere et al. (2004). Hum Reprod **19**:486–9*

OHSS patients. However, Daelemans et al. (2004) observed a significant enrichment in allele 680 as the severity of OHSS increased ($p = 0.034$). The authors suggested that the genotype in position 680 of the FSH receptor cannot predict which patient will develop OHSS, but could be a predictor of severity of OHSS symptoms among OHSS patients.

RECURRENT THYROTOXOCOSIS IN PREGNANCY DUE TO THYROTROPIN RECEPTOR MUTATION

A similar phenomenon has been described by Rodien et al. (1998), in which stimulation of the thyrotropin receptor occurred by chorionic gonadotrophin. A woman and her mother had *recurrent gestational hyperthyroidism* despite normal serum chorionic gonadotrophin concentration. Both women were heterozygous for missense mutation in the extracellular domain of the thyrotropin receptor. The mutant receptor was more sensitive than the wild-type receptor to hCG, thereby explaining the occurrence of hyperthyroidism despite the fact that chorionic gonadotrophin concentrations were low. The major difference between this case and the three cases of FSH receptor mutation is in the position of the amino acid substituted. The substitution of arginine for lysine is in a region of a receptor that constitutes the surface of interaction with thyrotropin, and arginine at position 183 may increase the stability of the illegitimate complex between hCG and thyrotropin receptor enough to cause signal transduction by the increased serum hCG concentrations present in pregnant women (Rodien et al., 1998).

REFERENCES

Aittomaki K, Dieguez-Lucena JI, Pakarinen P et al. (1995). Mutation in the follicle-stimulating hormone receptor gene causes hereditary hypergonadotropic ovarian failure. *Cell* **82**:959−68.

Daelemans C, Smits G, de Maerlelaer V et al. (2004). Prediction of severity of symptoms in iatrogenic ovarian hyperstimulation syndrome by follicle stimulating hormone receptor Ser680Asn polymorphism. *J Clin Endocrinol Metab* **89**:6310−15.

Dahl Lyons CA, Wheeler CA, Frishman GN et al. (1994). Early and late presentation of the ovarian hyperstimulation syndrome: two distinct entities with different risk factors. *Hum Reprod* **9**:792−9.

De Castro R, Ruiz R, Montoro L et al. (2003). Role of follicle-stimulating hormone receptor Ser680Asn polymorphism in the efficacy of follicle stimulating hormone. *Fertil Steril* **80**:571−6.

Delbaere A, Smits G, Olatunbosun O et al. (2004). New insights into the pathophysiology of ovarian hyperstimulation syndrome. What makes the difference between spontaneous and iatrogenic syndrome? *Hum Reprod* **19**:486−9.

Edwards RG & Rizquez F (Eds) (2003). *Modern Assisted Conception*. Cambridge UK: Biomedicine Online: Reporoductive Healthcare Ltd, pp. 66−70.

Gromoll J, Ried T, Holtgreve-Grez H, Nieschlag E et al. (1994). Localization of the human FSH receptor to chromosome 2p21 using a genomic probe comprising exon 10. *J Mol Endocrinol* **12**:265−71.

Gromoll J, Simoni M & Nieschlag E (1996). An activating mutation of the follicle-stimulating hormone receptor autonomously sustains spermatogenesis in a hypophysectomized man. *J Clin Endocrinol Metab* **81**:1367−70.

Kaiser UB (2003). The pathogenesis of the ovarian hyperstimulation syndrome. *N Engl J Med* **349**:729−32.

Laven JS, Mulders AG, Suryandari DA et al. (2003). Follicle stimulationg hormone receptor polymorphisms in women with normogonadotrophic anovulatory infertility. *Fertil Steril* **80**:986−92.

Montanelli L, Van Durme JJ, Smits G et al. (2004a). Modulation of ligand selectivity associated with activation of the transmembrane region of the human follitropin receptor. *Mol Endocrinol* **18**:2061−73.

Montanelli L, Delbaere A, Di Carlo C et al. (2004b). A mutation in the follicle-stimulating hormone receptor as a cause of familial spontaneous ovarian hyperstimulation syndrome. *J Clin Endocrinol Metab* **89**:1255−8.

Olijve W, de Boer W, Mulders JWM et al. (1996). Molecular biology and biochemistry of human recombinant folicle stimulationg hormone (Puregon®). *Mol Hum Reprod* **2**:371−82.

Perez Mayorga M, Gromoll J, Behre HM et al. (2000). Ovarian response to follicle stimulating hormone (FSH) stimulation depends on the FSH receptor genotype. *J Clin Endocrinol Metab* **85**:3365−9.

Rizk B & Abdalla H (2006). Reproductive physiology of the female. In (Rizk B, Abdalla H, Eds), *Infertility and Assisted Reproduction Technology*. Oxford, UK: Health Press, pp. 8−12.

Rizk B & Aboulghar MA (2005). Classification, pathophysiology and management of ovarian hyperstimulation syndrome. In: (Brinsden P, Ed.), *A Textbook of In-vitro Fertilization and Assisted Reproduction*, Third Edition. London: Parthenon Publishing, Chapter 12, pp. 217–58.

Rodien P, Bemont C & Sanson ML (1998). Familial gestational hyperthyroidism caused by a mutant thyrotropin receptor hypersensitive to human chorionic gonadotrophin. *N Eng J Med* **339**:1823–6.

Rousseau-Merck MF, Atger M, Loosfelt H et al. (1993). The chromosomal localization of the human follicle-stimulating hormone receptor (FSHR) gene on 2p21-p16 is similar to that of the luteinizing hormone receptor gene. *Genomics* **15**:222–4.

Simoni M, Gromoll J & Nieschlag E (1997). The follicle stimulating hormone receptor: biochemistry, molecular biology, physiology, and pathophysiology. *Endocr Rev* **18**:739–73.

Simoni M, Nieschlag E & Gromoll J (2002). Isoforms and single nucleotide polymorphisms of the FSH receptor gene: Implications for human reproduction. *Hum Reprod Update* **8**:413–21.

Smits G, Olatunbosun O, Delbaere A et al. (2003). Ovarian hyperstimulation syndrome due to a mutation in the follicle-stimulating hormone receptor. *N Eng J Med* **349**:760–6.

Sprengel R, Braun T, Nikolics K et al. (1990). The testicular receptor for follicle stimulating hormone: structure and functional expression of cloned cDNA. *Mol Endocrinol* **4**:525–30.

Sudo S, Kudo M, Wada S et al. (2002). Genetic and functional analyses of polymorphisms in the human FSH receptor gene. *Mol Hum Reprod* **8**:893–9.

Themmen HPN & Huhtaniemi IT (2000). Mutations of gonadotrophins and gonadotrophin receptors: elucidating the physiology and pathophysiology of pituitary-gonadal function. *Endocr Rev* **21**:551–83.

Vasseur C, Rodien P, Beau I et al. (2003). A chorionic gonadotrophin-sensitive mutation in the follicle-stimulating hormone receptor as a cause of familial gestational spontaneous ovarian hyperstimulation syndrome. *N Engl J Med* **349**:753–9.

Vlaeminck-Guillem V, Ho SC, Rodien P et al. (2002). Activation of the cAMP pathway by the TSH receptor involves switching of the ectodomain from a tethered inverse agonist to an agonist. *Mol Endocrinol* **16**:736–46.

Whithney EA, Layman LC, Chan PJ et al. (1995). The follicle-stimulating hormone receptor gene is polymorphic in premature ovarian failure and normal controls. *Fertil Steril* **64**:518–24.

V

COMPLICATIONS OF OVARIAN HYPERSTIMULATION SYNDROME

Complications of OHSS are well documented in the literature (Rizk, 1992, 1993a; Bergh and Lundkvist, 1992; Roest et al., 1996). Bergh and Lundkvist (1992) surveyed the 12 IVF clinics in the Nordic countries and documented OHSS requiring hospital care in 0.7% of 10 125 treatment cycles. Similarly, Roest et al. (1996) performed a retrospective analysis of 2,495 cycles at the single clinic in The Netherlands. Hospital admission was required in 0.7% of cycles due to severe OHSS. While vascular complications are the most dreaded, other complications, such as pulmonary, gastrointestinal and renal complications have very serious sequelae in severe cases (Rizk and Nawar, 2004; Rizk and Aboulghar, 2005).

FATAL CASES OF OVARIAN HYPERSTIMULATION SYNDROME

Since the introduction of gonadotrophins for ovulation induction, there have been a number of deaths directly and indirectly related to OHSS (Schenker and Weinstein, 1978). The incidence of mortality following OHSS has been estimated at 1 in 500 000 (Brinsden et al., 1995). In three large reports of IVF from the Nordic countries, The Netherlands and Australia, there have been no reports of death in 10 125, 2495 and 59 681 IVF treatment cycles, respectively (Bergh and Lundkvist, 1992; Roest et al., 1996; Venn et al., 2001). It is also reassuring that the Australian registry showed that the mortality in a cohort of IVF patients is significantly lower then that in the general female population of the same age (age standardized mortality ratio of 0.58 and 95%, confidence interval 0.48−0.65, Venn et al., 2001).

The first fatal cases were described in 1951 by Gotzsche (Esteban-Altirriba, 1961) and also in 1958 (Figueroa-Casas, 1958). Until 1961, 60 cases of hyperstimulation have been reported including two deaths in patients treated with pregnant mare serum gonadotrophins (PMSG) (Figueroa-Casas, 1958; Muller, 1962; Schenker and Weinstein, 1978).

Lunenfeld (1963) first reported on the use of human menopausal gonadotrophins for ovulation induction. Over the last four decades there have been a handful of reports of death due to OHSS but the majority of cases are not reported (Mozes et al., 1965; Cluroe and Synek, 1995; Beerendonk et al., 1998; Serour et al., 1998; Semba et al., 2000). These cases are extremely important from a clinical viewpoint, and therefore they deserve special mention.

Mozes et al. (1965) reported a patient's demise as a result of arterial thromboembolism associated with OHSS. The patient was 37 years old and had been treated for infertility. She was in a concentration camp during the war years. At that time, menstruation ceased and did not reappear until she reached the age of 17 in 1945. She got married at the age of 20 and a year later gave birth at full term following a normal pregnancy. She had amenhorrea and galactorrhea after her pregnancy and she was diagnosed with Chiari—Frommel syndrome. In 1964, she was treated with 28 ampoules of gonadotrophin therapy (Pergonal-500) using 2—3 ampoules per day, each containing 500 units of gonadotrophins. This treatment was followed by 30 000 IU of hCG. She became pregnant but had a missed abortion. A year later, she was treated with 60 ampoules of gonadotrophin using the same schedule of 2—3 ampoules per day. This time she was given 25 000 IU of hCG and she presented to the hospital with acute left hemiplegia, in shock and comatose, and had an occlusion of the left internal carotid artery. She died in the hospital the following day.

Cluroe and Synek (1995) reported a case of cerebral infarction from OHSS. Serour et al. (1998) reported a case of hepato-renal failure following moderate OHSS. The patient was a 39-year-old woman who developed moderate OHSS, after ovum pickup she became drowsy and never regained full consciousness. She deteriorated quickly over a 10-day period and died of hepato-renal failure. A retrospective review revealed a history of hepatitis C with residual liver function impairment. Beerendonk et al. (1998) reported four deaths in The Netherlands that occurred between 1985 and 1998.

Semba et al. (2000) reported an autopsy case of severe OHSS in a 28-year-old Japanese female. The patient developed bilateral chest pain and progressive dyspnea during the course of administration of human gonadotrophins. Pleural effusion and hypouresis clinically disappeared four days after the onset of the symptoms, but the patient died suddenly of rapid respiratory insufficiency. Autopsy revealed massive pulmonary edema, intra-alveolar hemorrhage and pleural effusion, without any evidence of pulmonary thromboembolism. Histopathological examination of the ovary demonstrated multiple well-developed follicle formations consistent with OHSS. This is the first autopsy report of a patient with severe OHSS.

We are aware of at least four cases in the UK over the last decade. All the reported cases were following IVF but it is most certain that there are an equal, if not larger number of cases following ovulation induction without IVF.

VASCULAR COMPLICATIONS

Cerebrovascular complications are by far the most serious in OHSS (Rizk, 2001, 2002) as they may result in death (Mozes et al., 1965), stroke (Rizk et al., 1990) or amputation of a limb (Mozes et al., 1965; Mancini et al., 2001).

Incidence of Vascular Complications

The incidence of thromboembolism could not be determined with accuracy because of the absence of registration for OHSS cases or their complications (Delvigne and Rozenberg, 2003; Rizk and Nawar, 2004). Three large series of OHSS studies from Belgium, Israel and Egypt reported thromboembolic complications. In Belgium during a period of four years, one case of cerebral thrombosis (0.8%) was documented among 128 cases of OHSS (87% moderate and severe). In Israel, over a period of 10 years, an incidence of 2.4% of thromboembolic complications was observed among 209 cases of severe forms of OHSS (Abramov et al., 1999a). Serour et al. (1998) reported 10% of thromboembolic phenomena among patients with severe OHSS. The authors studied in detail the complications of assisted reproductive technology in 3500 IVF cycles. Ovarian hyperstimulation occurred in its moderate form in 206 cycles (5.9%) and in its severe form in 60 cycles (1.7%). Deep vein thrombosis occurred in four patients (0.12%) and hemiparesis in two patients (0.06%). All cases in this series were associated with severe OHSS.

Localization of Thromboembolic Complications

Delvigne (2004) found 68 cases of thrombosis reported in the literature. Among these, 34.3% of the cases were *arterial* and 65.7% were *venous*. The *upper and lower body distribution* was interesting. Some 83% was localized in the *upper part* of the body and 17% in the *lower part*. Of the upper body thromboses, 60% were venous and 40% were arterial. Of the lower body thromboses, 81% were venous and 19% were arterial. There were as many patients with early and late OHSS complicated by thrombosis, and also as many singleton as multiple pregnancies complicated by thromboses.

Internal Jugular Venous Thrombosis and OHSS

Schanzer et al. (2000) reviewed the case reports involving jugular venous thrombosis associated with pregnancy and/or OHSS. Belaen et al. (2001) reported a case of internal jugular vein thrombosis after ovarian stimulation with gonadotrophins. Screening for hereditary hypercoagulability for this patient was negative. The patient was successfully treated with low-molecular-weight heparin and a twin pregnancy was diagnosed.

Thromboembolic Complications without Severe OHSS

To date, several important cases of thromboembolism have been reported in association with gonadotrophin stimulation without *severe* OHSS (Kligman et al., 1995; Germond et al., 1996; Stewart et al., 1997a; Aboulghar et al., 1998; Loret de Mola et al., 2000). Some of these cases occurred in patients with pre-disposing factors (Kligman et al., 1995; Stewart et al., 1997) and others in the presence of spontaneous OHSS (Todros et al., 1999). Aboulghar et al. (1998) described two patients who developed moderate OHSS without evidence of hemoconcentration. Both developed serious cerebrovascular thromboses resulting in hemiparesis, and were treated with anticoagulants and recovered. This report emphasizes the role of other factors that can result in vascular thrombosis and illustrates that cerebrovascular accidents may complicate moderate OHSS. Delvigne (2004) advised caution in all cases of OHSS since thrombosis complicated about 12% of moderate OHSS cases as well as about 12% of mild OHSS cases. Furthermore, thromboses could appear as late as 20 weeks gestation, even in the absence of hemoconcentration, and in severe cases the event occurred several weeks after OHSS (Delvigne and Rosenberg, 2003).

Stewart et al. (1997a) reported three cases of upper limb deep venous thrombosis in association with assisted conception, the cause of which was largely unexplained. The authors stressed that not only did these thromboses occur in unusual sites, but that they also occurred well after the assumed peak period of risk.

Loret de Mola et al. (2000) reported two cases of subclavian deep vein thrombosis associated with the use of recombinant follicle-stimulating hormone (Gonal-F) complicating mild OHSS. A case of cortical vein thrombosis presenting as intracranial hemorrhage was described in a patient with OHSS after IVF and embryo transfer (ET). Veno-occlusive disease of the brain could appear as a hemorrhagic lesion on magnetic resonance imaging (MRI), and this made the initial diagnosis of cortical vein thrombosis difficult. The patient developed deep vein thrombosis two weeks after the intracranial event, and the diagnosis of cortical vein thrombosis was made at the time of MRI study after the resolution of the hemorrhage. The patient actually developed generalized thrombosis as a complication of OHSS (Shan Tang et al., 2000). Although the initial MRI picture may be misleading, the diagnosis of thrombosis should always be kept in mind, as it is the commonest cause of intracranial lesions after OHSS.

Timing of Thromboses: Early and Late

Thrombosis following the development of OHSS can occur in the luteal phase but can also occur several weeks after the development of the syndrome (Rizk and Aboulghar, 2005). Ong et al. (1991) reported internal jugular vein thrombosis occurring more than six weeks after ovulation, and Mills et al. (1992) reported subclavian vein thrombosis seven weeks after egg

Table V.1 Pathogenesis of thromboembolism in OHSS

Hemoconcentration

Pelvic venous pressure

Hypercoagulable state

Thrombophilia factor

Personal or family history of thromboembolism without thrombophilia

Impaired vascular reactivity

collection for IVF. These two late complications suggest a generalized effect on the coagulation system that may persist for several weeks.

Etiopathology of Thromboembolic Complications

A number of factors have been implicated in the pathogenesis of thrombo-embolism following gonadotrophin therapy (Table V.1). These include: hemoconcentration, a hypercoagulable state, the presence of thrombophilia, pressure on pelvic vessels and impairment of vascular activity.

HEMOCONCENTRATION AND OHSS

Hemoconcentration is an important sign in severe OHSS (Rizk et al., 1990).

Hemoconcentration and increased hematocrit values, in the presence of normal coagulation parameters, were found in nine of 25 patients by Schenker and Weinstein (1978). Hemoconcentration was found in 95.2% of 209 patients affected by severe OHSS (Abramov et al., 1999) and in 71.1% of 128 patients affected by mild or moderate forms of OHSS (Delvigne et al., 1993).

Mechanical Factors and Thrombosis in OHSS

Venous compression due to enlarged ovaries and ascites, together with immobility, may contribute to pelvic and lower limb thromboses in patients with severe OHSS (Rizk 2001, 2002).

Hypercoagulable State

The term hypercoagulable state is used to refer to hematological changes that may result in increased risk of thrombogenesis. The natural assumption in assisted conception and ovulation induction cycles is that 'raised estrogen' concentration is to blame (Rizk 1993a, b).

Hyperestrogenism

Exogenous estrogens promote thrombogenesis in a dose-dependent fashion. Endogenous estrogens are usually considered the cause of the increased risk of thromboembolism in pregnancy. During pregnancy, hematological changes include increased concentrations of factor VII, VIII, IX, X and XII and fibrinogen. There is also reduced concentration of protein S and antithrombin III.

Kim et al. (1981) studied the response of blood coagulation parameters to elevated estradiol induced by hMG. They reported a rise in fibrinogen concentration which correlated with the estradiol rise as the cycle progressed. There were no significant changes in the prothrombin time or activated partial thromboplastin time. There was a significant rise in Von Willebrand factor and reduction of antithrombin III, indicating the presence of a relatively hypercoagulable state. All these measurements were conducted after hCG administration, and therefore considered not representative of the times at which many women appear to experience thromboembolic complications of treatment (Stewart et al., 1997b).

Aune et al. (1991) reported that ovarian stimulation for IVF induced a hypercoagulable state. They followed up 12 IVF cycles, measuring whole blood clotting time (WBCT), whole blood clot lysis time (CLT), antithrombin III, plasma fibrinogen and factor VII, both before stimulation and after hCG administration, at the peak of estradiol concentration. Their findings showed a significant increase in fibrinogen and reduction in antithrombin III concentration, and a significant increase in CLT over this time, implying a disruption of the balance of coagulation and thrombolysis leading to a relative increase in coagulability. In contrast, Lox et al. (1995) assessed coagulation parameters up to 14 days after hCG and found that none of the changes were out of their laboratory's normal ranges. Although they noted significant correlations of some factors with changes in estradiol, and in prothrombin time (PT) and partial prothrombin time (PTT), they concluded that these changes could not constitute a promotion of coagulability, challenging the findings of Aune et al. (1991).

Stewart et al. (1997b) proposed an interesting question. If hyperestrogenism alone is responsible for the risk of thromboembolic disease, then why are many of these cases diagnosed some time after the expected peak estradiol concentration that is usually the time of hCG administration? Stewart et al. (1997b) proposed several explanations to that question. The first explanation is that OHSS simply prolongs the risk period of thromboembolism; the second explanation is that prolonged hepatic dysfunction secondary to OHSS might contribute to the hypercoagulable state (Ryley et al., 1990; Mills et al., 1992; Stewart et al., 1997b). The third explanation relies on the fact that high endogenous estradiol may increase free protein S and therefore be thromboprotective, and hence explains delayed thrombogenesis if the fall in estradiol is prolonged in OHSS (Stewart et al., 1997b).

Hypercoagulable State in OHSS

Kodama et al. (1996) studied the plasma hemostatic markers in OHSS. They found that the levels of thrombin−antithrombin III and plasma α_2-antiplasmin complexes in the plasma began to rise within a few days after hCG administration, with significantly higher levels during the midluteal phase. In OHSS patients who became pregnant, elevation of these markers continued for three weeks after the onset of the disease. There were also some characteristic changes in OHSS cycles in other hemostatic markers, such as a decrease in the levels of antithrombin III and prekallikrein, and shortened activated partial thromboplastin time. The practice in that unit was to provide preoperative subcutaneous heparin (5000 IU, single dose) in women undergoing oocyte retrieval, and in women hospitalized with symptomatic OHSS (subcutaneous 5000 IU, twice daily). Balasch et al. (1996) found an increased expression of induced monocyte tissue factor by plasma from patients with severe OHSS. This increase in the procoagulant activity of blood monocytes, which is mediated principally by tissue factor expression, may be important in thrombotic events associated with the syndrome.

Increased levels of factor V, platelets, fibrinogen, profibrinolysin and fibrinolytic inhibitors were observed by Phillips et al. (1975). Thrombophlebitis occurred in two out of 25 patients. Kaaja et al. (1989) described deep venous thrombosis in a case of severe OHSS. They suggested that raised Von Willebrand factor could result from increased platelet adhesion potentiated by hemoconcentration, and therefore could be an impending marker for OHSS development. Todorow et al. (1993) performed a retrospective study to evaluate the changes in Von Willebrand factor in OHSS.

Kodama et al. (1997) studied the status of the plasma kinin system in patients with OHSS in order to investigate whether activation of the plasma kinin system correlates with increased blood coagulability. They concluded that activation of the plasma kinin system occurs specifically and occasionally in OHSS patients, and is associated with increased blood coagulability, and that, when an OHSS patient demonstrates a low value of plasma kinin, more careful management is required to prevent thromboembolic complications.

Thrombophilia and Thromboembolism in OHSS

Thrombophilias are important because they could potentiate the risk of thrombosis under conditions of relative hypercoagulability that occur in assisted conception, particularly when complicated with OHSS (Rizk, 1993a; Ryo et al., 1999). The major thrombophilias include factor V Leiden mutation, protein C, protein S and antithrombin III deficiencies and antiphospholipid syndrome (Table V.2).

Dulitzky et al. (2000) prospectively evaluated the prevalence of markers of thrombophilia in 20 women hospitalized for severe OHSS. The following markers were assessed: plasma levels of antithrombin III, protein S and protein C, antiphospholipid antibodies, factor V Leiden mutation, and mutation of the methyltetrahydrofolate reductase (MTHFR) gene. In patients with OHSS, 85% were carriers of one or more positive markers of thrombophilia. All the thrombotic events occurred in women who had more than one marker for thrombophilia (40%). Furthermore, 27% of controls were carriers of one marker of thrombophilia and none carried more than one marker.

Table V.2 Thrombophilia and OHSS

Author	Year	Thrombophilia factor
Kaaja et al.	1989	Low antithrombin III
Benifla et al.	1994	Decreased protein S activity
Hollemaert et al.	1996	Leiden factor V mutation
Hortskamp et al.	1996	Leiden factor V mutation
McGowan et al.	2003	Prothrombin 3'UTR and factor V Leiden mutation

In contrast, Delvigne et al. (2002) using a matched control study of 25 patients with OHSS and observed no increase in the prevalence in the markers of thrombophilia for several months after the OHSS resolved. Delvigne and Rozenberg (2003) suggested that these discordant results may be due to the different times of screening for the thrombophilia markers. Whereas Dulitzky et al. (2000) evaluated their patients in the acute phase of OHSS, Delvigne et al. studied the thrombophilia markers after the OHSS episode. During OHSS, the coexisting hyperestrogenemia may contribute to the decrease in antithrombin III or protein S levels.

Fabregues et al. (2004) conducted a case control study on prevalence of thrombophilia in women with severe OHSS and cost-effectiveness of screening. The cost of preventing one thrombotic event in a patient developing severe OHSS after IVF and having factor V Leiden or prothrombin G20210A mutations was calculated. None of the OHSS patients or controls had anti-thrombin, protein C, or free protein S deficiencies. All of them tested negative for antiphospholipid antibodies.

Todros et al. (1999) reported a case of spontaneous OHSS occurring in a pregnant woman carrying the Factor V Leiden mutation. Even though prophylactic treatment for thrombo-embolism was adopted by administering low-molecular-weight heparin, the pregnancy was complicated by thromboses of the left subclavian, axillary, humeral and internal jugular veins during the second trimester of gestation. The pregnancy was managed conservatively, and a healthy baby was delivered at term. In order to avoid unnecessary laparotomy the authors emphasized the importance of careful diagnosis in order to differentiate spontaneous OHSS from ovarian carcinoma, as well as the necessity to look for the presence of coagulation disorders in women affected by OHSS.

A 33-year-old female developed OHSS with thrombosis of the right internal jugular vein, subclavian vein and superior vein cava following IVF (Lamon et al., 2000). As pregnancy progressed, edema, pain and tingling sensation developed. CT scan confirmed thrombus with the right internal jugular and subclavian vein and a free floating tip in the superior vein cava. Following treatment with intravenous heparin and subcutaneous low-molecular-weight heparin until delivery, the symptoms improved.

Andrejevic et al. (2002) reported a 28-year-old patient with polycystic ovary syndrome who presented with fever and laboratory markers of inflammation. Intracardiac thrombosis was diagnosed in the presence of antiphospholipid antibodies. The authors suggested that primary antiphospholipid syndrome was possibly triggered by ovulation induction.

Elford et al. (2002) presented a case of a previously healthy woman who underwent in-vitro fertilization and experienced a middle cerebral artery thrombosis that was subsequently lysed with intra-arterial recombinant tissue plasminogen activator (rt-PA). To the authors' knowledge this was the first reported case of successful use of rt-PA to lyse a cerebral arterial thrombus resulting from severe OHSS. The patient made a nearly complete neurologic recovery and delivered a healthy infant at term, illustrating that intra-arterial thrombolysis can be used with relative safety even in very early pregnancy. Ulug et al. (2003) reported a case of bilateral internal jugular venous thrombosis following successful assisted conception in the absence of OHSS.

McGowan et al. (2003) reported a case of deep vein thrombosis followed by internal jugular vein thrombosis as a complication of IVF in a woman heterozygous for the prothrombin 3'UTR and factor V Leiden mutations. They suggested that neck pain and swelling in a pregnant woman, especially one that has undergone IVF, should be taken seriously and investigated with duplex scanning and/or MRI. Women with a personal or family history of thrombosis who are undergoing IVF should be made fully aware of the potential thrombotic risks, and should be considered for a thrombophilia screen.

Ou et al. (2003) reported a case of thromboembolism after ovarian stimulation and successful management of a woman with superior sagittal sinus thrombosis after IVF and embryo transfer. The authors recommended dose-adjusted heparinization as the first-line treatment of choice, while intravascular thrombolysis or operative thrombectomy is an aggressive but effective treatment. Continuation of pregnancy is considered safe without any increased risk of fetal congenital anomalies.

Nakauchi-Tanaka (2003) reported on a 31-year-old nulligravida woman who developed an acquired factor VIII inhibitor associated with severe OHSS. She developed hematuria, ecchymosis and intramuscular bleeding following the severe OHSS. Laboratory examinations showed a markedly prolonged activated partial thromboplastin time and a low level of factor VIII activity. Treatment with prothrombin complex concentrate and factor VIII inhibitor bypassing agent was successful in reducing the inhibitor, so that she delivered a healthy baby via spontaneous vaginal delivery. Acquired hemophilia is a life-threatening disorder. This was the first case report of acquired hemophilia in OHSS.

Personal or Family History of Thromboembolic Disease

Several cases of thromboembolic complications have been reported in patients who had either a personal or family history of thromboembolic disease without evidence of familial thrombophilia (Dalrymple et al., 1982–3; Boulier et al., 1989; Thill et al., 1994; Benshushan et al., 1995; Stewart et al., 1997a, b).

Impairment of Vascular Reactivity

Foong et al. (2002) performed measurement and quantification of the cutaneous arteriolar vasoconstrictor response using laser doppler fluximetry. Women with OHSS have impaired vascular reactivity when compared with normal women. Foong et al. (2002) suggested that OHSS is associated with reversible impairment of vascular reactivity that may contribute to the increased prevalence of thromboses.

RARE VASCULAR COMPLICATIONS ASSOCIATED WITH OHSS

Central Retinal Artery Occlusion

Turkistani et al. (2001) reported a case of severe OHSS presenting with central retinal artery occlusion.

Forearm Amputation

Mancini et al. (2001) reported a case of forearm amputation after ovarian stimulation for IVF-ET. The patient underwent many cycles of IVF-ET. She had a coagulation disorder as a result of OHSS, with thrombosis of the axillary vein recurring after thromboarterectomy and leading to the paradoxical result of the amputation of an arm.

Cerebral Infarction

Cerebral infarction represents the most serious complication of thrombo-embolism associated with OHSS (Neau et al., 1989; Rizk and Aboulghar, 1991; Yoshii et al., 1999; Dumont et al., 2000). The fatal case reported by Cluroe and Synek (1995) represents the worst of a spectrum of cases. More than 14 cases of stroke have been reported following OHSS. Six cases were treated with intravenous heparin and at least one case treated with interarterial recombinant tissue plasminogen activator (Elford et al., 2002).

Myocardial Infarction

Myocardial infarction associated with severe OHSS is extremely rare (Ludwig et al., 1999; Akdemir et al., 2002). Ludwig et al. (1999) reported the first case of myocardial infarction after ovarian hyperstimulation. A 35-year-old patient, 77 kg in weight, and a heavy smoker (30 cigarettes/day) underwent an IVF Intracytoplasmic Sperm Injection (ICSI) cycle. Decapeptyl depot 3.75 mg was administered and recombinant FSH 150 IU was started two weeks later.

The dose was increased to 225 IU on the fifth day and hCG 10 000 IU was given on the sixteenth day of stimulation. The serum estradiol level was 12 892 pmol/l on the day of hCG, and 16 oocytes were retrieved and three embryos were fertilized and transferred two days later. Human CG 5000 IU was given again on the day of transfer and micronized progesterone 600 mg was administered intravaginally each day. The patient returned at midnight to the emergency department with severe backache and dyspnea and a hematocrit of 48%. At the coronary care unit, 5000 IU of heparin and 500 mg of acetylsalicylate were given immediately, and a coronary angiogram demonstrated a distal occlusion of the left anterior descending coronary artery. Due to intracoronary thrombotic material, recannulization of the distal left anterior descending (LAD) artery by percutaneous transluminal coronary angioplasty was unsuccessful. A stent to the LAD artery only slightly improved the blood flow. The patient had an otherwise uncomplicated clinical course, and a follow-up coronary angiogram after 10 days and again after six months revealed no reanastomosis or thrombotic material, and the stented segment of the proximal LAD coronary artery remained open while the distal LAD coronary artery remained occluded. Results of all coagulation profiles were within normal limits and the patient did not become pregnant. Akdemir et al. (2002) reported a case of a patient with myocardial infraction associated with OHSS.

RESPIRATORY COMPLICATIONS

Respiratory complications can present with a variety of symptoms and signs in OHSS (Rizk, 1992, 1993b, 2001).

Abramov et al. (1999a) observed pulmonary complications in 7.2% of severe OHSS cases (Table V.3). Dyspnea and tachypnea were the most common symptoms appearing in 92% of these cases. A small proportion of patients that had pulmonary manifestations presented with complications, such as local pneumonia (4%), adult respiratory distress syndrome (2%) and pulmonary embolism (2%) (Abramov et al., 1999a). Pleural effusion was observed in 21% of 128 cases of OHSS in a Belgian multi-center study (Delvigne et al., 1993).

Unilateral Pleural Effusion

Jewelewicz and Van de Wiele (1975) reported the first case of pleural effusion as the sole presentation of OHSS following superovulation. Following the introduction of IVF, Kingsland et al. (1989) from the Hallam Medical Center reported the first case of right unilateral pleural effusion in an IVF patient. Wood et al. (1998) reported a case of symptomatic pleural effusion following an ICSI cycle in a patient who had previously undergone right hemicolectomy for Crohn's disease. The first aspirate removed 800 ml of serous fluid. The protein content was 53 mg/l which contrasts with our case

Table V.3 Pulmonary and extrapulmonary features of 209 patients hospitalized with severe OHSS in Israel from 1987 to 1996 *Reproduced with permission from Abramov et al. (1999a). Hum Reprod 71:645–51*

	No. (%) of patients
Pulmonary	
Dyspnea	193 (92)
Pneumonia	8 (4)
ARDS	5 (2)
Pulmonary embolism	4 (2)
Extrapulmonary	
Ascites	207 (99)
Gastrointestinal	112 (54)
Disturbances	
Oliguria	62 (30)
Peripheral edema	28 (13)
Peritoneal irritation	13 (6)
Acute renal failure	3 (1)

(Kingsland et al., 1989). Rabinerson et al. (2000) reported severe unilateral hydrothorax as the only manifestation of the OHSS. A 35-year-old woman presented with mild dyspnea two weeks after ovarian stimulation with hMG and hCG and IVF-ET. Chest X-ray revealed a large pleural effusion on the right side. Three consecutive thoracocenteses were needed to drain a total of 6800 cc of fluid. Following drainage, the respiratory symptoms disappeared. An uneventful pregnancy progressed.

Cordani et al. (2002) discussed a case of massive unilateral hydrothorax as the only clinical manifestation of OHSS. A decade later, we have described a case very similar to the first case following IVF (Gore et al., 2002) which we reported in the late 1980s and summarized the published literature regarding OHSS presenting only as pleural effusion (Table V.4).

Pathophysiology of Unilateral Pleural Effusion in OHSS

Several authors have investigated the pathophysiology of unilateral pleural effusions in severe OHSS, particularly in the absence of ascites (Kingsland et al., 1989; Friedler et al., 1998; Gore et al., 2002). It has been suggested that the diaphragmatic lymphatics are a route for the transfer of ascites into the pleural space in cases of cirrhosis and Meig's syndrome. Multiple macroscopic defects covered only with thin membranes have been directly observed in the tendinous portion of the diaphragm by laparoscopy and open thoracotomy.

Table V.4 Isolated pleural effusion as the only manifestation of OHSS
Reproduced with permission from Gore et al. (2002). Middle East Fertility Society Journal 7:211–13

Author and year of publication	Jewelewicz and Van de Wide, 1975	Kingsland et al., 1989	Daniel et al., 1995	Bassil et al., 1996	Wood et al., 1998	Friedler et al., 1998 (case 1)	Friedler et al., 1998 (case 2)	Man et al., 1997 (4 cases)	Arikan et al., 1997	Gore et al., 2002
Age	24	35	27	39	29	29	33	24–29	29	27
Peak follicular E2 level	180 mg/24 h	1221 nmol/24 h	1900 ng/ml	2650 pg/ml	3479 pg/ml	>3000 pg/ml	>3000 pg/ml	NM*	NM*	1840 pg/ml
No. of oocytes retrieved	none	7	none	11	18	22	19	NM*	NM*	none (IUI)**
Luteal support	none	none	none	progesterone	hCG	progesterone	progesterone	NM*	NM*	hcG and progesterone
Onset of OHSS hCG	13 days after hCG administration	10 days after oocyte retrieval	10 days after hCG administration	12 days after oocyte retrieval	6 days after oocyte retrieval	12 days after oocyte retrieval	5 days after oocyte retrieval	NM*	12 days after oocyte retrieval	10 days after hCG administration
Hydrothorax	right side	right side	right side	left side	right side	right side (recurrent)	right Side	right side (one left sided)	left side	right side (recurrent)
Fluid drained	none (resolved spontaneously)	3.5 l	2 l	2.5 l	4 l	1.7 l	4.5 l	1.2 l–2 l	4 l	10.4 l
Presence of ascites	none	none	none	none	none	minimal	none	none	minimal	none
Conception	in vivo	IVF-ET followed by miscarriage	in vivo	IVF-ET (twins)	none (after IVF-ET)	IVF-ET (twins)	none (after IVF-ET)	IVF-ET in one case (NM* for other cases)	IVF-ET (twins)	in vivo

* NM = not mentioned
** IUI = intrauterine insemination

There are documented cases of massive pleural effusion in patients who are undergoing peritoneal dialysis. Loret de Mola (1999) suggested that exposure to high pressure of ascites transforms these attenuated areas into blebs, which protrude into the thorax. The negative intrathoracic preferentially allows for the ascites to permeate through the open channels when the blebs rupture. These defects are more common on the right diaphragm, which explain the predominance of cases of right-sided pleural effusion reported in the literature (Gore et al., 2002).

Is the Pleural Effusion Transudate or Exudate?

Chemical analysis of the fluid obtained from pleurocentesis revealed both transudates (Daniel et al., 1995; Bassil et al., 1996; Friedler et al., 1998; Wood et al., 1998; Rabinerson et al., 2000) and exudates (Kingsland et al., 1989; Man et al., 1997; Gregory and Patton, 1999; Roden et al., 2000). This observation remains unexplained, as this may reflect the possibility of multiple mechanisms involved in the pathogenesis of isolated hydrothorax.

Adult Respiratory Distress Syndrome

Adult respiratory distress syndrome (ARDS) is defined as severe hypoxemia of acute clinical onset and bilateral scattered pulmonary infiltrates on a frontal chest radiograph (alveolar infiltrate) after exclusion of left atrial or pulmonary capillary hypertension (Delvigne and Rozenberg, 2003). Zosmer et al. (1987) reported the first case of ARDS complicating ovulation induction. The authors considered pulmonary capillary leakage induced by prostaglandin release, hypoalbuminemia and shift of dextran-40 molecules to the intralveolar space to be the most probable reason for the occurrence of this complication. Abramov et al. (1999a), in a series of cases of pulmonary complications following OHSS, noted that ARDS occurred after pronounced hydration. In their series, one patient with ARDS had dyspnea and 80% had a temperature of over 38 degrees. On auscultation, the patients had bilateral decrease of respiratory sounds in addition to the presence of bilateral pulmonary rauls.

Prostaglandins and cytokines may play a role in the pathophysiology of ARDS. The increase in vascular permeability results in a leakage of plasma and colloids resulting in pulmonary edema and atelectasis, which would be fatal. Schenker and Ezra (1994) reported 50% recovery without sequelae.

Renal Complications

Prerenal failure is a complication of hypovolemia secondary to fluid transudation in the peritoneal cavity. Balasch et al. (1990) reported a case of prerenal failure after treatment with indomethacin and advised against the use of prostaglandin synthetase inhibitors. Ovarian hyperstimulation syndrome in a renal transplant patient undergoing assisted conception treatment was reported (Khalaf et al., 2000). Ovarian enlargement secondary to OHSS resulted in obstruction in the transplanted kidney and deterioration of renal function. Conservative management was successful and a live twin birth was later achieved by replacement of two frozen—thawed embryos.

Liver Dysfunction

Abnormal liver functions tests occur in 25—40% of cases (Forman et al., 1990; Delvigne and Rozenberg, 2003; Fabregues et al., 1999). Sueldo et al. (1988) and Younis et al. (1988) were the first to report liver dysfunction in severe OHSS. Since then, abnormal hepatic function has been increasingly recognized as a complication of severe OHSS that may persist for over two months. It was interesting to note that, although the liver function tests were markedly abnormal, liver biopsy showed significant morphological abnormalities only at the ultrastructural level.

ETIOPATHOLOGY OF LIVER ABNORMALITIES IN OHSS

The relationship of serum pro-inflammatory cytokines and vascular endothelial growth factor with liver dysfunction in severe OHSS was studied (Rizk, 1993b; Southgate et al., 1999; Chen et al., 2000). Concentrations of IL-6 in the active phase of OHSS were significantly higher in the abnormal liver function tests group than in the normal liver function tests group. These results suggest that the IL-6 cytokine system may play a role in pathogenesis of liver dysfunction in severe OHSS. Abnormal liver function tests were associated with lower clinical pregnancy rates.

Elter et al. (2001) reported a case of hepatic dysfunction associated with moderate OHSS, suggesting that hepatic dysfunction is not limited to severe forms of OHSS. Liver function should be analyzed even in moderate cases.

Davis et al. (2002) reported a severe case of OHSS with liver dysfunction and malnutrition, in which the patient's albumin dropped to 9 g/l associated with liver function abnormalities: alanine aminotransferase 46 IU/l, alkaline phosphatase 706 IU/l, bilirubin 26 μmol/l and prothrombin time 19 s. The judicious use of paracentesis and commencement of total parenteral nutrition coincided with a rapid clinical improvement. One month after discharge, the patient was asymptomatic with normal liver function.

RECURRENT CHOLESTASIS

Recurrent cholestasis is unique to pregnancy and typically manifests during the last trimester. Characteristically, the first symptom is pruritus which is associated with serum bile acids and abnormal liver functions. The disease usually resolves spontaneously within a few days after delivery. A case of recurrent cholestasis during a twin pregnancy following IVF has been reported

(Midgley et al., 1999). It was proposed that the patient had a genetic predisposition to developing cholestasis on separate occasions, initially in the first trimester secondary to abnormally high estrogen concentration following OHSS and subsequently in the third trimester as is typical of obstetric cholestasis.

Gastrointestinal Complications

With the widespread use of ovulation induction for assisted conception, it is mandatory that general practitioners become aware that gastrointestinal symptoms may be the initial presentation of ovarian hyperstimulation (Rizk and Aboulghar, 1991, 2005). One such case presented to us with a cerebrovascular accident because such symptoms were ignored (Rizk et al., 1990).

Mesenteric Artery Occlusion in OHSS

Mesenteric resection after massive arterial infarction has been reported (Aurousseau et al., 1995).

Duodenal Ulcer Perforation

Uhler et al. (2001) reported the first case of perforated ulcer following severe OHSS. A 29-year-old nulligravid woman with polycystic ovarian syndrome underwent her first attempt at IVF in Chicago. A long protocol luteal phase GnRH agonist was used for pituitary—ovarian axis down-regulation followed by FSH for ovarian stimulation. On the tenth day of FSH administration, more than 10 follicles measured at least 18 mm in diameter on ultrasound, and the estradiol level was 4245 pg/ml on the day of hCG. Transvaginal ultrasound-guided follicular aspiration yielded 19 oocytes at 36 h after administration of 5000 IU of hCG. No fresh embryos were transferred and 11 cleaved embryos were cryopreserved. Two days later, the patient complained of abdominal distension, shortness of breath and mid to upper abdominal pain, and presented to her physician's office for the evaluation of possible OHSS. She was admitted to the hospital for observation and intravenous hydration. On hospital day 10, she underwent exploratory laparotomy and a posterior perforation of the posterior duodenum that required antrectomy gastrojejeunostomy and lateral tube duodenostomy for the control of the perforation. The pathology report confirmed chronic gastritis and *Helicobacter pylori*. The patient required prolonged assisted ventilation, and on hospital day 22 she required a tracheostomy tube placement, and then she was weaned to a tracheostomy collar of humidified air and her nutritional support was via a feeding tube. The patient was hospitalized for a total of 47 days and then transferred to a rehabilitation center for an additional 30 days before being discharged home. The patient had her tracheostomy removed during her stay at the first two-week rehabilitation center, and then was transferred to another rehabilitation center for her last two weeks for intensive physical and occupational therapy. She was finally discharged home 86 days after her IVF cycle. The authors felt that in this critically ill patient with OHSS, severe stress associated with invasive monitoring and multiple therapies in the intensive care unit, as well as *H. pylori* infection, were probably the most likely causal factors of her perforated duodenum. We are aware of a similar case in the UK that resulted in mortality following perforated duodenum and other associated complications from intensive monitoring.

OHSS COMPLICATED PERITONITIS DUE TO PERFORATED APPENDICITIS

Fujimoto et al. (2002) reported a case of peritonitis due to a perforated appendix. The patient presented with abdominal distension after ovarian stimulation with hMG followed by hCG to trigger ovulation. The patient developed massive ascites and swollen ovaries and was admitted with a diagnosis of OHSS. An intravenous infusion of serum albumin and low dose dopamine were administered to increase her fluid output. The dopamine failed to increase her urinary output, the abdominal symptoms deteriorated and paracentesis revealed infected foul-smelling fluid. An emergency laparotomy was performed and the final diagnosis was peritonitis due to perforated appendix and a right tubal pregnancy. Appendectomy, right salpingectomy and vigorous irrigation and drainage were performed. The authors caution that OHSS may not only mask typical manifestations of appendicitis, but could also compromise concurrent intraperitoneal infection.

BENIGN INTRACRANIAL HYPERTENSION

Lesny et al. (1999) reported a case of OHSS and benign intracranial hypertension in pregnancy after IVF/ET. Shortly after embryo transfer, the patient developed clinical signs of moderate OHSS with symptoms which were later diagnosed as benign intracranial hypertension (BIH). The BIH was treated effectively using repeated lumbar puncture and diuretics. Spontaneous labor and delivery occurred at 40 weeks' gestation. There was no neurological sequel and no recurrence of the BIH two years after the pregnancy. The possible link between OHSS and BIH as well as the risks of further pregnancy should be considered.

Mesothelial Cells Proliferation in Lymph Nodes after Severe OHSS

Endometriosis and endosalpingiosis are the most well known benign intranodal heterotopic inclusions. Leiomyomatosis, and intranodal inclusions of nevus and decidua are much less common (Colby, 1999). Van der Weiven et al. (2005) reported a rare case of ectopic mesothelial preformation in cervical lymph nodes after severe OHSS. They reported a rare case in which a 42-year-old woman underwent successful IVF and developed severe OHSS, and pathologically enlarged cervical lymph nodes. Familiarity with this event is important for the clinician, as well as for the pathologist, in order to prevent the misdiagnosis of malignancy.

FEBRILE MORBIDITY

Febrile morbidity is common during OHSS. Abramov et al. (1998a) performed the most comprehensive study to define the incidence of febrile morbidity and its causes in severe and critical OHSS. The authors reviewed the medical records of all OHSS patients hospitalized in 16 out of 19 tertiary medical centers in Israel between January 1987 and December 1996. They defined febrile morbidity as at least one temperature rise above 38°C, lasting ≥24 h. They identified 2902 patients who had 3305 hospitalizations as a result of OHSS, of whom 196 had severe and 13 critical OHSS. The incidence of febrile morbidity in these 209 patients was 82.3%. The causes of the infections are presented in Table V.5. The causative organisms encountered are presented in Table V.6. Interestingly, no infectious etiology could be found in 50.2% (105 patients). Hypoglobulinemia was observed in most patients. The ascitic and pleural fluids aspirated from these patients contained high globulin concentrations. Abramov et al. (1998a) concluded that infection-related febrile morbidity in severe and critical OHSS is high and may be related to immune deficiency that resulted from the loss of plasma globulins to the third space (Abramov et al., 1999b). Interestingly, non-infection-related febrile morbidity was possibly related to endogenous pyrogenic mechanisms (Abramov et al., 1998a).

OBSTETRIC COMPLICATIONS

Early Pregnancy Complications

Raziel et al. (2002) reported increased early pregnancy loss in IVF patients with severe OHSS (38% as compared to 15% in the control group). Abnormal hCG levels may occur in early pregnancy in patients with ovarian hyperstimulation syndrome. However, these abnormal levels do not predict poor outcome in pregnancies complicated by OHSS (Samuel and Grosskinsky, 2004); therefore, they are not helpful in the decision-making process to diagnose ectopic pregnancy or otherwise compromised pregnancies.

Late Pregnancy Complications

A higher prevalence of obstetric complications have been reported in pregnancies following IVF, mainly as a result of multiple pregnancy, but also independent of multiplicity (Rizk et al., 1991b; Tan et al., 1992). Selection of appropriate control groups is of paramount importance in

Table V.5 Febrile morbidity in patients with severe and critical
OHSS
*Reproduced with permission from Abramov et al. (1998a). Hum
Reprod **13**:3128–31*

	No. of patients (%)
Mean (±SD) febrile episodes/patient	2.3 ± 0.8
Mean (±SD) duration of febrile episodes (documented infections)	34.6 ± 8.2
UTI	
positive	35 (16.7)
probable	8 (3.8)
Pneumonia	
positive	4 (1.9)
probable	4 (1.9)
URTI	
positive	3 (1.4)
probable	4 (1.9)
Intravenous line phlebitis	
positive	2 (1.0)
probable	2 (1.0)
Cellulitis at an abdominal puncture sight	
positive	2 (1.0)
probable	0 (0.0)
Gluteal abscess at the site of progesterone injection	
positive	1 (0.5)
probable	0 (0.0
Postoperative wound infection	2 (1.0)
Peritonitis	0 (0.0)
Total infection rate	67 (32.1)
Antibiotic treatment	
Intravenous	9 (4.3)
Oral	58 (27.8)
Mean (±SD) duration of treatment (days)	5.2 ± 2.1
No. of documented infections	105 (50.2)
Total febrile morbidity	172 (82.3)

determining whether IVF pregnancies have a higher or lower rate of perinatal
complications (Brinsden and Rizk, 1992; Rizk et al., 1991c). Only a few studies
examined the pregnancy outcome specifically in IVF patients who developed
OHSS (Abramov et al., 1998b; Mathur and Jenkins, 2000). In the larger

Table V.6 Infective organisms isolated from patients with severe OHSS
*Reproduced with permission from Abramov et al. (1998). Hum Reprod **13**:3128–31*

Infection/organism	No. of patients (%)
UTI*	
Proteus mirabilis	12 (34.3)
Klebsiella pneumoniae	7 (20.0)
Pseudomonas aeruginosa	6 (17.1)
Escherichia coli	4 (11.4)
Morganella morganii	2 (5.7)
Proteus vulgaris	2 (5.7)
Staphylococcus aureus	1 (2.9)
Enterobacter cloacae	1 (2.9)
Pneumonia	
Pseudomonas aeruginosa	1 (25.0)
Klebsiella pneumoniae	1 (25.0)
Staphylococcus aureus	1 (25.0)
Streptococcus pneumoniae	1 (25.0)
URTI**	
Group A streptococcus	1 (33.3)
M/P viral	2 (66.7)
Intravenous line phlebitis	
Staphylococcus epidermidis	1 (50.0)
Pseudomonas aeruginosa	1 (50.0)
Cellulitis at an abdominal puncture site	
Staphylococcus aureus	1 (100)
Postoperative wound infection	
Staphylococcus aureus	1 (50)
Pseudomonas aeruginosa	1 (50)

* UTI = urinary tract infection
** URTI = upper respiratory tract infection

study by Abramov et al. (1998b), the control group was selected from international data, whereas in the smaller study by Mathur and Jenkins (2000) a contemporaneous control group was used. Abramov et al. (1998b) reported that, among IVF patients with severe and critical OHSS, pregnancy rates, multiple gestations, miscarriage, preterm premature rupture of the membranes,

Table V.7 Perinatal complications of IVF pregnancies associated with severe OHSS in 68 patients compared with all IVF pregnancies (international data) *Reproduced with permission from Abramov et al. (1998). Fertil Steril* **70**:1070—6

Perinatal complication	Number of patients with indicated complication	
	Severe OHSS (%)	*All IVF (%)*
Preterm PROM*	12 (17.7)	4.9
Pregnancy induced hypertension	9 (13.2)	6.0
Gestational diabetes	4 (5.9)	0.8
Oligohydramnios	3 (4.4)	NA**
Placental abruption	3 (4.4)	0.4
Discordant twins	1 (1.5)	NA
Intrauterine growth retardation	1 (1.5)	7.0
Chorioamnioitis	1 (1.5)	NA
Stillbirth	1 (1.5)	0.7
Thromboembolic phenomena	1 (1.5)	NA

* PROM = premature rupture of the fetal membranes
** NA = not available

prematurity and low birth weight rates are significantly higher than those reported previously for pregnancies after assisted conception (Table V.7).

REFERENCES

Aboulghar MA, Mansour RT, Serour GI et al. (1998). Moderate ovarian hyperstimulation syndrome complicated by deep cerebrovascular thrombosis. *Hum Reprod* **13**:2088—91.

Abramov Y, Elchalal U & Schenker JG (1998a). Febrile morbidity in severe and critical ovarian hyperstimulation syndrome: a multicentre study. *Hum Reprod* **13**:3128—31.

Abramov Y, Elchalal U & Schenker JG (1998b). Obstetric outcome of in-vitro fertilized pregnancies complicated by severe ovarian hyperstimulation syndrome: a multicenter study. *Fertil Steril* **70**:1070—6.

Abramov Y, Elchalal U & Schenker JG (1999a). Pulmonary manifestations of severe ovarian hyperstimulation syndrome: a multicenter study. *Fertil Steril* **71**:645—51.

Abramov Y, Naparstek Y, Elchalal U et al. (1999b). Plasma immunoglobulins in patients with severe ovarian hyperstimulation syndrome. *Fertil Steril* **71**:102—5.

Akdemir R, Uyan C & Emiroglu Y (2002). Acute myocardial infarction secondary thrombosis associated with ovarial hyperstimulation syndrome. *Int J Cardiol* **83**:187—9.

Andrejevic S, Bonaci-Nikolic B, Bukilica M et al. (2002). Intracardiac thrombosis and fever possibly triggered by ovulation induction in a patient with antiphospholipid antibodies. *Scand J Rheumatol* **31**:249—51.

Arikan G, Giuliani A, Gucer F et al. (1997). Rare manifestations of the ovarian hyperstimulation syndrome: a report of two cases. *Clin Exp Obstet Gynecol* **24**:154—6.

Aune B, Hoie KE, Oian P et al. (1991). Does ovarian stimulation for in-vitro fertilization induce a hypercoagulable state? *Hum Reprod* **6**:925−7.

Aurousseau MH, Samama MM, Belhassen A et al. (1995). Risk of thromboembolism in relation to an in-vitro fertilization programme: three case reports. *Hum Reprod* **10**:94−7.

Balasch J, Carmona F, Llach J et al. (1990). Acute prerenal failure and liver dysfunction in a patient with severe ovarian hyperstimulation syndrome. *Hum Reprod* **5**:3448−51.

Balasch J, Reverter JC, Fabregues F et al. (1996). Increased induced monocyte tissue factor expression by plasma from patients with severe ovarian hyperstimulation syndrome. *Fertil Steril* **66**:608−13.

Bassil S, DaCosta S, Toussaint Demylle D et al. (1996). A unilateral hydrothorax as the only manifestation of ovarian hyperstimulation syndrome: a case report. *Fertil Steril* **66**:1023−5.

Beerendonk CC, Van Dop PA, Braat DD et al. (1998). Ovarian hyperstimulation syndrome: facts and fallacies. *Obstet Gynecol Surv* **53**:439−49.

Belaen B, Geerinckx K, Vergauwe P & Thys J (2001). Internal jugular vein thrombosis after ovarian stimulation. *Hum Reprod* **16**:510−12.

Benifla JL, Conard J, Naouri M et al. (1994). Ovarian hyperstimulation syndrome and thrombosis. Apropos of a case of thrombosis of the internal jugular vein. Review of the literature. *J Gynecol Obstet Biol Reprod (Paris)* **23**:778−83.

Benshushan A, Shushan A, Palitiel O et al. (1995). Ovulation induction with clomiphene citrate complicated by deep vein thrombosis. *Eur J Obstet Gynecol Reprod Biol* **62**:261−2.

Bergh T & Lundkvist O (1992). Clinical complications during in-vitro fertilization treatment. *Hum Reprod* **7**:625−6.

Boulieu D, Ninet J, Pinede L et al. (1989). Thrombose veineuse précoce de siège inhabituel, en début de grossesse apres hyperstimulation ovarienne. *Contracept Fertil Sex* **17**:725−7.

Brinsden P & Rizk B (1992). The obstetric outcome of assisted conception treatment. *Assisted Reproduction Reviews* **2**:16−25.

Brinsden PR, Wada J, Tan SL et al. (1995). Diagnosis, prevention and management of ovarian hyperstimulation syndrome. *Br J Ostet Gynaecol* **102**:767−72.

Chen CD, Wu MY, Chen HF et al. (2000). Relationships of serum pro-inflammatory cytokines and vascular endothelial growth factor with liver dysfunction in severe ovarian hyperstimulation syndrome. *Hum Reprod* **15**:66−71.

Choktanasiri W & Rojanasakul A (1995). Acute arterial thrombosis after gamete intrafallopian transfer: a case report. *J Assist Reprod Genet* **12**:335−7.

Cordani S, Bancalari L, Maggiani R et al. (2002). Massive unilateral hydrothorax as the only clinical manifestation of ovarian hyperstimulation syndrome. *Monaldi Arch Chest Dis* **57**:314−17.

Cluroe AD & Synek BJ (1995). A fatal case of ovarian hyperstimulation syndrome with cerebral infarction. *Pathology* **27**:344−6.

Colby TV (1999). Benign mesothelial cells in lymph node. *Adv Anat Pathol* **6**:41−8.

Dalrymple JC, Smith DH, Sinosich MJ et al. (1982−3). Venous thrombosis with high estradiol levels following gonadotrophin therapy. *Infertility* **5**:239−45.

Daniel Y, Yaron Y, Oren M et al. (1995). Ovarian hyperstimulation syndrome manifests as acute unilateral hydrothorax. *Hum Reprod* **10**:1684−5.

Davis AJ, Pandher GK, Masson GM et al. (2002). A severe case of ovarian hyperstimulation syndrome with liver dysfunction and malnutrition. *Eur J Gastroenterol Hepatol* **14**:779−82.

Delvigne A (2004). Epidemiology and pathophysiology of ovarian hyperstimulation syndrome. In (Gerris J, Olivennes F, de Sutter P, Eds), *Assisted Reproductive Technologies: Quality and Safety*. New York: Parthenon Publishing, Chapter 12, pp. 149−62.

Delvigne A & Rozenberg S (2003). Review of clinical course and treatment of ovarian hyperstimulation syndrome (OHSS). *Hum Reprod Update* **9**:77−96.

Delvigne A, Demoulin A, Smitz J et al. (1993). The ovarian hyperstimulation syndrome in in-vitro fertilization: a Belgian multicenter study. I. Clinical and biological features. *Hum Reprod* **8**:1353−60.

Delvigne A, Kostyla K, DeLeener A et al. (2002). Metabolic characteristics of OHSS patients who developed ovarian hyperstimulation syndrome. *Hum Reprod* **17**:1994−6.

Dulitzky M, Cohen SB, Inbal A et al. (2000). Increased prevalence of thrombophilia among women with severe ovarian hyperstimulation syndrome. *Fertil Steril* **77**:463−7.

Dumont M, Combet A & Domenichini Y (1980). Cerebral arterial thrombosis following ovarian hyperstimulation and sextuplet pregnancy. *Nouv Presse Med* **13**:3628−9.

Elford K, Leader A, Wee R & Stys PK (2002). Stroke in ovarian hyperstimulation syndrome in early pregnancy treated with intra-arterial rt-PA. *Neurology* **59**:1270−2.

Elter K, Scoccia B & Nelson LR (2001). Hepatic dysfunction associated with moderate ovarian hyperstimulation syndrome: a case report. *J Reprod Med* **46**:765−8.

Esteban-Altirriba J (1961). Le syndrome d'hyperstimulation massive des ovaries. *Rev Française de Gynécologie et d'Obstetrique* **7−8**:555−64.

Fabregues F, Balasch J, Gines P et al. (1999). Ascites and liver test abnormalities during severe ovarian hyperstimulation syndrome. *Am J Gastroenterol* **94**:994−9.

Fabregues F, Tassies D, Reverter JC et al. (2004). Prevalence of thrombophilia in women with severe ovarian hyperstimulation syndrome and cost-effectiveness of screening. *Fertil Steril* **81**:989−95.

Figueroa-Casas P (1958). Reaccion ovariaa monstruosa a las gonadotrophines a proposito de un caso fatal. *Ann Cirug* **23**:116−18.

Foong LC, Bhagavath B, Kumar J & Ng SC (2002). Ovarian hyperstimulation syndrome is associated with reversible impairment of vascular reactivity. *Fertil Steril* **78**:1159−63.

Forman RG, Frydman R, Egan D et al. (1990). Severe ovarian hyperstimulation synodrome using agonists of gonadotropin-releasing hormone for in vitro fertilization: a European series and a proposal for prevention. *Fertil Steril* **53**:502−9.

Friedler S, Rachstein A, Bukovsky I et al. (1998). Unilateral hydrothorax as a sole and recurrent manifestation of ovarian hyperstimulation syndrome following in-vitro fertilization. *Hum Reprod* **13**:859−61.

Fujimoto A, Osuga Y, Yano T et al. (2002). Ovarian hyperstimulation syndrome complicated by peritonitis due to perforated appendicitis: case report. *Hum Reprod* **17**:966−7.

Germond M, Wirthner D, Thorin D et al. (1996). Aorto-subclavian thromboembolism: a rare complication associated with moderate ovarian hyperstimulation syndrome. *Hum Reprod* **11**:1173−6.

Gore L, Nawar MG, Rezk Y et al. (2002). Resistant unilateral hydrothorax as the sole manifestation of ovarian hyperstimulation syndrome. *Middle East Fertility Society Journal* **7**:149−53.

Gregory WT & Patton PE (1999). Isolated pleural effusion in severe ovarian hyperstimulation: a case report. *Am J Obstet Gynecol* **180**:1468−71.

Hollemaert S, Wautrecht JC, Capel P et al. (1996). Thrombosis associated with ovarian hyperstimulation syndrome in a carrier of the factor V Leiden mutation. *Thromb Haemost* **76**:275−7.

Horstkamp B, Lubke M, Kentenich H et al. (1994). Internal jugular vein thrombosis caused by resistance to activated protein C as complication of ovarian hyperstimulation after in-vitro fertilization. *Hum Reprod* **11**:280−2.

Jewelewicz R & Van de Wiele RL (1975). Acute hydrothorax as the only symptom of ovarian hyperstimulation syndrome. *Am J Obstet Gynecol* **121**:1121−2.

Kaaja R, Sieberg R, Titinen A et al. (1989). Severe ovarian hyperstimulation syndrome and deep venous thrombosis. *Lancet* **2**:1043−4.

Khalaf Y, Elkington N, Anderson H et al. (2000). Ovarian hyperstimulation syndrome and its effect on renal function in a renal transplant patient undergoing IVF treatment: case report. *Hum Reprod* **15**:1275−7.

Kim HC, Kemmann E, Shelden R et al. (1981). Response of blood coagulation parameters to elevated endogenous 17β-estradiol levels induced by human menopausal gonadotropin. *Am J Obstet Gynecol* **140**:807−10.

Kingsland C, Collins JV, Rizk B & Mason B (1989). Ovarian hyperstimulation presenting as acute hydrothorax after in-vitro fertilization. *Am J Obstet Gynecol* **16**:381−2.

Kligman I, Noyes N, Benadiva CA & Rosenwaks Z (1995). Massive deep vein thrombosis in a patient with antithrombin III deficiency undergoing ovarian stimulation for in vitro fertilization. *Fertil Steril* **63**:673−6.

Kodama H, Fukuda J, Karube H et al. (1996). Status of the coagulation and fibrinolytic systems in ovarian hyperstimulation syndrome. *Fertil Steril* **66**:417−24.

Kodama H, Takeda S, Fukuda J et al. (1997). Activation of plasma kinin system correlated with severe coagulation disorders in patients with ovarian hyperstimulation syndrome. *Hum Reprod* **12**:891−5.

Lamon D, Chang CK, Hruska L et al. (2000). Superior vena cava thrombosis after in-vitro fertilization: case report and review of the literature. *Ann Vasc Surg* **14**:283−5.

Lesny P, Maguiness SD, Hay DM et al. (1999). Ovarian hyperstimulation syndrome and benign intracranial hypertension in pregnancy after in-vitro fertilization and embryo transfer: case report. *Hum Reprod* **14**:1953−5.

Loret de Mola JR (1999). Pathophysiology of unilateral pleural effusions in the ovarian hyperstimulation syndrome. *Hum Reprod* **14**:272−3.

Loret de Mola JR, Kiwi R, Austin C & Goldfarb JM (2000). Subclavian deep vein thrombosis associated with the use of recombinant follicle-stimulating hormone (Gonal-F) complicating mild ovarian hyperstimulation syndrome. *Fertil Steril* **73**:1253−6.

Lox C, Dorsett J, Canez M et al. (1995). Hyperoestrogenism induced by menotropins alone or in conjunction with leuprolide acetate in in vitro fertilization cycles: the impact on homeostasis. *Fertil Steril* **63**:566−70.

Ludwig M, Tolg R, Richardt G et al. (1999). Myocardial infarction associated with ovarian hyperstimulation syndrome. *JAMA* **282**:632−3.

Lunenfeld B (1963). Treatment of anovulation by human gonadotrophins. *J Int Fed Gynecol Obstet* **1**:153−8.

Man A, Schwarz Y & Greif J (1997). Pleural effusion as a presenting symptom of ovarian hyperstimulation syndrome. *Eur Resp J* **10**:2425−6.

Mathur RS & Jenkins JM (2000). Is ovarian hyperstimulation syndrome associated with a poor obstetric outcome? *Int J Obstet Gynaecol.* **107**:943−6.

Mancini A, Milardi D, Di Pietro ML et al. (2001). A case of forearm amputation after ovarian stimulation for in-vitro fertilization-embryo transfer. *Fertil Steril* **76**:198−200.

Mathur RS, Akande AV, Keay SD et al. (2000). Distinction between early and late ovarian hyperstimulation syndrome. *Fertil Steril* **73**:901−7.

McGowan BM, Kay LA & Perry DJ (2003). Deep vein thrombosis followed by internal jugular vein thrombosis as a complication of in-vitro fertilization in a woman heterozygous for the prothrombin 3UTR and factor V Leiden mutations. *Am J Hematol* **73**:276−8.

Midgley DY, Khalaf Y, Braude PR et al. (1999). Recurrent cholestasis following ovarian hyperstimulation syndrome. *Hum Reprod* **14**:2249−51.

Mills MS, Eddowes HA, Fox R et al. (1992). Subclavian vein thrombosis; a late complication of ovarian hyperstimulation syndrome. *Hum Reprod* 7:370—1.

Mozes M, Bogowsky H, Anteby E et al. (1965). Thrombo-embolic phenomena after ovarian stimulation with human menopausal gonadotrophins. *Lancet* 2:1213—15.

Nakauchi-Tanaka T, Sohda S, Someya K et al. (2003). Acquired haemophilia due to factor VIII inhibitors in ovarian hyperstimulation syndrome: case report. *Hum Reprod* 18:506—8.

Neau JP, Marechaud M, Guitton P et al. (1989). Occlusion of the middle cerebral artery after induction of ovulation with gonadotrophins. *Rev Neurol (Paris)* 145:859—61.

Ong ACM, Eisen V, Rennie DP et al. (1991). The pathogenesis of the ovarian hyperstimulation syndrome (OHS): a possible role of ovarian renin. *Clin Endocrinol* 34:43—9.

Ou YC, Kao YL, Lai SL et al. (2003). Thromboembolism after ovarian stimulation: successful management of a woman with superior sagittal sinus thrombosis after IVF and embryo transfer: case report. *Hum Reprod* 18:2375—81.

Phillips LL, Glanstone W & Van de Wiele R (1975). Studies of the coagulation and fibrinolytic systems in hyperstimulation syndrome after administration of human gonadotrophin. *J Reprod Med* 14:138—43.

Rabinerson D, Shalev J, Royburt M et al. (2000). Severe unilateral hydrothorax as the only manifestation of the ovarian hyperstimulation syndrome. *Gynecol Obstet Invest* 49:140—2.

Raziel A, Friedler S, Schachter M et al. (2002). Increased early pregnancy loss in IVF patients with severe ovarian hyperstimulation syndrome. *Hum Reprod* 17:107—10.

Rizk B (1992). Ovarian hyperstimulation syndrome. In (Brinsden PR, Rainsbury PA, Eds), *A Textbook of In-vitro Fertilization and Assisted Reproduction*. Carnforth, UK: Parthenon Publishing, Chapter 23, pp. 369—84.

Rizk B (1993a). Prevention of ovarian hyperstimulation syndrome: the Ten Commandments. Presented at the 1993 European Society of Human Reproduction and Embryology Symposium, Tel Aviv, Israel, 1—2.

Rizk B (1993b). Ovarian hyperstimulation syndrome. In (Studd J, Ed.), *Progress in Obstetrics and Gynecology*. Edinburgh: Churchill Livingstone, Chapter 18, Vol. 11, pp. 311—49.

Rizk B (2001). Ovarian hyperstimulation syndrome: prediction, prevention and management. In (Rizk B, Devroey P, Meldrum DR, Eds), *Advances and Controversies in Ovulation Induction*. 34th ASRM Annual Postgraduate Program, Middle East Fertility Society Pre-Congress Course. ASRM, 57th Annual Meeting, Orlando, FL, pp. 23—46.

Rizk B (2002). Can OHSS in ART be eliminated? In (Rizk B, Meldrum D, Schoolcraft W, Eds), *A Clinical Step-by-Step Course for Assisted Reproductive Technologies*. 35th ASRM Annual Postgraduate Program, Middle East Fertility Society Pre-Congress Course. ASRM, 58th Annual Meeting, Seattle, WA, pp. 65—102.

Rizk B & Aboulghar M (1991). Modern management of ovarian hyperstimulation syndrome. *Hum Reprod* 6:1082—7.

Rizk B & Nawar MG (2001). Laparoscopic ovarian drilling for surgical induction of ovulation in polycystic ovarian syndrome. In (Allahbadia G, Ed.), *Manual of Ovulation Induction*. Mumbai, India: Rotunda Medical Technologies, Chapter 18, pp. 140—4.

Rizk B, & Nawar MG (2004). Ovarian hyperstimulation syndrome. In (Serhal P, Overton C, Eds), *Good Clinical Practice in Assisted Reproduction*. Cambridge, UK: Cambridge University Press, Chapter 8, pp. 146—6.

Rizk B, Meagher S & Fisher AM (1990). Ovarian hyperstimulation syndrome and cerebrovascular accidents. *Hum Reprod* 5:697—8.

Rizk B, Aboulghar MA, Mansour RT et al. (1991a). Severe ovarian hyperstimulation syndrome: analytical study of twenty-one cases. *Proceedings of the VII World Congress on In-vitro Fertilization and Assisted Procreations, Paris, Hum Reprod*, **5**: pp. 368−9.

Rizk B, Tan SL, Morcos S et al. (1991b). Heterotopic pregnancies after in-vitro fertilizations and embryo transfer. *Am J Obstet Gynecol* **164**:161−4.

Rizk B, Doyle P, Tan SL et al. (1991c). Perinatal outcome and congenital malformations in in-vitro fertilization babies from the Bourn Hallam Group. *Hum Reprod* **6**:1259−64.

Rizk B & Aboulghar MA (2005). Classification, pathophysiology and management of ovarian hyperstimulation syndrome. In (Brinsden P, Ed.), *A Textbook of In-vitro Fertilization and Assisted Reproduction*, Third Edition. London: Parthenon Publishing, Chapter 12, pp. 217−58.

Roden S, Juvin K, Homasson JP et al. (2000). An uncommon etiology of isolated pleural effusion. The ovarian hyperstimulation syndrome. *Chest* **118**:256−8.

Roest J, Mous H, Zeilmaker G et al. (1996). The incidence of major clinical complications in a Dutch transport IVF programme. *Hum Reprod Update* **2**:345−53.

Ryley NG, Froman R, Barlow D et al. (1990). Liver abnormality in ovarian hyperstimulation syndrome. *Hum Reprod* **5**:938−43.

Ryo E, Hagino D, Yano N et al. (1999). A case of ovarian hyperstimulation syndrome in which antithrombin III deficiency occurred because of its loss into ascites. *Fertil Steril* **71**:860−2.

Samuel MJ & Grosskinsky CM (2004). Abnormal human chorionic gonadotropin levels and normal pregnancy outcomes in the ovarian hyperstimulation syndrome. *J Reprod Med* **49**:8−12.

Schanzer A, Rockman CB, Jacobowits GR et al. (2000). Internal jugular vein thrombosis in association with the ovarian hyperstimulation syndrome. *J Vasc Surg* **31**:815−18.

Schenker JG (1999). Clinical aspects of ovarian hyperstimulation syndrome. *Eur J Obstet Gynecol Reprod Biol* **85**:13−20.

Schenker JG & Ezra Y (1994). Complications of assisted reproductive techniques. *Fertil Steril* **62**:658−64.

Schenker JG & Weinstein D (1978). Ovarian hyperstimulation syndrome: a current survey. *Fertil Steril* **30**:255−68.

Semba S, Moriya T, Youssef EM et al. (2000). An autopsy case of ovarian hyperstimulation syndrome with massive pulmonary edema and pleural effusion. *Pathol Int* **50**:549−52.

Serour GI, Aboulghar M, Mansour R et al. (1998). Complications of medically assisted conception in 3,500 cycles. *Fertil Steril* **70**:638−42.

Shan Tang O, Ng E, Wai Cheng P et al. (2000). Cortical vein thrombosis misinterpreted as intracranial hemorrhage in severe ovarian hyperstimulation syndrome. *Hum Reprod* **15**:1913−16.

Southgate HJ, Anderson SK, Lavies NG et al. (1999). Pseudocholinesterase deficiency: a dangerous unrecognized complication of the ovarian hyperstimulation syndrome. *Ann Clin Biochem* **36**:256−8.

Stewart JA, Hamilton PJ & Murdoch AP (1997a). Upper limb thrombosis associated with assisted conception treatment. *Hum Reprod* **12**:2174−5.

Stewart JA, Hamilton PJ & Murdoch AP (1997b). Thromboembolic disease associated with ovarian and assisted conception techniques. *Hum Reprod* **12**:2167−73.

Sueldo CE, Price HM, Bachenberg K et al. (1988). Transient liver function test abnormalities of ovarian hyperstimulation syndrome: a case report. *J Reprod Med* **33**:387−90.

Tan SL, Doyle P, Campbell S et al. (1992). Obstetric outcome of in-vitro fertilization pregnancies compared to naturally conceived pregnancies. *Am J Obstet and Gynecol* **167**:778−84.

Thill B, Rathat C, Akula A et al. (1994). Accidents thrombo-emboliques lors des fécondations in vitro. *Ann Fr Anesth Réanim* **13**:726−9.

Todorow S, Schricker ST, Siebzinruebl ER et al. (1993). Von Willebrand factor: an endothelial marker to monitor in vitro fertilization patients with ovaran hyperstimulation syndrome. *Hum Reprod* **8**:2039−49.

Todros T, Carmazzi CM, Bontempo S et al. (1999). Spontaneous ovarian hyperstimulation syndrome and deep vein thrombosis in pregnancy: case report. *Hum Reprod* **14**:2245−8.

Turkistani IM, Ghourab SA, Al-Sheikh OH et al. (2001). Central retinal artery occlusion associated with severe ovarian hyperstimulation syndrome. *Eur J Opthalmol* **11**:313−15.

Uhler ML, Budinger GR, Gabram SG & Zinaman J (2001). Perforated duodenal ulcer associated with ovarian hyperstimulation syndrome: case report. *Hum Reprod* **16**:174−6.

Ulug U, Aksoy E & Erden H (2003). Bilateral internal jugular venous thrombosis following successful assisted conception in the absence of ovarian hyperstimulation syndrome. *Eur J Obstet Gynecol Reprod Biol* **109**:231−3.

Van der Weiden RMF, Meijers CJH & Hegt VN (2005). Ectopic mesothelial cell proliferation in cervical lymph nodes after severe ovarian hyperstimulation syndrome. *Fertil Steril* **83**:739−41.

Venn A, Hemminki E, Watson L et al. (2001). Mortality in a cohort of IVF patients. *Hum Reprod* **16**:2691−6.

Wood N, Edozien L & Lieberman B (1998). Symptomatic unilateral pleural effusion as a presentation of ovarian hyperstimulation syndrome. *Hum Reprod* **13**:571−2.

Yoshii F, Ooki N, Shinohara Y et al. (1999). Multiple cerebral infarctions associated with ovarian hyperstimulation. *Neurology* **53**:225−7.

Younis JS, Zeevi D, Rabinowitz R et al. (1988). Transient liver function test abnormalities of ovarian hyperstimulation syndrome. *Fertil Steril* **50**:176−8.

Zosmer A, Katz Z, Lancet M et al. (1987). Adult respiratory distress syndrome complicating ovarian hyperstimulation syndrome. *Fertil Steril* **47**:524−6.

VI

PREDICTION OF OVARIAN HYPERSTIMULATION SYNDROME

PREDICTION OF OVARIAN HYPERSTIMULATION SYNDROME

The first priority in the management of ovarian hyperstimulation syndrome is precise prediction and active prevention (Rizk, 1992, 1993). An accurate and detailed history in addition to experienced ultrasound monitoring and endocrine evaluation (Rizk, 2001, 2002) are the cornerstones of a successful prediction and prevention program (Figure VI.1).

ENDOCRINE MONITORING

Serum Estradiol

A role for estrogen monitoring for the prediction and prevention of OHSS was suggested more than 30 years ago (Karam et al., 1973; Haning et al., 1985;

Fig. VI.1: Prediction of OHSS

Prediction of OHSS

1. **OHSS in a previous cycle**
2. **Polycystic Ovarian Syndrome**
3. **High serum estradiol, rapid slope of E2 and absolute value**
4. **Ultrasonography**
   Baseline PCO pattern
   PCO pattern of response to GnRH before gonadotropins
   Large number of follicles >20 on each ovary
5. **Doppler low intraovarian vascular resistance**
6. **Conception cycles, particularly multiple pregnancy**
7. **Young patients**
8. **Low Body Mass Index**

Rizk and Aboulghar, 1991). Over the last three decades, reproductive endocrinologists have been divided between those who valued the role of estrogen monitoring for prevention of OHSS (Rizk and Aboulghar, 1991, 2005; Smith and Cooke, 1991) and those who do not (Thomas et al., 2002). Haning et al. (1983) compared plasma 17β-estradiol, 24-h urinary estriol glucuronide and ultrasound as predictors of ovulation in 70 ovulation induction cycles. Plasma estradiol was the best predictor of the hyperstimulation score. No case of OHSS occurred when the plasma estradiol level was <1000 pg/ml, and the authors considered 4000 pg/ml to be the level above which hCG should be withheld, because OHSS occurred in all pregnancies when the estradiol level was >4000 pg/ml. Several authors reported severe OHSS with peak follicular plasma estradiol levels well below 1500 pg/ml. On the other hand, only a small fraction of patients with excessive estrogen concentrations will develop severe OHSS.

Two studies from southern California highlight how the prevalence of OHSS can vary among patients with similar estradiol levels. Asch et al. (1991) reported severe OHSS in 5 of 13 IVF cycles where the serum estradiol on the day of hCG was >6000 pg/ml. This gives a sensitivity of 83% and a specificity of 99%, although the positive predictive value was only 38%. When the number of eggs aspirated was >30, the sensitivity was 83%, the specificity was 67% but the positive predictive value was only 23%. The number of patients that met both criteria, estradiol >6000 pg/ml and >30 oocytes was not given but analysis predicted an 80% chance of developing OHSS (Morris et al., 1995). In order to determine the prediction of OHSS in patients meeting both criteria, and to assess the effects of pregnancy, Morris et al. (1995) compared two groups of patients, oocyte donors ($n = 72$) and IVF patients ($n = 67$). They studied 139 IVF cycles between 1990 and 1993 in which estradiol was over 4000 pg/ml, oocyte number >25, or both were elevated. There were no severe cases of OHSS in the oocyte-donor group but six cases occurred in the IVF group. In contrast to the results of Asch et al. (1991), they had only one OHSS case in 10 patients with estradiol concentration >6000 pg/ml and >30 oocytes (10%). The relative risk of OHSS in pregnancy was 12 with a confidence interval of 2.18−66.14. Morris et al. (1995) concluded that the risk of OHSS even at high levels of stimulation is lower than previously believed. They believed that oocyte donors had a very low risk of OHSS because of the absence of pregnancy.

VASCULAR ENDOTHELIAL GROWTH FACTOR

Vascular endothelial growth factor (VEGF) expression by luteinized granulosa cells has been demonstrated in vitro and its extent differs widely between individual patients (Rizk et al., 1997). The different mechanisms for reaching different results and conclusions regarding the levels of VEGF in serum has been elegantly discussed by Delvigne (2004). These reasons, which have been reviewed in detail in Chapter III, explain the variation in results among different investigators who ascertain VEGF levels in order to predict OHSS (Geva et al., 1999; D'Ambrogio et al., 1999; Enskog et al., 2001; Mathur et al., 2002). Even in the same patient, Tozer et al. (2004) observed a wide variation in follicular fluid levels of VEGF in follicles of the same size. There was also wide variability among different patients.

While Agrawal et al. (1999) and Artini et al. (1998) found increased levels of VEGF in follicular fluid to be predictive of the development of OHSS (Figures VI.2 and VI.3), other investigators have found that women at risk of developing OHSS have significantly lower levels of VEGF in follicular fluid, and that lower levels are associated with good prognosis in patients who are hyperresponders (Friedman et al., 1998; Pellicer et al., 1999; Quintana et al., 2001).

Agrawal et al. (1999) performed one of the earlier studies to explore the value of serum VEGF concentration during IVF cycles to predict the risk of OHSS. They studied 107 women undergoing IVF. Mild OHSS developed in 10 women, moderate OHSS in seven women, and severe OHSS in three women. Serum VEGF concentrations were higher in women in whom OHSS developed. The increase in the VEGF concentration that occurred between the day of hCG administration and the day of oocyte collection was termed the VEGF rise, and proved to be an important marker of OHSS (Figures VI.2 and VI.3). The VEGF rise was higher in women in whom OHSS developed. A higher VEGF predicted all cases of OHSS and moderate/severe cases of OHSS with a sensitivity of 100% and specificity of 60%. A likelihood ratio test demonstrated that, by adding the VEGF rise or the VEGF concentration on the day of oocyte collection to a regression model as a continuance variable to the number of follicles, the

Fig. VI.2: Serum VEGF concentrations in IVF cycles with mild OHSS, moderate or severe OHSS and without OHSS
*Reproduced with permission from Agrawal et al. (1999). Fertil Steril **71**:287–93*

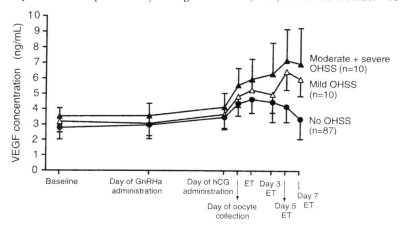

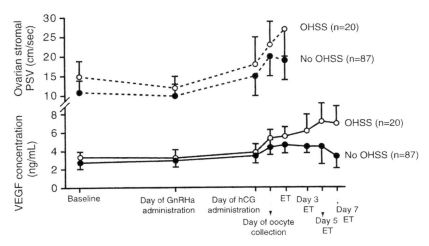

Fig. VI.3: Changes in serum VEGF concentrations and doppler blood flow velocity in patients with and without OHSS
*Reproduced with permission from Agrawal et al. (1999). Fertil Steril **71**:287–93*

estradiol concentration and the presence of polycystic ovaries significantly contributed to predicting the risk of OHSS.

Free Serum VEGF for the Prediction of OHSS

Ludwig et al. (1999) compared free serum VEGF levels in 10 patients who developed severe OHSS, and 15 control patients who did not develop OHSS. A positive predictive value of 75% and negative predictive value of 92% was obtained, using a cutoff level of 200 pg/ml on the day of hCG administration. The possible predictive role of free VEGF should be investigated further.

SERUM AND FOLLICULAR FLUID CYTOKINE LEVELS IN THE PREDICTION OF OHSS

Chen et al. (2000) examined the role of serum and follicular fluid cytokines and VEGF in the prediction of OHSS. The study group consisted of 12 women who developed moderate $(n = 7)$ or severe $(n = 5)$ OHSS. The authors chose two control groups which consisted of 12 high-risk and 12 low-risk women in whom OHSS did not develop. Serum was collected on the days of hCG, oocyte retrieval and embryo transfer, and then serum and follicular fluid concentrations of IL-6 and IL-8, TNFα and VEGF were determined. Follicular fluid concentration of IL-6 $(p = 0.026)$ at the time of oocyte retrieval and serum levels of IL-8 at the time of embryo transfer were significantly higher $(p = 0.017)$ in the OHSS group than in the control groups. Serum VEGF and TNFα levels were not statistically significant for either group when compared to controls. The authors concluded that follicular fluid IL-6 at the time of oocyte retrieval and serum IL-8 at the time of embryo transfer may serve as early predictors of this syndrome.

VON WILLEBRAND FACTOR

Todorow et al. (1993) were the first to suggest the possible involvement of von Willebrand factor (vWF) in the pathophysiology of OHSS. They performed a retrospective study to evaluate the possible role of endothelial and extracellular factors in the pathophysiology of the syndrome. Plasma changes of vWF were correlated with the clinical condition of the hyperstimulated patients. Basal values of patients who did and did not develop OHSS were not different. Mean values were significantly different in the two groups on the day preceding oocyte retrieval (Figure VI.4). A consistent increase in the OHSS group lasted after embryo transfer even into the late corpus luteum phase. The subtle changes in capillary permeability always preceded the clinical signs such as ascites, hemoconcentration, hypoproteinemia and pleural effusion. The authors considered that vWF provides an additional prognostic marker for early recognition and monitoring of OHSS.

Ogawa et al. (2001) retrospectively evaluated the vWF and VEGF serum levels on the days of oocyte retrieval and embryo transfer in 46 women who developed early-onset OHSS. Severe, moderate and mild OHSS occurred in 13, 14 and 19 patients respectively. There were inconsistent changes in the VEGF levels during oocyte retrieval and embryo transfer. However, the net increase in serum vWF showed an increase in absolute value at the time of embryo transfer that paralleled the severity of OHSS. The authors suggested that the rise of serum levels of vWF occurs prior to clinical manifestation of OHSS in patients with severe OHSS, but not in patients with mild OHSS.

Fig. VI.4: vWf antigen in IVF cycles: control vs. OHSS
Reproduced with permission from Todorow et al. (1993). Hum Reprod 8:2039–46

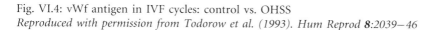

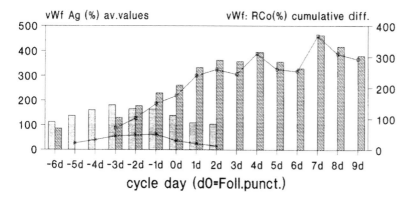

Inhibin-B

Enskog et al. (2000) found that peripheral blood concentrations of inhibin-B are elevated during gonadotrophin stimulation in patients who later develop OHSS, and inhibin-A concentrations are elevated after OHSS onset.

FOLLICULAR MONITORING BY ULTRASOUND

Ultrasound monitoring is the cornerstone of prediction of OHSS (Rizk, 1993).

Baseline Necklace Sign Appearance

The diagnosis of polycystic ovaries at ultrasound examination (the necklace sign) is essential for prediction of OHSS (Rizk and Smitz, 1992). It improved the prediction of OHSS to 79% in a Belgian multicenter study (Delvigne et al., 1993a, b).

Number and Size of Follicles During Ovarian Stimulation

Ultrasound is widely used for monitoring follicular development in assisted conception (Rizk and Nawar, 2004). The number, size and pattern of distribution of the follicles are important in the prediction of OHSS. Tal et al. (1985) found a positive correlation between the mean number of immature follicles and OHSS. One of the most-often-quoted articles in reference to prediction is that by Blankenstein et al. (1987). They stated that a decrease in the fraction of the mature follicles and an increase in the fraction of the very small follicles correlated with an increased risk of the development of severe OHSS.

Baseline Ovarian Volume and the Prediction of OHSS

Danninger et al. (1996) studied the baseline ovarian volume prior to stimulation, to investigate whether it would be a suitable predictor for the risk of OHSS. They performed three-dimensional volumetric ultrasound assessment of the ovaries prior to ovarian stimulation and on the day of hCG injection. There was a significant correlation between the baseline ovarian volume and the subsequent occurrence of OHSS. The authors suggested that volumetry of the ovaries could help to detect patients at risk. Lass et al. (2002) studied whether ovarian volume in the early follicular phase of WHO Group II anovulatory patients would predict the response to ovulation induction with gonadotrophins. They analyzed retrospective data from two prospective randomized multicenter studies, including 465 patients undergoing ovulation induction. WHO Group II anovulatory women with medium-sized or large ovaries undergoing low-dose gonadotrophin stimulation for ovulation induction would have a higher risk for OHSS than women with small ovaries.

Low Intra-vascular Ovarian Resistance

Moohan et al. (1997) assessed the intra-ovarian blood flow in relation to the severity of OHSS in 30 patients with OHSS after embryo transfer who also had sonographic evidence of ascites. The authors measured the resistance to blood flow within the ovaries of 11 patients with severe OHSS and 19 patients with mild OHSS by using transabdominal ultrasonography with color flow and pulsed Doppler imaging. The pulsatility index (PI), resistance index (RI) and the systolic–diastolic ratio, all measures of downstream vascular impedance, were significantly lower in severe OHSS patients. In patients with RI < 0.48, more than two thirds had pleural effusion. In patients with either PI < 0.75 or S-D < 1.92, pleural effusion was observed in more than one-half. The blood flow velocity did not differ significantly between the two groups despite the fact that there were changes in vascular impedance. A close correlation was observed between the OHSS severity and the intra-ovarian blood flow resistance. The authors suggested that measurements of intra-ovarian vascular resistance in patients undergoing controlled ovarian hyperstimulation may help in predicting those patients at particular risk of developing OHSS.

Genetic Prediction of OHSS: Severity, but not Occurrence

It is greatly hoped that studies on the FSH receptor genotype will be able to predict in advance patients at risk of developing OHSS. One such important study, evaluating FSH receptor genotype, concluded that it was not possible to predict which patients would develop OHSS but FSH receptor genotype could be a predictor of *severity* in OHSS patients (Daelemans et al., 2004).

Prediction of OHSS by One or More Risk Factors

The use of one or more risk factors for the prediction of OHSS has been extensively investigated (Delvigne et al., 1993a, b; Agrawal, 2003; D'Angelo et al., 2004). D'Angelo et al. (2004) assessed the value of different serum estradiol cut-off levels for predicting OHSS. They studied 40 women with OHSS and 40 control patients in a retrospective case-controlled study. Serum estradiol level of 3354 pg/ml on day 11 of ovarian stimulation gives a sensitivity and specificity of 85% for detection of women at risk of developing OHSS. Markers such as serum estradiol concentrations, the number of follicles on the day of hCG administration, the presence of polycystic ovaries (PCO) and the number of oocytes retrieved, each predicts less than a quarter of cases of the syndrome (Agrawal, 2003). On the other hand, a combination of pretreatment diagnosis of PCO, along with the number of follicles on the day of hCG administration and a "VEGF rise" in serum gives the highest prediction rate for the development of OHSS.

The considerable overlap of values for different parameters between OHSS and control patients makes any single variable inefficient for a reliable risk prediction (Delvigne, 2004). Multiple discriminate analysis, using a combination of variables, was studied in order to increase predictive power and decrease false negative prediction (Delvigne et al., 1993b). In their study of 128 OHSS patients and 256 controls, a prediction of 78.5%, with a corresponding false negative rate of 18.1%, was obtained for OHSS under post-retrieval conditions using log estradiol concentration, slope of log estradiol increment, gonadotrophin dosage, number of oocytes retrieved and LH/FSH ratio in the formula. However, effective prevention of OHSS implies the ability to withhold hCG injection, therefore, Delvigne et al. (1993a, b) devised a formula for the prediction of OHSS utilizing preoocyte retrieval conditions. That formula yielded a prediction rate of 76.1% with a false negative rate of 18.1%.

Ovarian Hyperstimulation Syndrome Information for Patients

Ovarian hyperstimulation syndrome (OHSS) is an uncommon complication that may result from the use of fertility injections during the course of treatment. It can occur in one to two of every 100 women undergoing treatment for infertility by in vitro fertilization. Awareness of symptoms is very important as a patient, because more interventions can be carried out earlier rather than later.

Patients at risk of ovarian hyperstimulation are young women with polycystic ovaries. Polycystic ovaries can be detected by ultrasound scans prior to the treatment cycle. If, during treatment, further ultrasound scans suggest that the ovaries are overresponding, then this matter would be discussed with you.

Usually the symptoms of OHSS occur a few days after the injection of hCG is given to help in releasing the eggs. The symptoms may worsen and last longer if a pregnancy occurs. In OHSS the ovaries are enlarged and swell, and finally, fluid leaks into the abdomen. The leakage of fluid results in dehydration and the risk of thrombosis or clotting in the veins, and rarely kidney damage. The symptoms we want you to look for are nausea and vomiting, abdominal discomfort and bloating, and abdominal swelling. If you become short of breath or develop extreme thirst and pass only small amounts of concentrated dark urine, you need to immediately contact the IVF center and explain these symptoms. During all times, you should drink plenty of clear fluids, such as Sprite. You can also drink milk and take Tylenol as a pain killer, and avoid strenuous physical activity. Keep with you at all times the hospital number for out of hours and emergency situations. The art and the science is to intervene early to prevent the situation from getting worse.

REFERENCES

Agrawal R, Tan SL, Wild S et al. (1999). Serum vascular endothelial growth factor concentrations in in-vitro fertilization cycles predict the risk of ovarian hyperstimulation syndrome. *Fertil Steril* **71**:278–93.

Agrawal R (2003). What's new in the pathogenesis and prevention of ovarian hyperstimulation syndrome? *Hum Fertil (Camb)* **3**:112–15.

Artini PG, Fasciani A, Monti M et al. (1998). Changes in vascular endothelial growth factor levels and the risk of ovarian hyperstimulation syndrome in women enrolled in an in vitro fertilization program. *Fertil Steril* **70**:560−4.

Asch RH, Li HP, Balmaceda JP et al. (1991). Severe ovarian hyperstimulation syndrome in assisted reproductive technology: definition of high risk groups *Hum Reprod* **6**:1395−9.

Blankenstein J, Shalev J, Saadon T et al. (1987). Ovarian hyperstimulation syndrome prediction by number and size of preovulatory ovarian follicles. *Fertil Steril* **47**:597−602.

Chen CD, Chen HF, Lu HF et al. (2000). Value of serum and follicular fluid cytokine profile in the prediction of moderate to severe ovarian hyperstimulation syndrome. *Hum Reprod* **15**:1037−42.

D'Ambrogio G, Fasciani A, Monti M et al. (1999). Serum vascular endothelial growth factor levels before starting gonadotrophin treatment in women who have developed moderate forms of ovarian hyperstimulation syndrome. *Gynecol Endocrinol* **13**:311−15.

D'Angelo A, Davies R, Salah E et al. (2004). Value of the serum estradiol level for preventing ovarian hyperstimulation syndrome: a retrospective case control study. *Fertil Steril* **81**:332−6.

Daelemans C, Smits G, de Maertelaer V et al. (2004). Prediction of severity of symptoms in iatrogenic ovarian hyperstimulation syndrome by follicle stimulation hormone receptor Ser 680 Asn polymorphism. *J Clin Endocrinol Metab* **89**:6310−15.

Danninger B, Brunner M, Obruca A et al. (1996). Prediction of ovarian hyperstimulation syndrome of baseline ovarian volume prior to stimulation. *Hum Reprod* **11**:1597−9.

Delvigne A (2004). Epidemiology and pathophysiology of ovarian hyperstimulation syndrome. In (Gerris G, Olivennes F, De Sutter P, Eds), *Assisted Reproductive Technologies: Quality and Safety*. New York: Parthenon Publishing, Chapter 12, pp. 149−62.

Delvigne A, Demoulin A, Smitz J et al. (1993a). The ovarian hyperstimulation syndrome in in-vitro fertilization: a Belgian multicenter study. I. Clinical and biological features. *Hum Reprod* **8**:1353−60.

Delvigne A, Dubois M, Battheu B et al. (1993b). The ovarian hyperstimulation syndrome in in-vitro fertilization: a Belgian multicenter study. II. Multiple discriminant analysis for risk prediction. *Hum Reprod* **8**:1361−6.

Enskog A, Nilsson L & Brannstrom M (2000). Peripheral blood concentrations of inhibin B are elevated during gonadotrophin stimulation in patients who later develop ovarian OHSS and inhibin A concentrations are elevated after OHSS onset. *Hum Reprod* **15**:532−8.

Enskog A, Nilsson L & Brannstrom M (2001). Plasma levels of free vascular endothelial growth factor (165) (VEGF 165) are not elevated during gonadotrophin stimulation in in-vitro fertilization (IVF) patients developing ovarian hyperstimulation syndrome (OHSS): results of a prospective cohort study with matched controls. *Eur J Obstet Gynecol Reprod Biol* **96**:196−201.

Friedman CI, Seifer DB, Kennard EA et al. (1998). Elevated level of follicular fluid vascular endothelial growth factor is a marker of diminished pregnancy potential. *Fertil Steril* **64**:268−72.

Geva E, Amit A, Lessing JB et al. (1999). Follicular fluid levels of vascular endothelial growth factor. Are they predictive markers for ovarian hyperstimulation syndrome? *J Reprod Med* **44**:91−6.

Haning RV Jr, Austin CW, Carlson IH et al. (1983). Plasma estradiol is superior to ultrasound and urinary estriol glucuronide as a predictor of ovarian hyperstimulation during induction of ovulation with menotropins. *Fertil Steril* **40**:31−6.

Haning RV, Strawn EY & Nolten WE (1985). Pathophysiology of the ovarian hyperstimulation syndrome. *Obstet Gynecol* **66**:220−4.

Karam KS, Taymor ML & Berger MJ (1973). Estrogen monitoring and the prevention of ovarian overstimulation during gonadotrophin therapy. *Am J Obstet Gynecol* **115**:972−7.

Lass A, Vassiliev A, Decosterd G et al. (2002). Relationship of baseline ovarian volume to ovarian response in World Health Organization Group II anovulatory patients who underwent ovulation induction with gonadotropins. *Fertil Steril* **78**:265−9.

Ludwig M, Jelkmann W, Bauer O et al. (1999). Prediction of severe ovarian hyperstimulation syndrome by free serum vascular endothelial growth factor concentration on the day of human chorionic gonadotrophin administration. *Hum Reprod* **14**:2437−41.

Mathur R, Hayman G, Bansal A et al. (2002). Serum vascular endothelial growth factor levels are poorly predictive of subsequent ovarian hyperstimulation syndrome in highly responsive women undergoing assisted conception. *Fertil Steril* **78**:1154−58.

Moohan JM, Curcio K, Leoni M et al. (1997). Low intraovarian vascular resistance: a marker for severe ovarian hyperstimulation syndrome. *Fertil Steril* **57**:728−32.

Morris RS, Paulson RJ, Sauer MV et al. (1995). Predictive value of serum oestradiol concentrations and oocyte number in severe ovarian hyperstimulation syndrome. *Hum Reprod* **10**:811−14.

Ogawa S, Minakami H, Araki S et al. (2001). A rise of the serum level of von Willebrand factor occurs before clinical manifestation of the severe form of ovarian hyperstimulation syndrome. *J Assist Reprod Genet* **18**:114−19.

Pellicer A, Albert C, Mercader A et al. (1999). The pathogenesis of ovarian hyperstimulation syndrome: in vivo studies investigating the role of interleukin-1β, interleukin-6 and vascular endothelial growth factor. *Fertil Steril* **71**:482−9.

Quintana R, Kopcow L, Marconi G et al. (2001). Relationship of ovarian stimulation response with vascular endothelial growth factor and degree of granulosa cell apoptosis. *Hum Reprod* **16**:1814−18.

Rizk B (1992). Ovarian hyperstimulation syndrome. In (Brinsden PR, Rainsbury PA, Eds), *A Textbook of In-vitro Fertilization and Assisted Reproduction*. Carnforth, UK: Parthenon Publishing, pp. 369−83.

Rizk B (1993). Ovarian hyperstimulation syndrome. In (Studd J, Ed.), *Progress in Obstetrics and Gynecology*. Edinburgh: Churchill Livingstone, Vol.11, Chapter 18, pp. 311−49.

Rizk B (2001). Ovarian hyperstimulation syndrome: prediction, prevention and management. In (Rizk B, Devroey P, Meldrum DR, Eds), *Advances and Controversies In Ovulation Induction*. 34th ASRM Annual Postgraduate Program, Middle East Fertility Society Precongress Course. ASRM, 57th Annual Meeting, Orlando, FL, pp. 23−46. Published by the American Society for Reproductive Medicine.

Rizk B (2002). Can OHSS in ART be eliminated? In (Rizk B, Meldrum D, Schoolcraft W, Eds), *A Clinical Step-by-Step Course for Assisted Reproductive Technologies*. 35th ASRM Annual Postgraduate Program, Middle East Fertility Society Precongress Course. ASRM, 58th Annual Meeting, Seattle, WA, pp. 65−102. Published by the American Society for Reproductive Medicine.

Rizk B & Aboulghar M (1991). Modern management of ovarian hyperstimulation syndrome. *Hum Reprod* **6**:1082−7.

Rizk B & Aboulghar MA (2005). Classification, pathophysiology and management of ovarian hyperstimulation syndrome. In (Brinsden P, Ed.), *A Textbook of In-vitro Fertilization and Assisted Reproduction*, Third Edition. London: Parthenon Publishing, Chapter 12, pp. 217−58.

Rizk B & Nawar MG (2004). Ovarian Hyperstimulation Syndrome. In (Serhal P, Overton C, Eds), *Good Clinical Practice in Assisted Reproduction*. Cambridge, UK: Cambridge University Press, Chapter 8, pp. 146−66.

Rizk B & Smitz J (1992). Ovarian hyperstimulation syndrome after superovulation for IVF and related procedures. *Hum Reprod* **7**:320−7.

Rizk B, Aboulghar MA, Smitz J et al. (1997). The role of vascular endothelial growth factor and interleukins in the pathogenesis of severe ovarian hyperstimulation syndrome. *Hum Reprod Update* **3**:255—66.

Smith BH & Cooke ID (1991). Ovarian hyperstimulation: actual and theoretical risks. Comment. *BMJ* **302**:127—8.

Tal J, Faz B, Samberg I et al. (1985). Ultrasonographic and clinical correlates of menotrophin versus sequential clomiphene citrate: menotrophin therapy for induction of ovulation. *Fertil Steril* **45**:342—9.

Thomas K, Searle T, Quinn A et al. (2002). The value of routine estradiol monitoring in assisted conception cycles. *Acta Obstet Gynecol Scand* **81**:554—5.

Todorow S, Schricker S, Siebzehnruebl E et al. (1993). Von Willebrand factor: an endothelial marker to monitor in-vitro fertilization patients with ovarian hyperstimulation syndrome. *Hum Reprod* **8**:2039—46.

Tozer AJ, Iles RK, Iammarrone E et al. (2004). The effects of 'coasting' on follicular fluid concentrations of vascular endothelial growth factor in women at risk of developing ovarian hyperstimulation syndrome. *Hum Reprod* **19**:522—8.

VII

PREVENTION OF OVARIAN HYPERSTIMULATION SYNDROME

Rizk (1993a, b) suggested the "Ten Commandments" for the prevention of OHSS. Today, the list has expanded to two lists of "Ten Commandments". The first list addresses the primary prevention of OHSS, which include options before stimulation, such as ovarian diathermy, and during stimulation, such as using low-dose gonadotrophins (Figure VII.1). The second list addresses the secondary prevention of OHSS, which includes withholding or delaying hCG, use of a LH or GnRH agonist in place of hCG for triggering ovulation and progesterone for luteal phase support (Figure VII.2).

PRIMARY PREVENTION OF OHSS

Identification of Patients at Risk of OHSS before Stimulation

It would be impossible to completely prevent OHSS without careful assessment of patients to identify those who are at significant risk (Rizk and Abdalla, 2006). I cannot overemphasize the role of the tools used for prediction to be able to achieve primary prevention of OHSS.

Fig. VII.1: Primary prevention of OHSS

Primary Prevention of OHSS

1. **Prediction of OHSS from history, exam and ultrasound**
2. **Laparoscopic ovarian drilling in PCOS patients**
3. **Metformin in PCOS patients**
4. **Octreotide in PCOS patients**
5. **Low dose gonadotropins in PCOS patients**
6. **GnRH antagonist protocol**
7. **Recombinant LH to trigger ovulation**
8. **GnRH agonist to trigger ovulation**
9. **In vitro maturation of oocytes**
10. **Replacement of only one embryo**

Secondary Prevention of OHSS

The Ten Commandments

1. Witholding hCG ± continuation of GnRH-a/GnRH antagonist
2. Coasting or delaying hCG: currently most popular method
3. Use of GnRH-a to trigger ovulation
4. Follicular aspiration
5. Gradual and slow hMG protocol in PCOS and laparoscopic drilling
6. Cryopreservation and replacement of frozen-thawed embryos at a subsequent cycle
7. Selective oocyte retrieval in spontaneous conception
8. Albumin, administration at time of retrieval
9. Glucocorticoid administration
10. Progesterone for luteal phase support

Fig. VII.2: Secondary prevention of OHSS: the "Ten Commandments"

Ovulation Induction in PCOS Patients

1. Weight Loss in patients with BMI ≥ 28
2. Clomiphene Citrate for ovulation induction
3. Clomiphene Citrate and Metformin
4. Clomiphene Citrate and Dexamethasone treatment
5. Aromatase Inhibitors
6. Low dose step-up FSH injections
7. Low dose step-down FSH injections
8. Laparoscopic Ovarian Drilling
9. In-Vitro Fertilization
10. In-vitro Maturation of oocytes

Fig. VII.3: Ovulation induction in PCOS patients

STIMULATION PROTOCOLS TO AVOID OHSS

Prevention of OHSS in PCOS Patients

Rizk and Smitz (1992) highlighted that ovarian stimulation for patients with PCOS carries the highest risk for development of the severe forms of OHSS. Similar observations have been made by almost all investigators over the last decade (MacDougall et al., 1993; Delvigne et al., 1993; Aboulghar et al., 1996a). Today, this is one of the major challenges in PCOS patients. Several approaches have been used (Figure VII.3) starting with such lifestyle modifications as weight loss and metformin treatment, moving on to low-dose gonadotropins and ending with laparoscopic ovarian drilling and assisted reproductive technology (ART) (Rizk, 1992, 1993a, 2001, 2002).

Lifestyle Modification in PCOS patients

A recent pilot prospective randomized placebo-controlled trial on the effect of lifestyle modification and metformin therapy on ovulation and androgen concentration in women with PCOS was performed (Hoeger et al., 2004). In the study, 30 overweight or obese women with PCOS were randomized to one of four 48-week interventions. The interventions were: metformin, 850 mg two times per day; lifestyle modification plus metformin, 850 mg two times per day; lifestyle modification plus placebo; or placebo alone. The authors concluded that weight reduction might play the most significant role in the restoration of ovulation in obese women with PCOS.

Low-dose Gonadotrophins in PCOS Patients

LOW-DOSE OVARIAN STIMULATION IN NON-IVF CYCLES

Prevention of OHSS in this group of patients is rather difficult because of the narrow margin between the dose required to induce reasonable stimulation and the dose that may result in the development of OHSS (Figure VII.4). The original work on the low-dose protocol was reported by Seibel et al. (1984) in Boston and was soon followed by fine modifications of the dose and the protocol. The low-dose gonadotropin protocol was successfully used in the treatment of patients with PCOS to achieve satisfactory ovulation and pregnancy rates and reduce the risk of developing OHSS (Seibel et al., 1984; Polson et al., 1987; Buvat et al., 1989; Shoham et al., 1991; Homburg et al., 1995; Rizk and Thorneycroft, 1996).

Both low-dose step-up (Figure VII.5) and step-down protocols (Figure VII.6) have been used with similar ovulation and pregnancy rates and OHSS rates (Table VII.1). Two randomized trials comparing the low-dose step-up with the low-dose step-down protocol have demonstrated similar successful results (Table VII.2).

LOW-DOSE FSH IN PCOS

The induction of ovulation was reported successfully using recombinant FSH in patients with PCOS (Hornnes et al., 1993). Hedon et al. (1998) found significantly fewer follicles larger than 10 mm and a lower estradiol level in the chronic low-dose compared with the conventional regimen. Aboulghar et al. (1996b) compared the low-dose recombinant FSH and hMG protocols in the treatment of patients with a history of severe OHSS. The recombinant FSH low-dose protocol proved to be as effective as the low-dose hMG protocol in producing reasonable ovulation and pregnancies in PCOS patients with a history of severe OHSS; the protocol was safe with regard to the risk of developing OHSS. Rosenwaks (2003) highly recommended a very gentle stimulation approach as the key component of prevention of OHSS. This involves lower gonadotrophin dosage and hCG dosage as well. Bayram et al. (2001) performed a meta-analysis on the safety and effectiveness in terms of ovulation, pregnancy, multiple pregnancy, miscarriage, and OHSS of recombinant FSH

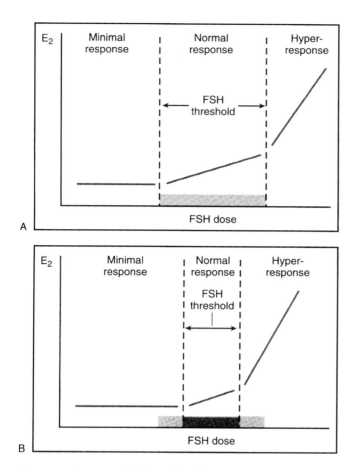

Fig. VII.4: Conceptualized model of granulosa cell responses to a range of follicle stimulating hormone (FSH) doses administered during ovulation induction in normal women (A) and women with PCOS (B)
Reproduced with permission from Chang (2004). In (Strauss, Barbieri, Eds), Yen and Jaffe's Reproductive Endocrinology: Physiology, Pathophysiology and Clinical Management, 5th ed. Philadelphia: Elsevier, Saunders, Chapter 19, p. 613

Fig. VII.5: Continuous low-dose step-up protocol (adapted from Macklon et al., 1999)
Reproduced with permission from Edwards and Risquez (Eds) (2003). Modern Assisted Conception, Reproductive Biomedicine Online: Reproductive Healthcare Ltd, p. 98

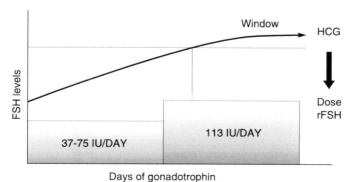

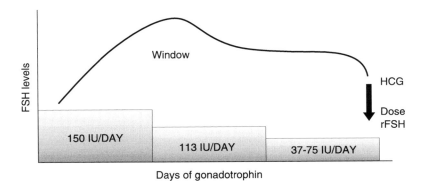

Fig. VII.6: Continuous low-dose step-down protocol (adapted from Macklon et al., 1999)
Reproduced with permission from Edwards, Risquez (Eds) (2003). Modern Assisted Conception, Reproductive Biomedicine Online: Reproductive Healthcare Ltd, p. 98.

Table VII.1 Comparison of ovarian response and clinical outcome following the low-dose step-up and step-down regimens for gonadotropin induction of ovulation
Reproduced with permission from Fauser and Macklon (2004). Medical approaches to ovarian stimulation for infertility. In (Strauss, Barbieri, Eds), Yen and Jaffe's Reproductive Endocrinology. Philadelphia: Elsevier, Saunders, Chapter 31, pp. 965–1012

	Low-dose step-up			*Step-down*
	Hamilton-Fairley (1991)	*Hull (1991)*	*Balen et al. (1994)*	*Van Santbrink et al. (1995)*
No. patients	100	144	103	82
No. cycles	401	459	603	234
Duration of treatment (days)	14	NR*	NR	11
Ampules per cycle	19	NR	NR	14
Ovulation rate (%)	72	74	68	91
Monofollicular cycles:				
% ovulatory cycles	73	NR	NR	62
% of all started cycles	55	NR	NR	56
Pregnancy rate				
per started cycle	11	11	14	16
per ovulatory cycle	16	15	20	17
Cumulative pregnancy rate (%)	55	NR	73	47
Multiple pregnancy rate (%)	4	11	18	8
Ongoing singleton pregnancy rate (%)	7	10	9	12
OHSS rate (%)	1	NR	1	2

* NR = not recorded

Table VII.2 Randomized studies comparing the low-dose step up with the step-down protocol for ovulation induction
Reproduced with permission from Fauser and Macklon (2004). In (Strauss, Barbieri, Eds), Yen and Jaffe's Reproductive Endocrinology, 5th ed. Philadelphia: Elsevier and Saunders, Chapter 31, pp. 965–1012

	Van Santbrink and Fauser (1997)			Christin-Maitre and Hughes(2003)		
	Step-up	Step-down	p-value	Step-up	Step-down	p-value
Median duration of treatment (days)	18	9	0.003	15	10	<0.001
Monofollicular growth	56%	88%	0.04	68%	32%	<0.0001
Overall ovulation rate	84%	89%	NS*	70%	61%	<0.02

* NS = not significant

(rFSH) versus urinary FSH (uFSH) in women with clomiphene-resistant PCOS. Four randomized trials comparing rFSH vs. uFSH were identified and no significant differences were demonstrated for the outcome. The odds ratio for the ovulation rate was 1.19 (95% confidence interval (CI), 0.78–1.80), pregnancy rate 0.95 (95% CI, 0.64–1.41), miscarriage rate 1.26 (95% CI, 0.59–2.70), multiple pregnancy rate 0.44 (95% CI, 0.16–1.21) and OHSS 1.55 (95% CI, 0.50–4.84). Similarly, in the only randomized trial that compared chronic low-dose vs. conventional regimen with rFSH, no significant differences were found.

LOW-DOSE OVARIAN STIMULATION FOR IVF

If ovarian hyperstimulation is performed for IVF, it is recommended to start with lower doses of hMG or FSH if the patient has had previous OHSS or is at high risk (Rizk et al., 1991a, b; Marci, 2001). In general, the starting dose of gonadotrophins in the United States is higher than the starting dose in Europe (Rizk, 2001, 2002). A useful example to illustrate this concept (Figure VII.7) was presented by Professor Johan Smitz from Belgium to demonstrate the impact of lowering the dose (Rizk and Smitz, 1992). It must be mentioned that lowering the dose could in some cases result in an unsuccessful IVF cycle so the situation is more difficult than ovarian stimulation without IVF.

In general, we recommend starting at a dose of 150 IU/day for IVF stimulation in young PCOS patients. If the patients have become hyperstimulated on this dose in a previous cycle, we would start at 100–112.5 IU/day. If the patient is 40 years old or older, we recommend a starting dose of 225 IU/day, and to consider reducing the dose to 150 IU/day.

LIMITED OVARIAN STIMULATION

A different approach whereby the hCG was administered when the leading follicle reached a diameter of 12 mm was reported by El-Sheikh et al. (2001). In a prospective study, with the patients serving as their own control,

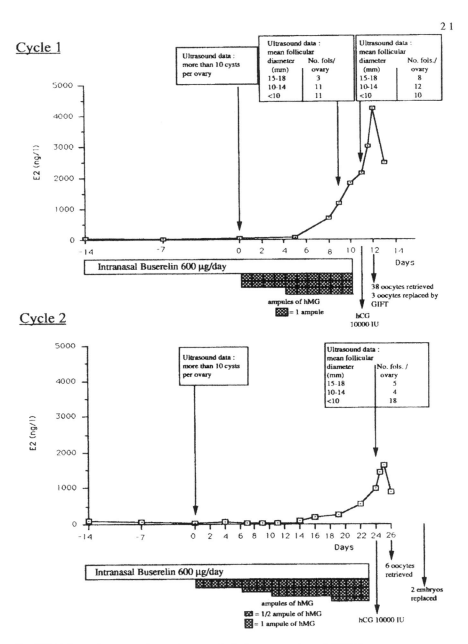

Fig. VII.7: Low-dose gonadotropins may help in prevention of OHSS
Reproduced with permission from Rizk and Smitz (1992). Hum Reprod 7:320–7

20 patients with a history of severe OHSS have undergone a second IVF cycle with what is termed as "limited ovarian stimulation." All patients produced mature oocytes and fertilization and eight clinical pregnancies were achieved. None of the patients experienced symptoms of severe OHSS or required hospitalization.

Table VII.3 Meta-analysis of metformin for ovulation induction in PCOS
Reproduced with permission from Lord et al. (2003). Cochrane database systematic review

	Odds ratios	95% confidence intervals
Metformin versus placebo		
ovulation rate	3.8	2.3–6.7*
pregnancy rate	2.8	0.9–9.0
Metformin and CC** versus CC alone		
ovulation rate	4.4	2.4–8.2*
pregnancy rate	4.4	2.0–9.9

* Statistically significant difference
** CC = clomiphene citrate

Metformin in PCOS Patients

Metformin is widely used for the treatment of insulin resistance in women with PCOS. A Cochrane review (Table VII.3), based on 14 randomized clinical trials, including 543 human subjects with biochemical and/or ultrasound evidence for PCOS, was recently published (Lord et al., 2005). DeLeo et al. (1999) performed a prospective randomized trial on 21 women with clomiphene-resistant PCOS which demonstrated that metformin use results in a reduction of intra-ovarian androgens by reducing hyperinsulinism. This leads to a reduction in estradiol and favors orderly follicular growth in response to exogenous gonadotrophins. Therefore, it is possible that in obese PCOS patients undergoing IVF, the addition of metformin might decrease the incidence of OHSS.

Aromatase Inhibitors in PCOS Patients

Aromatase inhibitors have been successfully used for ovulation induction in women with polycystic ovarian syndrome (Mitwally and Casper, 2000, 2001). The favorable pregnancy outcome and low multiple gestation rate of aromatase inhibitors for ovarian stimulation is encouraging for the development of these agents as first-line ovulation induction agents (Mitwally et al., 2005). However, there has been recent concern about anomalies in pregnancies following cycles where aromatase inhibitors were used.

Ketoconazole in PCOS Patients and OHSS

Parsanezhad et al. (2003) performed a prospective randomized double-blind, placebo-controlled trial to evaluate the role of ketoconazole in the prevention of OHSS in PCOS women undergoing ovarian stimulation with gonadotrophins at Shiraz University, Iran. Fifty patients were randomly assigned to receive two ampoules of hMG on day two or three of the cycle and ketoconazole, 50 mg every 48 h starting on the first day of hMG treatment, and 51 patients received hMG plus placebo tablets. Ketoconazole did not prevent OHSS in patients with PCOS undergoing ovarian stimulation. It reduced the rate of folliculogenesis and steroidogenesis.

OCTREOTIDE AND OHSS

Morris et al. (1999) performed a prospective double-blind, placebo-controlled crossover trial to determine whether octreotide is effective for ovulation induction and/or prevention of OHSS in PCOS patients with clomiphene resistance. Octreotide was no more effective than placebo for clomiphene-resistant patients; however, it reduced estradiol levels and number of follicles when combined with urinary FSH. No cases of OHSS occurred in either group. The authors concluded that octreotide may reduce the incidence of OHSS in PCOS patients.

Pentoxifylline in the Prevention of OHSS

Pentoxifylline is a methylxanthine phosphodiesterase inhibitor that has been utilized in a variety of areas in assisted reproductive technology (Yovich, 1993; Rizk et al., 1995; Fountain et al., 1995). Pentoxifylline inhibits tumor necrosis factor alpha synthesis. Serin et al. (2002) conducted a study into whether pentoxifylline would prevent OHSS in the rabbit model. Despite an observed decrease in ovarian weight and number of ovulations in OHSS in the rabbit model, pentoxifylline did not prevent ascites formation.

LAPAROSCOPIC OVARIAN DRILLING IN PCOS PATIENTS

Laparoscopic ovarian drilling has been used successfully for prevention of OHSS in patients with polycystic ovaries (Rizk and Nawar, 2001). Both ovarian diathermy and laser vaporization have been used immediately prior to the commencement of ovarian stimulation in patients at risk of OHSS. Ovarian diathermy has been performed in either one or both ovaries (Figure VII.8). Transvaginal ovarian drilling has also been reported in patients with PCOS undergoing assisted reproductive technology. It has been suggested that transvaginal ovarian drilling has been effective in improving IVF results in difficult cases, and is less invasive and expensive when compared with laparoscopic ovarian drilling (Ferraretti et al., 2001).

How Does Ovarian Drilling Work?

Stein and Leventhal (1935) were the first to perform ovarian wedge resection for the treatment of anovulation and infertility associated with PCOS. Many

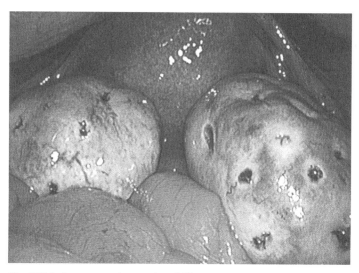

Fig. VII.8: Laparoscopic ovarian drilling in PCOS patients
Reproduced with permission of Goldberg and Falcone (2000). Atlas of Endoscopic Techniques in Gynecology. Edinburgh: Saunders, Chapter 13, p. 61

investigators postulated different mechanisms for resumption of ovulation (Rizk and Nawar, 2001). Stein and Leventhal (1935) proposed that wedge resection decreased the crowding of the ovarian cortex by cysts, allowing the progression of normal follicles to the surface. Gjönnaess (1984) pioneered the treatment of electrocautery by laparoscopy, and suggested that cautery of the ovary destroyed a substance that inhibits ovulation. Gjönnaess and Norman (1987) studied the endocrine effects of electrocautery in PCOS patients and observed decreased androgen production with a subsequent decline in LH secretion. Daniell and Miller (1989) performed laparoscopic laser vaporization of the ovaries and postulated that removal of androgenic fluid is the underlying mechanism by which ovulation is enhanced. Kovacs et al. (1991) observed a transient production of inhibin resulting in increased FSH. Balen and Jacobs (1991) suggested that production of putative gonadotrophin surge attenuating factor from the ovary might be restored after electrocautery. A postoperative surge of LH and FSH followed by a normal pattern of gonadotrophin secretion and gonadotrophin surge attenuating factor was observed following surgery (Balen and Jacobs, 1991).

How Can You Perform Ovarian Drilling?

Stein and Leventhal (1935) pioneered wedge resection for the treatment of infertility associated with amenorrhea, hyperandrogenism and polycystic ovaries. Following the introduction of laparoscopy, a wide variety of techniques have been used (Rizk and Nawar, 2001). Laparoscopic ovarian electrocautery was pioneered by Gjönnaess in 1984. Since then, unipolar and bipolar diathermy, as well as carbon dioxide (CO_2), potassium titanyl phosphate

(KTP), neodymium–yttrium–aluminum–garnet (Nd:Yag) and argon lasers have been utilized. The principles of microsurgery should be adhered to during the use of any technique of ovarian drilling. The introduction of microlaparoscopy has made the procedure less invasive, and therefore safer (Rizk, 2001, 2002; Risquez et al., 1993; Almeida and Rizk, 1998; Rizk and Nawar, 2001).

The technique is relatively straightforward: a triple puncture laparoscopy is usually performed and the ovary is grasped by the ovarian ligament. A variety of instruments have been used for many years with tremendous variation in the literature regarding the three variables involved, which are the number of ovarian punctures, the duration of diathermy and the wattage used (Rizk and Nawar, 2001). Gjönnaess increased the number of punctures to the ovary from three, initially, to four then five then finally eight. The length of each diathermy was 3 s and the wattage used was 200–300 W (Gjönnaess, 1984, 1994; Gjönnaess and Norman, 1987). Armar and Lachelin (1993) performed 3–4 cauteries for each ovary, Kovacs (1998) cauterized the ovary 10 or more times, Balen and Jacobs (1994) suggested that unilateral cautery of one ovary at four sites, at 40 W for 4 s, resulted in ovulation in three of four patients. Interestingly, ovulation occurred in both ovaries. Naether and Fischer (1993) recommended adjusting the number of cauteries according to the ovarian size and other clinical factors. Microlaparoscopic scissors (2 mm) have been used in an attempt to minimize adhesion formation, and the cautery size was 3–4 mm in diameter and 5 mm in depth (Almeida and Rizk, 1998).

Daniell and Miller (1989) recommended 25 W continuous mode laser to vaporize all the subcapsule follicles. They vaporized 20 to 40 sites in each ovary. Ostrzenski (1992) performed laparoscopic CO_2 laser ovarian wedge resection with excellent results and minimal adhesion formation. Feste (1990) used a sapphire tip at 25 W to perforate the ovarian stroma 15 to 20 times. Classic vaporization of the ovarian capsule using an argon laser beam was compared with simple perforation and subcapsule destruction in a Belgian study by Verhelst et al. in 1993.

How Aggressive Should Ovarian Drilling Be?

Different authors have differing opinions on the extent of destruction necessary to desensitize PCOS to exogenous gonadotrophins. While Balen (1999) suggested that minimal destruction is necessary to sensitize the ovaries, Rimington (1997) found that, in order to avoid OHSS, a considerable amount of healthy ovarian tissue destruction is required.

Complications of Ovarian Drilling

The risk of ovarian adhesions and, rarely, ovarian atrophy are of concern (Adashi et al., 1981). This is particularly true if a macrosurgical rather than a microsurgical approach is used. The need for general anesthesia for standard laparoscopy is another drawback. Most recently, Almeida and Rizk (1998) reported the first case of microlaparoscopic ovarian drilling under local anesthesia in a patient with PCOS. This minimally invasive procedure might be the way to proceed in the future.

Laparoscopic Ovarian Drilling in Non-IVF PCOS Patients

Rizk and Nawar (2001) reviewed the treatment of PCOS by ovarian drilling using electrosurgery (Table VII.4) and laser treatment (Table VII.5). Similar ovulation and pregnancy rates were observed. The pregnancy rates varied from 20% to 60%.

Fukaya et al. (1995) studied 26 infertile patients with PCOS who previously had OHSS after ovarian stimulation with hMG and who failed to conceive. All patients were treated by KTP and Nd:Yag laser. After laser vaporization, spontaneous ovulation was confirmed in six patients. In the remaining 20 patients not ovulating spontaneously after laser vaporization, ovulation was successfully induced by using clomiphene citrate (three patients) or hMG (17 patients), in contrast to the difficult ovulation induction prior to laser treatment. Nineteen clinical pregnancies (73%) were confirmed after laser treatment. Of the patients treated with hMG, mild OHSS occurred in only three patients. Fukaya et al. (1995) concluded that laser vaporization of the ovaries is promising for the prevention of OHSS in patients who previously had this syndrome.

Table VII.4 Ovulation and pregnancy rates following electrocautery treatment of PCOS
Reproduced with permission from Rizk and Nawar (2001).
Laparoscopic ovarian drilling for surgical induction of ovulation in polycystic ovarian syndrome. In (Allahbadia G, Ed.), Manual of Ovulation Induction. Rotunda Medical Technologies, Mumbai, India, Chapter 18, pp. 140–4

Author	Year	No. of women treated	Ovulation	Pregnancy
Farhi et al.	1995	22	41%	
Gjöannaess	1994	252	201 (92%)	145 (58%)
Gjöannaess	1984	65	57 (88%)	24 (37%)
Naether et al.	1993	133		73 (55%)
Naether and Fisher	1993	199		
Tütinen et al.	1993	10	3 (30%)	2 (20%)
Kovacs et al.	1991	10	7 (70%)	3 (30%)
Abdel Gadir et al.	1990a	29	71%	10 (34%)
Rizk and Abdalla	2000	7	86%	58%

Table VII.5 Ovulation and pregnancy rates following laser treatment
of PCOS
*Reproduced with permission from Rizk and Nawar (2001). Laparoscopic
ovarian drilling for surgical induction of ovulation in polycystic ovarian
syndrome. In (Allahbadia G, Ed.), Manual of Ovulation Induction.
Mumbai, India, Rotunda Medical Technologies, Chapter 18, pp. 140–4*

Author	Year	No. of women treated	Ovulation	Pregnancy
Heylen et al.	1994	44	35 (80%)	24 (55%)
Verhelst et al.	1993	17	14 (82%)	11 (65%)
Ostrzenski	1992	12		75%
Gurgan et al.	1992	40		20 (50%)
Keckstein et al.	1990	19		8 (42%)
		11	60 (70%)	3 (27%)
Daniell and Miller	1989	85		48 (56%)

Abdel Gadir et al. (1990a, b) compared gonadotrophin therapy with
ovarian drilling in PCOS patients. The pregnancy rates were similar but the
miscarriage rate was lower in PCOS patients.

Cochrane Review

Farquhar et al. (2001) reviewed 15 clinical trials addressing laparoscopic
drilling by diathermy or laser for ovulation induction in anovulatory PCOS.
The main outcomes of the meta-analysis were ovulation and pregnancy rates.
The miscarriage rate, multiple pregnancy rate and OHSS were secondary outcomes. The pregnancy rate following ovarian drilling compared with gonadotrophins differed according to the length of follow-up. Overall the pooled odds
ratio (OR) was not statistically significant (OR = 1.27; 95% CI, 0.77–1.98).
Multiple pregnancy rates were reduced in the ovarian drilling arms of the four
trials where there was a direct comparison to gonadotrophins (OR = 0.16; 95%
CI, 0.03–0.98). There was no difference in the miscarriage rates in the drilling
group when compared to gonadotrophins in these trials (OR = 0.61; 95% CI,
0.17–2.16). Farquhar et al. (2001) concluded that there is insufficient evidence
that there is a difference in cumulative pregnancy rates between laparoscopic
ovarian drilling after 6–12 months follow-up and 3–6 cycles of gonadotrophins
as a primary treatment for subfertile patients with anovulation and PCOS.
Multiple pregnancy rates are considerably reduced in women who conceive
following laparoscopic ovarian drilling.

Laparoscopic Ovarian Drilling in PCOS Patients Before IVF

Laparoscopic ovarian drilling has been used for treating patients suffering from
PCOS before starting their IVF stimulation (Rimington et al., 1997; Egbase

et al., 1998; Tozer et al., 2001). The laparoscopic drilling in three trials was performed on both ovaries and on only one ovary in one trial. Electrocautery and laser vaporization were used.

Rimington et al. (1997) performed a prospective randomized study on 50 patients undergoing IVF. Patients who failed to become pregnant in the previous trial, or whose cycle had been cancelled because of high OHSS risk, were randomized in two groups. In the first group, 25 women were stimulated by long protocol pituitary desensitization followed by gonadotrophin stimulation and IVF. In the second group, 25 patients underwent laparoscopic cautery after pituitary desensitization followed by gonadotrophin stimulation and IVF. The pregnancy and miscarriage rates were identical; however, five cycles were cancelled because of OHSS risk compared to none in the laparoscopic-electrocautery group. Moderate OHSS occurred in four patients in the first group compared to one patient in the second group.

Egbase et al. (1998) performed unilateral ovarian diathermy on three patients with clinical and sonographic features of PCOS who previously had severe OHSS requiring hospitalization. Two of the patients conceived and none developed OHSS.

Tozer et al. (2001) performed a retrospective comparative study on 31 women with clomiphene-resistant PCOS. In 15 women (Group A), 22 cycles of IVF were performed preceded by laparoscopic ovarian diathermy. In 16 patients (Group B), 25 cycles of IVF were performed. The incidence of severe OHSS was higher in Group B than Group A (4.2% vs. 0%). There was also a trend for a lower miscarriage rate and higher pregnancy rate in the laparascopic ovarian diathermy group.

GnRH ANTAGONIST AS AN ALTERNATIVE TO THE LONG AGONIST PROTOCOL

Modern GnRH antagonists such as Cetrorelix and Ganirelix reliably prevent premature LH surges in controlled ovarian hyperstimulation for assisted reproduction (European Orgalutran Study Group, 2000; European–Middle East Orgalutron Study Group, 2001; Fluker et al., 2001; Felberbaum and Diedrich, 2003). GnRH antagonists have helped to overcome some major disadvantages of GnRH agonists, especially of the long protocol, which is currently the standard for ovarian stimulation. However, several studies have indicated a slight reduction in pregnancy rate compared to the GnRH agonist. If the GnRH antagonist is associated with a lower risk of OHSS, that could be a significant advantage (Howles, 2002). In three clinical trials, the incidence of OHSS was reduced using a GnRH antagonist compared with a GnRH agonist long luteal protocol (Albano et al., 2000; Ludwig et al., 2000; Olivennes et al., 2000). In a Cochrane review (Table VII.6), the efficacy of GnRH antagonists was compared to the long agonist protocol in assisted conception (Al-Inany and Aboulghar, 2002). At the time of the review, five published randomized controlled trials fulfilled the inclusion criteria. In four studies,

Table VII.6 Meta-analysis comparing GnRH anatagonist vs.
GnRH agonist co-treatment for ovarian hyperstimulation for IVF
Reproduced with permission from Al-Inany and Aboulghar (2002).
Cochrane Review. Hum Reprod **17**:874–85

	Odds ratio	95% confidence interval
Prevention of premature LH surge	1.8	0.8–4.2
Clinical pregnancy rate/cycle	0.8	0.6–0.99*
Miscarriage rate	1.0	0.5–2.0
Duration of ovarian hyperstimulation	1.1	−1.5−−0.8
Amount of gonadotropins used	−3.3	−5.2−−1.5*
OHSS	0.5	0.2–1.2

* Statistically significant difference

the multiple low-dose 0.25 mg antagonist regimen was used, and in one study a single high-dose (3 mg) antagonist regimen was investigated. In all five trials, reference treatment included a long protocol of GnRH agonist (buserelin, leuprorelin or triptorelin) starting in the mid-luteal phase of the preceding cycle. In comparison with the long GnRH agonist protocol, the overall odds ratio for the prevention of premature surge was 1.76 (95% CI, 0.75–4.16), which was not statistically significant (Table VII.6). There were significantly fewer pregnancies in the GnRH antagonist group (OR = 0.79; 95%CI, 0.63–0.99). There was no statistically significant reduction in the occurrence of severe OHSS (relative risk (RR) = 0.50; OR = 0.79; 95% CI, 0.22–1.18). It is interesting, however, that, except for the study by Ludwig et al. (2000), which was not included in this meta-analysis, none of the five studies was primarily designed to determine the difference in OHSS occurrence between the two protocols. In this prospective randomized study, there were 85 patients and 188 patients for stimulation in the GnRH agonist and the GnRH antagonist groups respectively. The incidence of OHSS was significantly lower in the Cetrorelix group vs. the buserelin group: 1.1% vs. 6.5% respectively (Ludwig et al., 2000). Furthermore, the patients studied were normo-responders and, in two studies, PCOS patients were excluded (Albano et al., 2000; Olivennes et al., 2000).

Ludwig et al. (2001) performed a meta-analysis to evaluate whether there is a reduction in OHSS and/or pregnancy rates associated with the use of two GnRH antagonists, Cetrorelix and Ganirelix. A significant reduction of OHSS was observed in the Cetrorelix studies, (OR = 0.2; 95% CI, 0.10–0.54) but no reduction for Ganirelix (OR = 1.13; 95% CI, 0.24–5.31). The incidences of OHSS degree III cases was reduced in the Cetrorelix protocols as compared with the long protocol to a nearly significant degree (OR = 0.26; 95% CI, 0.07–1.0). Ganirelix did not reduce the incidence of OHSS degree III at all (OR = 1.08; 95% CI, 0.27–4.38). The pregnancy rate in the Cetrorelix studies was not significantly different from the long GnRH agonist protocol (OR = 0.91; 95% CI, 0.68–1.22). The pregnancy rate in the Ganirelix protocols was significantly lower compared to the long GnRH agonist protocol (OR = 0.76; 95% CI, 0.59–0.98). Ludwig et al. (2001) concluded that Cetrorelix and not Ganirelix will reduce the incidence of OHSS, and that Cetrorelix not Ganirelix will result in the same pregnancy rates as the long GnRH agonist protocol. At this point I believe that the final word has not been said in relation to the development of OHSS in GnRH antagonist cycles, and that further studies, some of which have recently been published, will clarify this situation (Ragni et al., 2005).

NATURAL CYCLE IVF

IVF without ovarian stimulation avoids the potential complications of OHSS. However, premature LH surge, cycle cancellation and low pregnancy rates have decreased its popularity. The development of GnRH antagonists has revived the natural cycle IVF by preventing premature LH surges (Figure VII.9; Rongieres-Bertrand, 1999).

SINGLE EMBRYO TRANSFER

The incidence of OHSS is directly related to hCG levels, which in turn is also increased in multiple pregnancies. The severity of OHSS is enhanced by the number of gestational sacs (Mathur et al., 2000). Avoiding multiple pregnancies is a legitimate way to prevent the occurrence of late, severe OHSS. This could in fact be achieved by a single-embryo transfer policy (Gerris and Van Royen, 2000; Gerris et al., 2002, 2004). Transferring a single zona-free day-5 blastocyst allows further time for observation, and offers the patient with moderate OHSS an optimal chance for a singleton pregnancy, while avoiding the complications of OHSS (Kinget, 2002).

Fig. VII.9: Cetrorelix single dose in a natural cycle with minimal stimulation
Reproduced with permission from Olivennes F, Fanchin R, Bertrand C et al. (2001). GnRH antagonist in single dose applications. Infertility and Reproductive Medicine Clinics of North America **12***:119–28. Philadelphia: W.B. Saunders Company*

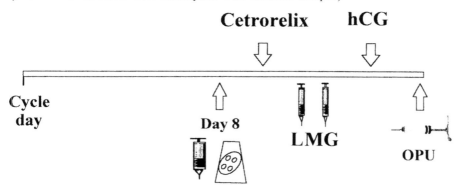

In-vitro Maturation of Oocytes

The first in-vitro maturation of human oocytes and the first fertilization of an in-vitro matured (IVM) oocyte were reported by Edwards (1965) and Edwards et al. (1969), respectively. Today, more than 300 babies have been reported after IVM followed by assisted reproduction treatment, and more than 100 healthy babies from unstimulated cycles in PCOS patients (Mikkelsen, 2004; LeDu et al., 2005) (Table VII.7). Successful in vitro culture of immature oocytes could possibly replace controlled ovarian hyperstimulation. Since ovarian stimulation is not required for IVM, this approach is both safer and cheaper for women with PCOS. The indications for IVM include women requiring IVF who have PCOS, those with poor-quality embryos in repeated IVF cycles for no apparent reason and poor responders to high gonadotrophin stimulation (Tan and Child, 2002). The pregnancy rate following IVM is correlated with the number of antral follicles present, the peak ovarian stromal blood flow velocity at the baseline ultrasound scan, the number of immature oocytes retrieved, the absence of a dominant follicle and endometrial thickness at embryo transfer (Tan and Child, 2002).

The first birth was achieved by Veeck et al. (1983), although in this case the immature oocytes were retrieved during a cycle in which ovarian stimulation was used. Other teams have reported live birth following IVM of oocytes retrieved from non-stimulated cycles (Cha et al., 1991; Trounson et al., 1994; Barnes et al., 1995; Chian and Tan, 2002). A triplet birth after donation of oocytes obtained by aspiration of follicles recovered at the time of oophorectomy during a Cesarean section was reported by Cha et al. (1991). The first pregnancy achieved in PCOS patients from immature oocytes retrieved by puncture during non-stimulated cycles was reported by Trounson et al. (1994). LeDu et al. (2005) reported the French experience of IVM in which 45 cycles of IVM was performed in 33 PCOS patients (Table VII.7). A total of 509 oocyte-cumulus complexes were obtained; 276 oocytes matured in 24 h and 45 in 48 h. The normal fertilization rate for oocytes matured in 24 h and 48 h was 69.5% and 73.3%, respectively. The clinical pregnancy rate was 20% per retrieval and 22.5% per transfer. The role of IVM in the management of patients with PCOS is increasing, and deserves further investigation in the context of randomized controlled trials.

Is There an Ideal Protocol for Prevention of OHSS?

Rizk (2002) proposed the following protocol as an ideal protocol for the prevention of OHSS (Table VII.8). I suggest that, to minimize the risk of OHSS, pretreatment with OCP and low-dose gonadotrophin is initiated, GnRH antagonist used to prevent LH surge, GnRH agonist used to trigger ovulation and progesterone for luteal phase support. I emphasize that no comparison of pregnancy rates has been performed between this protocol and more conventional protocols. Simply put, you may see a drop in pregnancy rate if you adopt any or all of the above. However, it would be estimated that the

Table VII.7 Biological data and birth reports after in-vitro maturation from unstimulated cycles in polycystic ovarian syndrome patients
*Reproduced with permission from Le Du et al. (2005). Hum Reprod **20**:420–4.*

		Immature oocytes		Maturation		Fertilization		Transfers		Pregnancies		
	Cycles	Total	Mean	Total	%	Total	%	(n)	Embryos	Biochemical	Ongoing	Births
Trounson et al. (1994)	9	308	13.4	169	60.4		41	13	17	1		1
Barnes et al. (1995)	3				57.6		62	2	4	1		1
Barnes et al. (1996)	9	165	16.5	102	60.0	27	26					0
Cha and Chan (1998)		832		499	60.0	364	73	64	306	16		16
Chian et al. (1999a)	3	17		13	76.5	10	77	4	10	2	2	4
Chian et al. (1999b)	25	249		209	84.0					10	5	
Chian et al. (2000)	24	183		142	77.6	125	88	24	63	8	6	6
Cha et al. (2000)	94	1139	13.6	708	62.0	481	75	85	416	23		20
Mikkelsen and Lindenberg (2001)	12	81		36	44	25	69	30	53	7		0
Child et al. (2001)	68		11.3				79	67	217	20		10
Chian et al. (2001)	1	63		22		15		1	3			2
Abdul-Jalil et al. (2001)	1	12		6	50	4	67	1	3			2
Child et al. (2002)	107	1102	10.3	834	75	652	78	107		28	23	17
Nagele et al. (2002)	1	16		11		7	64	1	3	1		1
Son et al. (2002)	1	61		40	65.6	38	95	1	3	2		2
Kyono et al. (2002)	1	12		12				1	3	2		2
Lin et al. (2003)	33	762	23.1	548	71.9	383	69.5	33	125	12		12
Le Du (2005)	45	509	11.4	321	63.0		70	40	103	11	6	5 (+1)

Table VII.8 Is there an ideal protocol for the prevention of OHSS?

Pretreatment with oral contraceptive pills

Low-dose gonadotropins

GnRH antagonist to prevent LH surge

GnRH agonist to trigger ovulation

Progesterone for luteal phase support

incidence of severe OHSS would decrease from 1%–2% to 0.5%–0.8%. It has to be mentioned that with any protocol there is still a 0.5% chance of OHSS unless a more liberal policy for cancellation is adopted.

SECONDARY PREVENTION OF OHSS

Preventive Measures During Controlled Ovarian Stimulation

Withholding hCG

Rizk and Aboulghar (1991) found that withholding hCG was the most commonly used method of preventing OHSS in patients predicted to be at high risk of developing the syndrome. Strict criteria for withholding hCG will lower and possibly abolish the incidence of OHSS, but at the expense of canceling the cycle. Today, cancelation of the IVF cycle is the least-favorite approach among clinicians except for extreme situations. Rizk and Nawar (2004) highlighted that the cancelation of the IVF cycle creates a frustrating situation for both the physician and the patient. In ovulation induction cycles when GnRH antagonists or agonists are not used, Delvigne and Rozenberg (2000b) advise caution since a spontaneous LH peak may occur, resulting in a pregnancy that may be associated with OHSS complications.

At What Point Should hCG Be Withheld?

The serum estradiol levels above which hCG should be withheld vary widely among different centers (Rizk et al., 1991a, b). Schenker and Weinstein (1978) withheld hCG when serum estradiol levels exceeded 800 pg/ml. Blankstein et al. (1987) suggested 1700 pg/ml, and Haning et al. (1983) accepted 4000 pg/ml as the upper limit.

Withholding hCG and Continuation of GnRH Agonist or Antagonist

Forman et al. (1990) suggested that hCG should be withheld if the serum estradiol level exceeded 2000 pg/ml in association with a total of more than 15 follicles, each more than 12 mm in mean diameter. GnRH-a was continued and hMG commenced at a lower dosage after a further period of desensitization. An interesting case report, where the patient was at high risk of severe OHSS, was treated by a high dose of GnRH antagonist in addition to discontinuation of gonadotrophins and withholding hCG (de Jong et al., 1998).

I and others believe that, when guidelines for withholding hCG are suggested, more than one parameter should be considered, namely the presence of polycystic ovaries on ultrasound, occurrence of OHSS in previous cycles, serum estradiol level of ≥3500 pg/ml, the slope of the estradiol rise and the presence of 20 or more follicles (Rizk and Aboulghar, 1991, 1999, 2005; Aboulghar and Mansour, 2003).

Coasting or Delaying hCG Administration

PHILOSOPHY OF COASTING

Coasting introduced a new philosophy in ovarian stimulation. It has demonstrated that you can switch off the exogenous gonadotrophin supply without an immediate detrimental effect on follicular development and granulosa cell function. Withholding hMG and delaying hCG has been attempted for two decades. Serum estradiol levels at the time of ovulation triggering has been thought of as a predictor of the risk of developing OHSS. It has therefore been proposed to postpone hCG administration to allow the serum estradiol levels to drop below a certain threshold. This has been termed "coasting" or "controlled drift period."

Coasting has been employed in ovulation induction since the late 1980s and early 1990s (Rizk, in press; Rabinovici et al., 1987; Urman et al., 1992). Shortly afterwards, coasting was used to prevent severe OHSS in IVF cycles (Sher et al., 1993). Currently, coasting is the most popular method among physicians to prevent OHSS (Delvigne and Rozenberg, 2001). More than 15 studies (Tables VII.9–VII.11) have been published and several reviews have critically evaluated the effect of coasting on OHSS (Delvigne and Rozenberg, 2002a, b; Aboulghar and Mansour, 2003; Rizk and Aboulghar, 2005). The differences between the American approach and the European approach for prevention of OHSS has generated scientific discussion (Rizk, in press). It is generally perceived that the American approach is more aggressive, using a higher dose of gonadotrophins, retrieving a large number of oocytes, and replacing a larger number of embryos, resulting in a significantly higher number of multiple pregnancies that has attracted significant media attention with serious criticism (Adamson et al., 2005). That approach is changing but is still very tardy compared with Europe, and is at least a decade behind Europe. However, coasting will continue to play a major role in both the United States and Europe.

ADVANTAGES OF COASTING

Coasting is currently the most popular method for prevention of OHSS because of many advantages (Delvigne et al., 2001; Delvigne and Rozenberg, 2002a, b; Grace et al., 2005). First, this method has the great attraction of the cycle not being cancelled. Second, fresh embryos are still being transferred in contrast to cryopreservation. Finally, no additional gonadotrophins or medications are used (Delvigne, 2004).

HOW DOES COASTING WORK?

It is well-established that high estradiol levels are associated with OHSS; however, it is very unlikely that the high estradiol levels are the cause of OHSS. Therefore, reduction of the estradiol levels themselves is not the main goal of coasting (Dhont et al., 1998; Aboulghar and Mansour, 2003). Coasting may diminish the functional granulosa cell cohort, resulting in the gradual decline in the circulating estradiol levels but, more importantly, reduction of the chemical mediators that augment capillary permeability as vascular endothelial

Table VII.9 Population characteristics of the study, design and selection criteria used for coasting
Reproduced with permission from Delvigne & Rozenberg (2002b). Hum Rep Update **8:**291–6

Study (n)	Mean age (years) ± SD (range)	Selection criteria E_2 (pg/ml), additional criteria	Design/control group(s)
Sher et al. (1995) (51)	37.3 (28–42)	E_2 >3000, follicle number > 29 and 30% follicles ≥ 15 mm	descriptive/NA*
Benadiva et al. (1997) (22)	34.5 ± 3.6	E_2 ≥3000	retrospective/cryopreserved patients
Tortoriello et al. (1998) (44)	32.6 ± 0.7	E_2 >3000, follicle number ≥ 5 ≥ 16 mm and two follicles ≥19 mm	retrospective/subgroup of coasted vs. two control groups
Dhont et al. (1998) (120)	NA	E_2 ≥ 2500, follicle number ≥ 20	retrospective/historical cohort
Lee et al. (1998) (20)	NA	E_2 ≥ 2777 and many immature follicles of which less than three follicles >18 mm	retrospective/IVF patients
Fluker et al. (1999) (63)	32.2 ± NA	E_2 rose rapidly and generally > 3000	descriptive/NA
Waldenstrom et al. (1999) (65)	31.5 (23–39)	'very high' E_2 and >25 'large' follicles of which the three largest ≥ 17 mm	descriptive/NA
Egbase et al. (1999) (15)	33.5 ± 2.8	E_2 > 6000 and >15 follicles/ovary and two or more > 18 mm	prospective randomized early follicular aspiration
Dechaud et al. (2000) (14)	NA	E_2 ≥5000 and/or > 20 follicles of which three or more follicles ≥ 18 mm without abdominal pain	descriptive/NA
Ohata et al. (2000) (5)	32 (25–37)	≥ 30% follicles ≥ 16 mm and severe OHSS in a previous cycle	descriptive/NA
Aboulghar et al. (2000) (24)	29.9 ± 4.6	E_2 >3000 and >20 follicles with a dominant follicle ≥ 16 mm	retrospective/historical group
Al-Shawaf et al. (2001) (50)	32.5 ± 4.5 (23–41)	>20 follicles and 25% ≥ 15 mm, E_2 >3596	prospective/observational normal cycle

* NA = not available

Table VII.10 IVF data for the coasted cycle. The E_2 data are in pg/ml. Means (ranges) or $\pm$ SD are given
*Reproduced with permission from Delvigne Rozenberg (2002). Hum Rep Update **8**:291–6*

Study	E_2 day of coasting	E_2 day of hCG retrieved	ΔE_2	Coasting duration	Oocytes	Fertilization rate (%)	Pregnancy rate (%)**
Sher et al. (1995)	NA*	2163 (560–2920)	5487	6.1 (3–11)	21	69	41[a]
Benadiva et al. (1997)	3803 ± 731	2206 ± 731	1597	1.9 ± 0.9	15 ± 6.5	62.2	63.6[b]
Tortoriello et al. (1998)	4015 ± 112	2407 ± 130	2475	2.6 ± 0.3	15.8 ± 1.2	59.8	44.45[a]
Dhont et al. (1998)	3834 ± 872	2348 ± 472.2	1486	1.94 ± 0.8	19.7 ± 0.6	NA	37.5[b]
Lee et al. (1998)	NA	NA	NA	2.8 ± 1.3	NA	63	40[c]
Fluker et al. (1999)	NA	2832 ± 129	2245	5.3 ± 0.2	10.8 ± 0.5	71	36.5[b]
Waldenstrom et al. (1999)	>6483 (3541–7764) 4471 (2821–7353)	1569 (472–2507)	4576	4.3 (3–6)	10 (3–21)	61	42[b]
Egbase et al. (1999)	10055 ± 965	1410 ± 246	NA	4.9 ± 1.6	9.6 ± 3.2	58.4 ± 2.1	33.3
Dechaud et al. (2000)	5761	3596	NA	1.6 (1–3)	15	36.7	30[a]
Ohata et al. (2000)	NA	1242.6 (425–1800)	NA	4 (3–6)	9.2 (6–15)	NA	20[b]
Aboulghar et al. (2000)	7150 ± 1050	4640 ± 1100	NA	2.92 ± 0.92	16 ± 3.5	59	35[a]
Al-Shawaf et al. (2001)	NA	NA	NA	3.4 ± 1.6	11.0 ± 5.5 (0–22)	55.1	40[b]

* NA = not available
[a] Pregnancy rate/retrieval
[b] Pregnancy rate/cycle
[c] Pregnancy rate/embryo transfer

Table VII.11 Clinical description of registered OHSS cases
Reproduced with permission from Delvigne & Rozenberg (2002). Hum Rep Update **8:**291–6

Study (no. coasted patients)	No. patients with ascites	Hemoconcentration	Comment/OHSS classification
Sher et al. (1995) (51)	12	0	
Benadiva et al. (1997) (22)	NA*	NA	1 moderate/classification not defined
Tortoriello et al. (1998) (44)	6 (5 clinically and 1 at ultrasound)	3	
Dhont et al. (1998) (120)	NA	1	5.8% moderate (involving ascites) and severe OHSS
Lee et al. (1998) (20)	4 (2 paracentesis)	NA	4 severe OHSS (distress with ovarian enlargement and ascites)
Fluker et al. (1999) (63)	1	1	Cumulated results of two groups (classical and modified coasting $n = 93$); 9/93 had nausea and vomiting, 2 had ascites
Waldenstrom et al. (1999) (65)	<300 ml: 6/61 300–800 ml: 3/61 >800 ml: 2/61	2/61	1 paracentesis
Egbase et al. (1999) (15)	3	NA	3 additional cases of moderate OHSS when using the classification of Schenker
Dechaud et al. (2000) (14)	NA	0/10	refers only to severe forms of OHSS
Ohata et al. (2000) (5)	5	0	ascites at ultrasound
Aboulghar et al. (2000) (24)	4	0	ascites at ultrasound (moderate according to the classification of Golan)
Al-Shawaf et al. (2001) (50)	1**/50	NA	2 moderate according to the classification of Navot
Total	46/283	7/378	
%	16.3	2.8	

* NA = not available
** This patient was excluded because of a protocol violation

growth factor (VEGF) (Rizk et al., 1997). In an interesting study from Spain, Garcia-Velasco et al. (2004) suggested that coasting acts through down-regulation of VEGF gene expression and protein secretion. The fact that medium and small follicles are more likely to undergo atretic changes is of crucial relevance in both steroid and vasoactive mediator secretion. They also observed that a significantly higher percentage of granulosa lutein cells become apoptotic after coasting. This difference is even greater for immature follicles. During coasting, estradiol levels initially increased because dominant follicles may continue their growth despite the lack of hormonal stimulus, whereas intermediate follicles may undergo atresia.

The characteristics of granulosa cells in the follicles of women undergoing coasting in controlled ovarian stimulation for IVF has recently been characterized (Tozer et al., 2004a). The effect of withholding gonadotrophins during controlled ovarian stimulation in women at risk of developing OHSS was recently evaluated (Tozer et al., 2004b). Individual follicles of variable sizes were assessed in relation to the granulosa cell number, oocyte retrieved, fertilization and embryo quality. The authors acknowledged that the ideal control group of women would be those identified to be at risk of developing OHSS but not coasted. However, this was not ethically possible since coasting has been successfully used to prevent severe OHSS in their unit for several years (Al-Shawaf et al., 2001). The control group was selected from optimally responsive women that excluded all poor and hyper-responders. Twenty-two women who had been coasted and the control group of optimally responding women were studied in detail. At the time of oocyte retrieval, the follicular fluid from four to six individual follicles of different sizes was collected for VEGF analysis. The authors observed wide variations of follicular fluid levels of VEGF in follicles of the same size, both in different patients and in the same patient, which reflects the unique and individual composition of each follicular environment. Despite these wide variations, VEGF levels in the follicular fluid of follicles in the coasted group were constantly lower than the VEGF follicular fluid levels in the control group.

VEGF concentration in follicular fluid may depend on the quality and number of granulosa cells (Van Blerkom et al., 1997). As discussed above, a negative correlation was observed between follicular fluid VEGF and granulosa cell number, which was independent of follicle size (Tozer et al., 2004b). Greater granulosa cell numbers have been associated with more competent follicles (McNatty et al., 1979) and lower follicular fluid VEGF levels with more oocytes (Friedman et al., 1998) and better embryo quality (Barroso et al., 1999). Tozer et al. (2004b) suggested that this correlation, which was more significant in the coasted group, may be due to the differential effect of gonadotrophin withdrawal on individual follicles in favor of those follicles with greater number of granulosa cells and/or that are more competent. The study did not confirm or refute VEGF as the cornerstone of OHSS pathophysiology, but established that VEGF follicular fluid concentrations in highly responsive women who have undergone coasting are significantly lower than in the control group of women studied.

PHYSICIAN ATTITUDES TOWARDS COASTING

There is no question about the popularity of coasting in Europe and the United States. Delvigne and Rozenberg (2001) assessed whether physicians would modify their preventive attitude in relation to clinical factors and to the estradiol response. They constructed case scenarios with three levels of risk factors for OHSS. At random, three out of the 12 artificially constructed case scenarios were sent to 573 physicians who are members of the European Society for Human Reproduction and Embryology (ESHRE). Among the selected preventive measures, coasting was by far the most popular choice (60%), followed by the use of intravenous albumin; or hydroxyethyl starch solution (36%) and cryopreservation of all embryos (33%).

COASTING IN NON-IVF CYCLES

Several authors have reported successful reduction of severe OHSS by delaying hCG or coasting. Rabinovici et al. (1987) from Israel were the first to report their experience with rescue of 12 gonadotrophin-induced cycles that were liable to develop hyperstimulation. Treatment with hMG was stopped in 12 patients who either had overt biochemical overstimulation or were at an increased risk of hyperstimulation. The duration of the pause in treatment ranged from 2 to 10 days. In nine patients, including the six who were overstimulated, the plasma estradiol levels declined despite the continuing growth of most follicles. None of these patients conceived following hCG. The pregnancies occurred in three patients whose estradiol levels continued to rise until the day of hCG. They therefore concluded that, although rescue of the overstimulated cycles is sometimes possible, resulting conceptions seem to be associated with a continuing rise of estradiol during the period of treatment pause.

Urman et al. (1992) from Canada studied 40 cycles in 32 patients with PCOS. The authors used a controlled drift period to avoid cancellation. The clinical pregnancy rate per cycle was 25% (10 out of 40). OHSS occurred in 2.5% (1 out of 40). The authors did not share the same conclusion about the relation between pregnancy and the rise of estradiol suggested by Rabinovici and colleagues.

A more recent Canadian study was published by Fluker et al. (1999). The patients considered for this study were 51 women undergoing superovulation who had estradiol levels of $>3000\,pg/ml$. In 4 of the 51 women, excessive follicular diameter was observed with the presence of 8 to 10 follicles $\geq 18\,mm$ ($n=2$) or more than 30 follicles $>10\,mm$ ($n=2$). For religious reasons, none of the four women would consider converting to IVF. The cycles were canceled and hCG administration was withheld. Among the remaining 47 women who received the hCG, serum estradiol levels continued to rise for at least one day after the onset of the coasting period, then gradually reached a plateau on the second day and began to fall precipitously on the third day (Figure VII.10). Human gonadotrophin was administered on the evening of the third to the fifth day (mean 3.4 days). The fall from peak E_2 levels of 2824 pg/ml to final levels of 1246 pg/ml on the day of hCG administration represents a mean

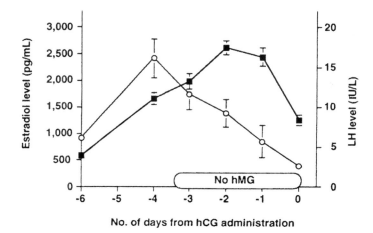

Fig. VII.10: Serum estradiol and LH concentrations before and during the coasting period in superovulation cycles
*Reproduced with permission from Fluker et al. (1999). Fertil Steril **71**:294–301*

reduction in serum estradiol concentrations of 56%. Mean LH levels rose near the onset of the coasting period and decreased spontaneously, while follicular growth continued. Moderate OHSS occurred in three (6%) of the 47 women to whom hCG was administered. A small amount of ascites was noted sonographically and ovaries were enlarged to 6–10 cm. This was not accompanied by significant abnormalities in renal function or hemotologic parameters. Spontaneous resolution occurred with bed rest at home. Eleven pregnancies occurred among the 47 women (23.4%), including eight singletons, one twin, one triplet, and one ectopic pregnancy.

COASTING IN GnRH AGONIST IVF CYCLES

An extensive literature has been published on the role of coasting to prevent hyperstimulation in GnRH agonist IVF cycles (Rizk, in press). Rizk and Smitz (1992) observed that the GnRH agonist is associated with a higher incidence of OHSS. In most of the published studies, the long agonist protocol was used, with the exception of a study by Dhont (1998) when the short protocol was used (Tables VII.9–VII.11).

The credit for the first observation study on coasting in IVF goes to the west coast of the United States in San Francisco. Sher et al. (1993) suggested that prolonged coasting in GnRH-a/hMG/FSH cycles could prevent the life-endangering complications of OHSS. They withheld gonadotrophins in 17 patients whose serum estradiol exceeded 6000 pg/ml, and continued daily GnRH-a until estradiol levels had fallen below 3000 pg/ml. HCG (10 000 IU) was administered to trigger ovulation. The estradiol levels continued to rise rapidly in the 48 h following the initiation of the coasting period, then plateaued and began to fall 96–168 h after the gonadotrophins were stopped. The coasting period lasted between four and nine days and the day of hCG administration fell on cycle days 12–16. Six of the 17 cycles (35%)

produced viable pregnancies. All 17 patients developed signs of grade 2 or 3 OHSS but none developed severe OHSS. In 1995, the same authors treated 51 women at risk of developing OHSS by coasting and also waited until the estradiol level dropped to below 3000 pg/ml (Sher et al., 1995). The clinical pregnancy rate was 41% per oocyte retrieval (21 out of 51). None of the patients developed severe OHSS; however, the mean number of embryos transferred was 5.4 which was extremely high.

Ben-Nun et al. (1993) conducted a pilot study of 66 patients at risk of developing OHSS. These patients were coasted and hCG was given when the estradiol level reached 2500 pg/ml. Four of the 66 patients developed OHSS.

Finding a control group for patients undergoing coasting is not an easy task. In an attempt to use an acceptable control group, Benadiva et al. (1997) therefore compared coasting to cryopreservation. Gonadotrophins were withheld in 22 patients at risk of OHSS. HCG was administered when the estradiol levels dropped to ≤3000 pg/ml. The control group consisted of 26 patients in which no fresh embryo transfer was performed, and all the embryos were cryopreserved and transferred during a subsequent unstimulated cycle. Fertilization and delivery rates were not significantly different between the two groups and Benadiva concluded that coasting could produce high pregnancy rates without the need for multiple frozen/thawed cycles.

In a large retrospective study from Belgium, 120 women at risk of developing OHSS were included (Dhont et al., 1998). These patients were coasted when the estradiol levels exceeded 2500 pg/ml, and hCG was withheld and then administered when the estradiol levels dropped below 2500 pg/ml. The authors compared the outcome to those of 120 matched OHSS high-risk patients who did not undergo coasting. Coasting significantly decreased the incidence of moderate and severe OHSS.

Lee et al. (1998) carried out a pilot study of coasting in 20 patients at risk of OHSS. The mean duration of coasting was three days. HCG was administered on the day that the serum estradiol levels began to fall and four of the 20 patients developed severe OHSS despite coasting. The authors concluded that the hCG administration was too early to prevent OHSS.

Tortoriello et al. (1998a) studied three groups of IVF patients. The first group consisted of highly responsive coasted patients. The second group consisted of equally responsive patients who did not undergo coasting. The control group consisted of age-matched normally responsive patients. The rates of moderate and severe OHSS did not differ statistically among the three groups. No patient in group three developed OHSS. Moderate OHSS was diagnosed in one patient from group one on the basis of sonographically demonstrable minimal ascites. One patient in group two was a singleton pregnancy who developed critical OHSS with severe hemoconcentration, oliguria, and a large pleural effusion that required seven days of hospitalization.

Two subsets of coasted patients were also compared to assess the effect of estradiol levels at the time they met the criteria for hCG. Subset one was identical to group one, consisting of those 22 coasted patients who achieved an estradiol level between 3000 and 3999 pg/ml at the time they met the criteria. Subset two consisted of the remaining 22 coasted patients excluded from the comparison analysis who achieved estradiol levels of >4000 pg/ml at the time they met the criteria. The two subsets did not differ regarding age, FSH levels, instance of polycystic ovaries, number of oocytes retrieved or oocyte maturity, fertilization and cleavage. These patients on average coasted approximately one day longer than the less-responsive subset ($p=0.0463$). The authors observed a significantly higher implantation rate, and the trends suggested a higher clinical and multiple pregnancy rate. There were no significant differences in severe or moderate OHSS among the two subsets. However, all three of the patients who developed severe OHSS were in subset two, and two of them were hospitalized for two days (Tortoriello et al., 1998a).

The estradiol and progesterone levels in all 44 coasted patients were significantly reduced by the end of coast periods lasting longer than two days. Linear regression analysis demonstrated a statistically significant positive relationship between the duration of coasting and peak estradiol level achieved ($p<0.0001$), as well as a significant negative relationship between coasted duration and the total number of mature oocytes retrieved ($p=0.036$). Logistic regression analysis of coast interval duration also suggested an inverse relation with the clinical pregnancy rate ($p=0.09$).

Tortortiello et al. (1998b) also observed severe OHSS despite coasting as gonadotrophins were withheld when serum estradiol levels were 14 700 pmol/l. An important but not surprising finding was that there was a higher than expected incidence of severe OHSS (33%) when coasting was started with serum estradiol levels $>29\,000$ pmol/l and a large number of follicles with diameter larger than 18 mm.

In a study from Sweden, Waldenstrom et al. (1999) performed a multi-center trial of coasting on 65 IVF cycles considered to be severely hyper-stimulated. HCG was given when the estradiol levels fell below 10 000 pmol/l. The mean duration of coasting was 4.3 days, 4 cycles were cancelled. The pregnancy rate was 42% and the implantation rate was 31%, and only one patient developed severe OHSS.

In an interesting Canadian study, Fluker et al. (1999) studied two groups of IVF patients undergoing coasting with mature and immature follicles. In the first group ($n=63$), estradiol concentration rose rapidly and exceeded 3000 pg/ml. Exogenous gonadotropins were withheld to allow estradiol concentrations to decrease by at least 25% before hCG administration. Each subject met the follicular criteria for hCG administration and oocyte retrieval, ≥3 follicles of ≥18 mm before or during the coasting period. Oocyte retrieval occurred 34 h later. The luteal phase was supported with micronized progesterone at a dosage of 200 mg twice daily. In the second group ($n=30$) estradiol concentrations rose rapidly in the presence of numerous intermediate size follicles. In anticipation of overstimulation, the HMG dosage was reduced. This was followed by an abrupt and inadvertent decline in estradiol concentrations before the attainment of appropriate follicular maturity. Gonadotrophin treatment was then reinstituted to restimulate follicular growth. The hCG, 10 000 IU, was administered once three or more follicles ≥ 3 mm were achieved. Oocyte retrieval was performed as per the routine protocol. The mean age, etiology and duration of infertility was similar between the two groups. The average duration of rise was longer in the first group, 3.3 days, than in the second group, 1.37 days, in keeping with the larger follicles and more established steroid oogenesis (Fluker et al., 1999). Clinical pregnancies occurred in 23 of the 63 cycles (36.5%) and in 12 of 30 cycles (40%). The implantation rate per embryo was 14.3% and 17.8%, respectively. Eleven women (12%) had evidence of moderate OHSS, which was managed conservatively at home. One woman (1.1%) from the second group was hospitalized with severe OHSS that required treatment with paracentesis and intravenous albumin. The authors noted that their implantation rates compared favorably with those of Sher et al. (1993), 15.4% versus 9.5%, respectively, as did the clinical pregnancy rates, 37.5% versus 41%, respectively, despite the difference in the number of embryos transferred, 2.9 versus 5.4, respectively. The authors suggested that IVF cycles do not have to be markedly overstimulated to have enough reserve to withstand the coasting period. Rather, a limited period of coasting before the administration of hCG may improve the margin of safety and still be well tolerated, even in cycles in which the response is only slightly increased. The approach in the IVF cycles in the study by Fluker et al. (1999) was different from those in the studies by Sher et al. (1993, 1995). In the two clinical studies by Sher et al. (1993, 1995) the estradiol levels were >6000 pg/ml, or had >30 follicles and received hCG after their estradiol levels decreased to <3000 pg/ml. In contrast, the more conservative approach to stimulation in the study by Fluker et al. (1999), resulted in lower peak estradiol levels and a less precipitous decline in estradiol concentration. As a result, only 18 of 93 patients undergoing IVF in their study had estradiol levels of >6000 pg/ml and 28 received hCG, even though their estradiol levels remained >3000 pg/ml. Fluker et al. (1999) highlighted that the only women in whom severe OHSS developed in their study had an estradiol level of 2762 pg/ml, which is below the limit suggested by most investigators as a safe point to give hCG and have success with coasting.

Aboulghar et al. (2000) performed a "hybrid" study. In a prospective randomized study the authors evaluated the incidence of OHSS in 49 high-risk patients using a reduced hMG dose in one arm and continuation of the same dose in the other arm before coasting. There were no cases of severe OHSS in either group after coasting; however, the duration of coasting was significantly reduced when the dose of hMG was reduced. A historical control group was used to compare the two subsets of the coasted patients. The incidence of severe OHSS in the historical control group was 25%, as compared with 17% in the coasted group (Aboulghar et al., 2000).

In a study from Japan, Ohata et al. (2000) performed coasting in five patients with PCOS who had been previously hospitalized due to severe OHSS in a previous IVF cycle. Coasting was effective in preventing OHSS in these patients.

Grochowski et al. (2001) performed a coasting study on 112 hyperstimulated IVF patients when the estradiol level was over 3000 pg/ml and the leading follicle's diameter was ≥18 mm. Fertilization failed in six patients. All the embryos were frozen in another 10 patients. The pregnancy rate was 30.4% and the implantation rate was 18.1%. Moderate OHSS occurred in six patients and severe OHSS occurred in another two patients.

Al-Shawaf et al. (2001) performed a modified coasting protocol in patients at risk of severe OHSS based on ultrasound monitoring. Serum estradiol levels were measured only in patients with >20 follicles on ultrasound. Moderate OHSS occurred in three patients (0.7%) and severe OHSS in one patient (0.2%). Pregnancy rates were 39.6% and 40% in cycles where the gonadotrophin dose was reduced or withheld, respectively.

Al-Shawaf et al. (2002) determined that measuring serum FSH in addition to estradiol levels during coasting could assist in predicting the point at which the serum estradiol level had declined to a sufficiently safe point for hCG administration.

When to Initiate Coasting?

EARLY COASTING

Egbase et al. (2002) performed a pilot study to determine the impact of withholding gonadotrophins at an earlier stage in patients at risk of developing OHSS. The background of the study was their observation that OHSS still occurred despite coasting in patients with excessive follicular response and high estradiol levels. In this trial, they withheld gonadotrophins for a fixed period of three days once the lead follicle was 15 mm with continuation of pituitary downregulation. They investigated 102 obese patients with PCOS in whom there was evidence of excessive follicular response, more than 10 follicles per ovary and serum estradiol levels >1500 but <3000 pg/ml. The mean serum estradiol level on coasting day 1 was 1943 pg/ml and 2169 pg/ml on the day of hCG administration. Normal fertilization and cleavage rates were observed and the clinical pregnancy rate was 45%. There were no cases of severe OHSS. Four patients suffered pregnancy-associated late-onset moderate OHSS. The authors concluded that early withholding of gonadotrophins in patients with excessive follicular response at risk of developing severe OHSS is consistent with good embryological and clinical outcome in IVF cycles.

VERY EARLY COASTING

In a recent study presented at the American Society for Reproductive Medicine, very early coasting was attempted in order to prevent OHSS (Lukaszuk et al., 2005). The authors studied 27 patients who had experienced OHSS in previous ICSI cycles. For the next ICSI procedure, they were randomized into two groups: 12 patients underwent ovarian stimulation and received 225 IU hMG for two days followed by two days without hMG and then resumed stimulation. The second group received standard doses of stimulation without interruption of their hMG injections. The authors observed that very early coasting resulted in no cases of OHSS compared to six cases in the control group. They suggested that a multi-center trial could determine the value of this approach.

Levinsohn-Tavor et al. (2003) appraised the three factors that should be considered for the initiation of coasting. Plasma estradiol concentration, which reflects the total functional granulosa cell population, the number of ovarian follicles, which predicts the potential for further granulosa cell population and estradiol rise, and, finally, the diameter of the leading follicles, are the three key issues.

Most publications addressing coasting show that an estradiol concentration of 2500 to 3000 pg/ml was the value most commonly chosen by the clinicians (Sher et al., 1995; Benadiva et al., 1997; Dhont et al., 1998; Lee et al., 1998; Tortoriello et al., 1998; Fluker et al., 1999; Al-Shawaf et al., 2001). The relatively low threshold for coasting has been shown to effectively reduce the incidence of OHSS without compromising the cycle outcome (Levinsohn-Tavor et al., 2003) High cutoff levels around 6000 pg/ml are associated with a higher incidence of OHSS and the need for longer periods of coasting (Waldenstrom et al., 1999).

Since the first study by Rabinovici et al. (1987), it has been demonstrated that, even after withholding gonadotrophins, a subsequent rise in serum estradiol for one or two days still occurs (Sher et al., 1995; Fluker et al., 1999; Egbase et al., 2000) (Figure VII.10). In one of the earlier studies when coasting was initiated at a plasma estradiol value of over 3000 pg/ml, the plasma estradiol increased to over 6000 pg/ml during the coasting period.

WHEN TO ADMINISTER hCG AND END COASTING?

The timing of hCG administration at the end of coasting is a matter of great clinical significance in terms of avoidance of OHSS and successful outcome. Administration of hCG when the estradiol level drops below 2500 to 3000 pg/ml has been termed to be effective in lowering the risk of OHSS (Sher et al., 1995; Benadiva et al., 1997; Dhont et al., 1998; Tortoriello et al., 1998; Al-Shawaf et al., 2001). Dhont et al. (1998) compared a coasting group with a control group. Both had a similar maximum estradiol level (3830 pg/ml) and number of follicles ($n = 24$). On the day of hCG administration estradiol levels were 2348 pg/ml in the coasted group compared with 3833 pg/ml in the control group. Only one patient in the coasted group developed severe OHSS compared with nine patients in the control group.

Levinsohn-Tavor et al. (2003) advised that when an appropriate threshold for administering hCG is attained, serum estradiol should be followed and not allowed to fall too low below the threshold. I fully agree with this excellent clinical remark. However, the greatest difficulty that we have encountered is the significant drop in the estradiol level that can occur in one day. Our group encountered two patients whose estradiol level was above 4000 pg/ml during coasting and dropped to below 1000 pg/ml over a 24 h period, with a detrimental effect on the quality of oocytes and pregnancy outcome (Grace et al., 2005). Waldenstrom et al. (1999) reported two cases in which they delayed hCG for an additional two days after the serum estradiol level had dropped below the threshold level of 2724 pg/ml, which led to bleeding and cycle cancellation. In three other cases, serum estradiol was allowed to fall below the threshold value, resulting in the retrieval of one to three oocytes of poor quality.

THE DURATION OF COASTING

How many days of coasting can be carried out without compromising the outcome of ovarian stimulation? The number of recorded days of coasting has varied between 1 and 11 days (Table VII.10). The effect of the duration of coasting has remained controversial. While some studies suggested that gonadotrophins could be withheld for 10 or more days without compromise of the outcome, others have reported a decrease in pregnancy rate when the duration has exceeded four days (Tortoriello et al., 1998a; Ulug et al., 2002; Isaza et al., 2002; Grace et al., 2005).

Ulug et al. (2002) carried out a retrospective study to define the optimal interval of coasting in patients at high risk of developing OHSS. In their study, patients were characterized according to the number of days between the cessation of gonadotrophins and hCG administration. Overall, out of 207 patients coasted, coasting lasted one day in 39 cycles, two days in 61 cycles, three days in 49 cycles, and ≥four days in the remaining 59 cycles. Patients in whom coasting lasted ≥four days had significantly reduced implantation and pregnancy rates compared to patients with a shorter coasting interval. The authors concluded that coasting for more than four days appears to reduce implantation and pregnancy rates where oocyte and embryo quality did not appear to be affected. The authors suggested that, in patients who needed coasting for more than three days, cryopreservation of the embryos should be considered.

Moreno et al. (2004) performed a retrospective study of 132 patients who demonstrated a high response to ovarian stimulation with estradiol >4500 pg/ml and/or more than 20 follicles >17 mm, and who were coasted due to the high risk of developing OHSS. The authors investigated the impact of the duration of coasting on IVF cycle outcome. In addition, serum progesterone and LH were measured to investigate whether premature luteinization was present in the cycles, and whether it might be related to coasting duration. A significant difference in implantation rate was observed when coasting was required for more than four days, together with a trend towards a high cancellation rate. Premature luteinization was significantly elevated in women undergoing coasting compared with control women, 34 versus 15.6% ($p < 0.05$). In the majority of patients who showed premature luteinization, coasting lasted three days. The authors concluded that prolonged coasting may affect the endometrium in relation to the implantation window. These findings may explain why some patients undergoing extended coasting demonstrate a lower implantation rate compared with controls.

COASTING IN GnRH ANTAGONIST IVF CYCLES

The use of GnRH antagonists has simplified the IVF cycle for many patients who were not used to using GnRH agonist from the luteal phase of the cycle preceding their IVF cycle. Most of the data on coasting in IVF come from the GnRH agonist long protocol, but as the use of the GnRH antagonist becomes more commonplace, cases of coasting in GnRH antagonist cycles are being reported. Delvigne et al. (2001) reported two cases in which coasting was used in a stimulation regimen that included GnRH antagonist and gonadotrophins. The first case had an estradiol level of 7851 pg/ml on day 16 of the cycle, and the second patient had a level of 6701 pg/ml on day 13 of her cycle. The first patient increased her level of estradiol on the first day after coasting and had a rapid and clinically significant 83% decrease in the level of estradiol. The second patient experienced a more progressive decrease of estradiol, but her estradiol level did not increase after hMG administration was stopped. Neither patient developed OHSS. The authors suggested that coasting could be used when the stimulation involves hMG and GnRH antagonist.

Another interesting case comes from Belgium where a 23-year-old patient with PCOS was referred to the Center for Reproductive Medicine in Brussels because of a high risk of developing OHSS. She exhibited a rising LH following ovulation induction with a low-dose step-up protocol using gonadotrophins (Fatemi et al., 2002). The patient was counseled to perform a rescue IVF cycle and was coasted using 0.25 mg of ganirelix. The serum estradiol concentrations decreased and the LH peak was successfully suppressed. No OHSS occurred and a twin pregnancy resulted after the transfer of two embryos.

HOW SUCCESSFUL IS COASTING IN ELIMINATING OHSS?

Coasting is very successful in decreasing if not eliminating OHSS (Grace et al., 2005). There is no question that coasting has had a tremendous impact on the clinical management of OHSS. Most investigators have included it at least as part of their approach to prevent this syndrome. From an evidence-based medicine point of view, there is a sparcity of data in terms of prospective randomized trials. The reason for this is obvious, I and others believe it would be difficult to have a randomized clinical trial in which one of the arms would not be coasted and therefore subjected to the risk of severe OHSS. Therefore, many investigators have included a control group or perhaps another modality of OHSS prevention (Rizk, in press).

COCHRANE REVIEW

D'Angelo and Amso (2002a) performed a Cochrane review on coasting for the prevention of OHSS. They identified 13 studies but only one trial met the inclusion criteria, therefore it was concluded that there was insufficient evidence available to determine whether coasting was an effective strategy in preventing OHSS. In the only prospective study, 15 patients were included in each study arm comparing coasting with unilateral follicular aspiration, a technique that is seldom used. The Cochrane review stressed the absence of high-quality studies, which limited to a great extent the conclusions that could be drawn.

IS THERE A PROBLEM WITH COASTING?

The greatest concern about adopting a policy of coasting or withholding gonadotrophins is a decrease in the quality or number of oocytes and a subsequent drop in the pregnancy rate. Aboulghar et al. (1997) studied oocyte quality in patients with severe OHSS. They reported that the inferior quality and maturity of oocytes in OHSS reduced the fertilization rate, but did not affect the quality or the number of embryos transferred, or the pregnancy rate. The effect on oocyte quality could be due to the prevalence of polycystic ovaries in this group of patients.

The literature is divided between those who believe that coasting has some negative impact on oocyte quality (Grace et al., 2005; Rizk, in press) and those who believe that coasting has no impact on the quality of oocytes (Delvigne et al., 2002; Isaza et al., 2002). The criteria used for the initiation and determination of coasting that has been published in the literature is very heterogeneous. This probably explains some of the differences between the reports. In 2002, Ulug et al. found that coasting for four or more days reduces implantation and pregnancy rates, while oocyte quality does not appear to be affected. Isaza et al., in 2002, compared cycle outcome in recipients of oocyte donation from donors who underwent coasting and donors who did not. The outcome of oocyte donation from donors undergoing coasting was not impaired, with similar implantation and pregnancy rates. If the duration of coasting was longer than four days, a significant decrease in implantation and pregnancy rates was found. Delvigne et al. (2002) performed a retrospective cohort study of 157 patients compared with a controlled group of 208 IVF cycles, which had reached serum estradiol levels of at least 4000 pg/ml without being coasted. In the group of coasted cycles, the question of whether indirect parameters related to coasting had an effect on IVF outcome was also analyzed. The authors observed that patients who had undergone coasting had higher maximum estradiol levels and greater numbers of large follicles ($p<0.001$) and lower oocyte recovery rates ($p<0.001$) than the control group. The IVF outcomes were similar between the two groups. The authors also observed that, within the group of patients who had undergone coasting, no significant relationship was observed between the number of coasting days, the estradiol levels on the day of hCG, or the fallen estradiol level and the outcome, whether measured in terms of oocyte quality, pregnancy rate or OHSS occurrence.

In a recent study we have observed a decline in the implantation and pregnancy rates in IVF cycles in those women who underwent coasting (Grace et al., 2005). The decrease in implantation and pregnancy rates was not statistically significant. The clinical pregnancy rate for the non-coasted patients was 34.4% per cycle (22 out of 64) compared with 20% per cycle (6 out of 30). However, in the subset of patients who received a lower dose of hCG (5000 versus 10 000 IU), the difference was statistically significant. The pregnancy rate was 9% per cycle (1 out of 11) compared with 34.4% ($p=0.04$). In the reported publications, ovulation was induced in three studies by administering 5000 units of hCG (Waldenstrom et al., 1999; Dechaud et al., 2000; Ohata et al., 2000), but more often with 10 000 units (Sher et al., 1995; Dhont et al., 1998; Tortoriello et al., 1998a; Egbase et al., 1999; Fluker et al., 1999; Aboulghar et al., 2000; Al-Shawaf et al., 2001). The fertilization rate was significantly lower compared to the non-coasted group (59.4% vs. 73.9%, respectively). The rate of cell division was also significantly slower and the mean and median cumulative embryo index (EI) and the mean number of blastomeres was also significantly lower ($p < 0.0001$). In our experience, coasting abolished severe OHSS. However, the clinical pregnancy rate was significantly lower in the coasted patients who received a lower dose of hCG. Therefore, the question is raised: should we adjust our expectations and accept a safer but less successful outcome? That question has to be asked every time this clinical scenario arises.

COASTING: CONCLUSIONS

Coasting is the most popular method for preventing OHSS. Prospective randomized studies regarding its efficacy are limited because it is unacceptable to have a control group subjected to the risk of severe hyperstimulation syndrome. The exact point at which coasting should start or finish varies from one group to another, which limits the ability to compare outcomes. Levinsohn-Tavor et al. (2003), after a critical review of the data in the different protocols, recommended avoiding certain pitfalls in the coasting protocol in order to achieve the best formula. Coasting should be initiated when the serum estradiol exceeds 3000 pg/ml, but not unless the leading follicles reach a diameter of 15–18 mm. The duration of coasting should be limited to less than four days to avoid a decrease in implantation and pregnancy rates that would occur after longer periods of coasting.

Opinion is divided about the impact of coasting on pregnancy outcome. In my opinion, there is no question that, by utilization of this approach, many cases of severe OHSS can be prevented. I believe that such a policy is useful; however, I also believe that the application of coasting to the point of complete prevention will result in a decrease in the number and the quality of oocytes and a lower pregnancy rate.

DECREASE IN HCG DOSAGE

It is amazing that there is only one clinical trial published in the literature regarding the impact of the dose of hCG on the occurrence of OHSS. Abdalla et al. (1987) reported a significantly lower successful oocyte recovery in patients who received 2000 IU of hCG (77.3%) compared with patients who received either 5000 IU of hCG (95.5%) or 10 000 IU of hCG (98.1%), $p < 0.001$.

It is very interesting to review the details of the first article on the classification of OHSS (Rabau et al., 1967). The authors listed seven cases with mild OHSS and another seven cases with severe OHSS, and the dose of hCG that was used ranged from 10 000 to 29 000 IU. Most of the patients received around 25 000 IU, which is an amazingly high dose by today's standards. During that period, the first report to suggest that hCG administration after ovarian stimulation with hMG resulted in pregnancy with simultaneous ovarian cyst formation was published by Pascetto and Montanino in 1964. The authors administered a total of 25 000 IU of hCG for their ovarian stimulation protocol. Schenker and Weinstein (1978) in their review summarized their experience in the 1960s and 1970s with some fascinating remarks about hCG administration. The dose and timing of hCG varied from 1000 to 25 000 IU or more, and from one to several doses, which could either overlap or not overlap with the administration of hMG. They found similar ovulation rates following any dosage of hCG but the pregnancy rate was highest after 6000 to 15 000 IU. Very interestingly, they noted the frequency of OHSS to be lower in patients given 1000–5000 IU or more than 25 000 IU, than in patients given 6000–25 000 IU. Data on the regimens of hCG which did not overlap hMG showed a significantly lower incidence of OHSS than when hCG overlapped (Thompson and Hansen, 1970; Schenker and Weinstein, 1978).

In the routine IVF cases, most centers in the United States administer one dose of hCG at 10 000 IU, whereas, in Europe, some centers administer 5000 only, while others administer 10 000 IU. In the past, some authorities have recommended a dosage of up to 25 000 IU to induce ovulation (Lunenfeld and Insler, 1978). I recommend a dose of 10 000 IU to trigger ovulation. If there are clinical or endocrinological suspicions of OHSS, I reduce the dose of hCG by one-third to one-half. I believe that this could at least help in decreasing the severity of OHSS.

RECOMBINANT hCG

Recombinant hCG, at a dose of 250 μg, is as effective as 10 000 IU urinary hCG in triggering ovulation. It also has the advantage of subcutaneous administration (Rizk and Abdalla, 2006). The pregnancy and implantation rates and the incidence of OHSS were comparable between recombinant and urinary hCG (Chang et al., 2001; Driscoll et al., 2000; European Recombinant Human Chorionic Gonadotrophin Group, 2000). Induction of ovulation in WHO group II anovulatory women undergoing ovulation induction using recombinant FSH produced comparable results between 250 μg recombinant hCG and 5000 IU urinary hCG (International Recombinant Human Chorionic Gonadotrophin Study Group, 2001).

Alternatives to hCG

The Use of GnRH-Agonist to Trigger Ovulation

Alternatives to hCG have been explored for the last two decades (Rizk et al., 1991a, 2002). These include GnRH agonists, native GnRH, and recombinant LH. GnRH agonist has been used to trigger ovulation in assisted conception for 15 years. The widespread use of the long protocol of pituitary down-regulation has practically limited its use to a minority of cycles where gonadotrophins only are used. If the next decade witnesses a significant increase in GnRH antagonist cycles, then the use of the GnRH agonist will be revisited extensively.

IN GONADOTROPHIN CYCLES

The use of GnRH agonists to trigger ovulation has been investigated since the late 1980s. Gonen et al. (1990) and Itskovitz et al. (1991) used the initial flare-up effect of the agonist to achieve ovulation and subsequent pregnancies. In patients at risk of OHSS, intranasal buserelin (200 mg three times at 8 h intervals) was used to trigger ovulation, and a 22% pregnancy rate resulted without any cases of OHSS. Imoedemhe et al. (1991) used GnRH-a in 38 women considered at risk of OHSS, having serum estradiol levels of > 4000 pg/ml, with 11 pregnancies and no cases of OHSS. Emperaire and Ruffie (1991) utilized buserelin 200 µg 3 × at 8 h intervals in a series of 126 cycles in 48 patients with primary infertility treated with gonadotrophins for anovulation. In the 37 cycles where buserelin was used, no OHSS occurred despite high preovulatory levels of serum estradiol. The pregnancy rate per cycle was 21.6% using buserelin, compared with 16.8% when hCG was used. Van der Meer et al. (1993) could not prevent OHSS by using GnRH agonist to trigger ovulation. Gerris et al. (1995) triggered ovulation in hMG stimulated cycles by using GnRH agonist and observed a high frequency of luteal phase insufficiency. OHSS could not be prevented by using this approach. The major limitation of the use of GnRH agonist is that it could not be used in cycles where ovarian stimulation with hMG was performed after pituitary desensitization using GnRH agonist (Rizk, 2001, 2002).

Revel and Casper (2001) carefully analyzed the use of GnRH agonist instead of hCG to trigger ovulation in cycles where gonadotrophins and clomiphene citrate have been used for ovulation induction. They evaluated the efficacy of GnRH agonist and pursued the concept of whether GnRH agonist would prevent OHSS. They analyzed the data from uncontrolled clinical trials as well as controlled studies comparing GnRH agonist with hCG in terms of its ability to trigger the LH surge (Tables VII.12, VII.13) or to prevent OHSS (Tables VII.14, VII.15). In uncontrolled studies when GnRH agonist was used to trigger ovulation, the incidence of OHSS was 0.9% (3 out of 334) (Table VII.14). In controlled studies, the incidence of OHSS was 1.5% in the hCG group, compared with 0.7% in the GnRH agonist group (Table VII.15). It appears therefore that GnRH agonist is as effective as hCG in triggering ovulation in gonadotrophin-only cycles with only half the incidence of OHSS.

IN GnRH-ANTAGONIST/GONADOTROPHIN CYCLES

Rizk (2002) reviewed the approaches that have been successfully used to induce the final stages of oocyte meiosis maturation in GnRH antagonist and gonadotrophin cycles. These include hCG, GnRH agonist, native GnRH, recombinant LH and withdrawal of GnRH antagonist. GnRH agonist has been successfully shown to induce these final stages of oocyte maturation in monkeys and humans, Felberbaum et al. (1995) and Olivennes et al. (1996) elegantly demonstrated ovulation triggering by GnRH agonist after GnRH antagonist treatment.

Table VII.12 Effectiveness of GnRH agonist in uncontrolled studies
Reproduced with permission from Revel and Casper (2001). Infertility and Reproductive Medicine Clinics of North America **12**:*105–18*

Study	Criteria	No.	LH surge, no. (%)*	Pregnancy rate per ET no. (%)**
Lanzone et al. (1989)		8	8 (100)	–
Emperaire and Ruffie (1991)	$E_2^\dagger > 1200$ pg/ml	126	–	27 (22)
Imoedemhe et al. (1991)	$E_2 > 4000$ pg/ml	27	–	11 (29)
Itskovitz et al. (1991)		12	12 (100)	4 (29)
Tulchinsky et al. (1991)	pilot study	13	11 (85)	4 (36)
van der Meer et al. (1993)	pilot study	48	44 (92)	10 (23)
Balasch et al. (1994)	cycles that would otherwise have been cancelled	23	17 (74)	4 (17)
Shalev et al. (1994)	$E_2 > 3500$ pg/ml	12	–	6 (50)
All		261	88%	29%

* LH = luteinizing hormone
** ET = embryo transfer
† E_2 = 17β-estradiol

Table VII.13 Effectiveness of GnRH agonist versus hCG in controlled studies
Reproduced with permission from Revel and Casper (2001). Infertility and Reproductive Medicine Clinics of North America **12**:*105–18*

Study	Stimulation*	No.	LH surge, no. (%)	Pregnancies no. (%)	No.	LH surge, no. (%)	Pregnancies, no. (%)	p
Gonen et al. (1990)	CC–hMG	9	9 (100)	0	9	9	3 (33)	NS**
Segal and Casper (1992)	CC–hMG	95	–	19 (19)	84	–	18 (20)	NS
Scott et al. (1994)	CC	21	21 (100)	–	21	21 (100)	–	NS
Kulikowski et al. (1995)	CC–hMG	34	–	3 (9)	32	–	4 (13)	NS
Gerris et al. (1995)	hMG	10	10	–	19	–	–	
Schmit-Sarosi et al. (1995)	CC	15	8 (53)	2 (13)	11	11 (100)	3 (27)	<0.01
Shalev et al. (1995a)	CC	106	–	14 (13)	104	–	3 (12)	NS
Shalev et al. (1995b)	hMG	68	–	18 (27)	72	–	11 (15)	NS
Romen et al. (1997)	FSH	416	413 (99)	71 (17)	345	342 (99)	93 (27)	0.0007
All		753	461/471 (98)	127/734 (16.7)	676	402/405 (99)	144/657 (22)	<0.05

* LH = luteinizing hormone; CC = clomiphene citrate; HmG = human menopausal gonadotropin; FSH = follicle-stimulating hormone
** NS = not significant

Table VII.14 Uncontrolled studies to determine whether GnRH agonists for triggering ovulation prevent OHSS
Reproduced with permission from Revel and Casper (2001). Infertility and Reproductive Medicine Clinics of North America **12**:*105–18*

Study	Criteria	No. cycles	No. with OHSS	Comments
Emperaire and Ruffie (1991)	$E_2^* > 1200$ pg/ml or > 3 follicles of 17 mm	37	10	
Imoedemhe et al. (1991)	$E_2 > 4000$ pg/ml	36	0	
Itskovitch et al. (1991)	E_2 5000–13000 pg/ml	8	0	
Van der Meer et al. (1993)	–	48	3	mild to moderate
Balasch et al. (1994)	cycles to be cancelled owing to high risk	23	0	
Balasch et al. (1995)		30	0	
Lanzone et al. (1989)	PCOS	40	0	some GnRh agonist, some hCG
Lewit et al. (1995)	High risk?	80	0	
Shalev et al. (1994)	$E_2 > 3500$ pg/ml, no of follicles > 20	12	0	not IVF
Total		334	3(0.9%)	

* $E_2 = 17\beta$-estradiol

Table VII.15 Controlled studies to determine whether GnRH agonist for triggering ovulation prevents OHSS
Reproduced with permission from Revel and Casper (2001). Infertility and Reproductive Medicine Clinics of North America **12**:*105–18*

Study	Criteria	GnRH		HCG		Comments
		No.	OHSS	No.	OHSS	
Gonen et al. (1990)		9	0	9	0	
Segal and Casper (1992)	randomized	84	0	95	0	
Gerris et al. (1995)	controlled	28	1	10	0	on native GnRH
Kulikowski et al. (1995)	non-randomized	48	0	34	4	moderate OHSS
Shalev et al. (1995b)	randomized	72	4	84	8	not significant
Shalev et al. (1995a)	randomized	104	0	106	0	clomiphene cycles
Romeu et al. (1997)	prospective, non-randomized	345	0	416	0	FSH, IUI
Penarrubia et al. (1998)	prospective, non-randomized	26	0	26	0	2 doses of hCG and of LH
All		716	5 (0.7%)	780	12 (1.5%)	significant, $p = 0.047$ (z test)

Focusing on OHSS prevention, recent studies suggested the safe use of GnRH agonist to trigger ovulation in women who underwent ovulation induction with recombinant FSH and the GnRH antagonist. Itskovitz-Eldor et al. (2000) reported the use of a single bolus of GnRH agonist (decapeptyl) 0.2 mg to trigger ovulation in women at risk for OHSS after treatment with recombinant FSH and ganirelix. All women had serum estradiol levels greater than 3000 pg/ml and more than 20 follicles; none developed signs or symptoms of OHSS and four conceived.

Bracero et al. (2001) studied 19 women who underwent controlled ovarian hyperstimulation for IVF using gonadotrophins and ganirelix, 0.5 mg. All 19 patients had serum estradiol greater than 3000 pg/ml with 20 or more follicles more than 15 mm in diameter. In eight patients, leuprolide acetate, 1 mg, was given twice, 12 h apart, and in 11 women, hCG, 10 000 IU, was administered and oocytes were retrieved 36 h later. In the first group, none of the patients developed symptoms or signs of OHSS, whereas two of the 11 patients in the second group developed mild OHSS, $p = 0.05$. The authors concluded that leuprolide acetate instead of hCG should be used for triggering ovulation to prevent OHSS in cycles where gonadotrophins and GnRH antagonist has been used.

More recently, several prospective randomized trials evaluated the use of GnRH agonist to trigger final oocyte maturation instead of hCG in patients undergoing IVF with GnRH antagonists. Humaidan et al. (2005) recently evaluated the use of an agonist as an alternative to hCG in 122 patients undergoing IVF. The authors used buserelin 0.5 mg subcutaneously to trigger ovulation. A significantly lower pregnancy rate was reported in the agonist arm. This might be associated with discontinuation of luteal support in the presence of a positive pregnancy test.

Kolibianakis et al. (2005) randomized 106 patients to receive either 10 000 IU urinary hCG or 0.2 mg triptorelin for triggering final oocyte maturation. Ovarian stimulation for IVF was performed using recombinant FSH at a fixed dose of 200 IU, and GnRH antagonist was started on the sixth day of ovarian stimulation. Luteal phase support was established using micronized vaginal progesterone and oral estradiol. The authors observed no significant differences in the number of cumulus–oocyte complexes, metaphase II oocytes, fertilization rates or the number and quality of embryos replaced. However, a significantly lower probability of ongoing pregnancy rate in the GnRH agonist arm prompted discontinuation of the trial (OR = 0.11; 95% CI, 0.02–0.52).

Recombinant Human LH to Trigger Ovulation

hCG is a promoter of OHSS whereas an endogenous LH surge rarely causes OHSS (Rizk and Smitz, 1992). The idea of using leuteinizing hormone is an old idea, not a new one. The only recent development is the development of recombinant LH. In 1970, Vande Wiele et al. substituted purified human pituitary LH (hLH) for hCG. They administered hLH in multiple injections over a 24 h period, mimicking the normal LH surge. Human LH maintained the corpus luteum, and by repeated injections prolonged its functional life beyond 14 days. The authors experienced no severe cases of OHSS; however, Schenker and Weinstein (1978) cautioned that the clinical experience with hLH was very limited. Jewelewicz (1972) reported a case of quintuplet pregnancy after ovulation induction with hMG and hLH.

In the experimental animal model, Gomez et al. (2004) compared the capacity of LH, FSH and hCG to trigger ovulation, and also studied their effects on vascular permeability and the expression of VEGF in the ovaries. As discussed in detail in Chapter III, they stimulated immature female rats with 10 IU of pregnant mare serum gonadotrophin (PMSG) for four days and thereafter ovulation was triggered by using 10 IU of hCG, 10 IU of FSH, 10 IU LH, 60 IU of LH or normal saline. All the hormones utilized were equally effective at triggering ovulation, and significantly different from the control injection. However, only 10 IU of LH resulted in a significantly lower vascular permeability and VEGF expression. Gomez et al. (2004) concluded that a lower dose of LH (10 IU vs. 60 IU) prevented the undesired changes in vascular permeability and the risk of OHSS. However, the authors encouraged clinicians to determine the optimal dosage of LH needed to trigger ovulation in women and at the same time to abolish OHSS. We believe that this is a very important issue, because the clinical trials of recombinant LH have also suggested a lower OHSS rate associated with a lower pregnancy rate, which will be discussed in the next section. The success in determining the optimal dose or doses of LH could be a significant step towards eliminating OHSS while retaining the pregnancy rate.

Considering the significant differences between hCG and recombinant human luteinizing hormone (r-hLH) and its impact on OHSS, this is the time to revolutionize the triggering of ovulation (Emperaire and Edwards, 2004). A European prospective randomized double-blind multicenter study evaluated the safety and minimal effective dose of recombinant LH in patients undergoing IVF compared with 5000 IU of urinary hCG (European Recombinant LH Study Group, 2001). The study showed that a single dose of r-hLH was effective in inducing final follicular maturation and early luteinization in IVF patients, and a dose between 15 000 and 30 000 IU was equivalent to 5000 IU of hCG. There were no statistically significant differences between urinary hCG (u-hCG) and r-hLH administration in the number of oocytes retrieved, oocyte nuclear maturity, oocyte potential for fertilization, the number of embryos, clinical and biochemical pregnancies and the implantation rate of the embryos. In terms of safety, r-hLH was well-tolerated at doses of up to 30 000 IU. Moderate OHSS occurred in 12.4% of patients who received u-hCG and 12.0% who received two injections of r-hLH. Interestingly, there was no moderate or severe OHSS in those patients who received a single dose of r-hLH of 30 000 IU (European Recombinant LH Study Group, 2001). A single dose of r-hLH resulted in a highly significant reduction in OHSS.

A recent double-blind large multicenter randomized study (Trial 21447), which compared the implantation and pregnancy rates following triggering ovulation by r-hLH versus hCG, was discussed in a letter to the editor by Aboulghar and Al-Inany (2005) in response to an article advocating the use of LH to trigger ovulation (Emperaire and Edwards, 2004). The study is as yet unpublished (Aboulghar and Al-Inany, 2005). A total of 437 patients were randomly allocated in a 2 to 1 ratio to either the r-hLH treatment group (291 patients) or the u-hCG treatment group (146 patients). The two groups were matched for age, height, weight, BMI, race and smoking habits at baseline. The mean ages were 31.1 ± 4.5 years and 30.5 ± 4.5 years, mean height 164 ± 7 cm and 161 ± 7 cm, mean body weight 65.3 ± 11.4 kg and 66.0 ± 11.8 kg, the mean BMI was 24.4 ± 4.2 kg/m^2 and 24.4 ± 4.1 kg/m^2 in the r-hLH and u-hCG groups respectively. The majority of patients in the study population were Caucasian (95.9 and 97.9 in the r-hLH and the u-hCG groups, respectively) and the majority did not smoke (78.0% and 82.2%, respectively). The results of Trial 21447 showed that a clinically significant OHSS (severe and all cases) was significantly lower in the r-hLH compared to the u-HCG group ($p = 0.001$), however the pregnancy rates and the clinical pregnancy rates were significantly lower in the r-hLH group compared to the u-hCG group ($p = 0.018$ and $p = 0.023$, respectively). In order for the r-hLH to be as effective as hCG, the dose should be increased. However, the cost/benefit ratio may not be beneficial. The study has not yet been published and the manufacturer of r-hLH decided not to register the high dose used for triggering ovulation (Aboulghar and Al-Inany, 2005). Unfortunately the clear advantage of r-hLH in reducing the incidence of OHSS which was demonstrated by the European Recombinant LH Study Group (2001) cannot be yet utilized in clinical practice because of the lower pregnancy rates after triggering ovulation with r-hLH (Aboulghar and Al-Inany, 2005).

Emperaire (2005) did not accept the findings of this unpublished study for at least four reasons. First, the debate upon the safety and efficiency of recombinant LH vs. hCG to trigger ovulation is important enough that it could not be ignored because of the results of an unpublished trial; and he also wondered why the trial was not published if the design was correct and prospectively performed. Second, the results are restricted only to the triggering of ovulation for IVF after GnRH agonist desensitization and cannot be extended to other types of stimulation (Emperaire and Edwards, 2004), or it could be used in IVF cycles where GnRH antagonists have been utilized. This second point has led to a reply by Aboulghar and Al-Inany (2005), where they quoted a significantly lower pregnancy rate when GnRH agonist was used instead of hCG to trigger ovulation in GnRH antagonist cycles, leading to the discontuation of clinical trials (Humaidan et al., 2005; Kolibianakis et al., 2005). A third but important point that Emperaire (2005) discussed was the fact that OHSS was significantly reduced when recombinant LH was used instead of hCG ($p < 0.001$). On the other hand the significance of a lower pregnancy and clinical pregnancy rate appears to be statistically much weaker ($p < 0.018$ and $p < 0.023$, respectively). Fourth, and finally, the dose of recombinant LH could be subject to further testing to determine the most optimal regimen. He observed that, in primates, two doses of 2500 IU rLH given 12 h apart were more efficient than a single double-dose (Zelinski-Wooten et al., 1991).

Native GnRH to Trigger Ovulation

Native GnRH has also been investigated for triggering ovulation instead of hCG in cycles stimulated by hCG. Gerris et al. (1995) compared intravenously administered gonadotropin hormone (100 and 500 μg), GnRH agonist (buserelin, 500 μg) and human chorionic gonadotrophin (10 000 IU). Endogenous LH surges occurred in all cycles of patients treated with GnRH or GnRH agonists. The rise was slowest but highest in the group of patients treated with GnRH agonist (500 μg) compared with GnRH both at the 100 and 500 μg doses ($p < 0.0001$). Although the serum estradiol was similar in all groups, day 8 estradiol was significantly higher in the hCG group. Luteal phase insufficiency, defined as cycles with progesterone concentrations of <8.0 ng/ml, occurred more frequently in patients whose ovulation was triggered by GnRH or GnRH agonist despite progesterone supplementation. Clinically, day 8 luteal scores showed more conspicuous OHSS in the hCG group ($p = 0.292$). The authors concluded that ovulation occurs and pregnancies can be achieved following endogenous LH surge induced by GnRH and its agonist. A high frequency of *luteal insufficiency* occurs in such cycles even with luteal supplementation. Finally, OHSS cannot be *totally prevented* by this approach although cycles with an endogenous LH surge, in general, result in fewer subclinical instances of ovarian hyperstimulation.

INTRAVENOUS ADMINISTRATION OF MACROMOLECULES AT THE TIME OF OOCYTE RETRIEVAL

Intravenous Albumin Administration

Experience in subjects with different forms of third space fluid accumulation have shown that albumin is effective in preventing and correcting hemodynamic instability. Using a similar approach, in an effort to increase the oncotic pressure and to reverse the leakage of fluids from the intravascular space, high-risk subjects for severe OHSS were treated with albumin. Asch et al. (1993) were the first to suggest that intravenous albumin during follicular aspiration could be potentially useful to prevent OHSS. The authors proposed that the role of albumin in prevention of OHSS is multifactorial. First, it acts to sequester vasoactive substances released from the corpora lutea. Albumin has a half-life of 10–15 days. Patients generally develop OHSS symptoms 3–10 days after hCG injection, regardless of the embryo transfer. Timely administration of albumin, during oocyte retrieval and immediately following, may serve to bind and inactivate this factor. Second, albumin also serves to sequester any additional substances which may have been synthesized as a result of OHSS. Finally, the oncotic properties of albumin also serve to maintain intravascular volume and prevent the ensuing effects of hypovolemia, ascites and hemoconcentration.

Following the first clinical trial by Asch et al. (1991) a series of publications for and against the efficacy of albumin were published (Table VII.16). Several investigators have conducted prospective trials and agreed with their conclusion (Shoham et al., 1994; Shalev et al., 1995a, b). Other authors have disagreed with the conclusion (Ng et al., 1995; Mukherje et al., 1995; Shaker et al., 1996; Lewitt et al., 1996).

Cochrane Database Review of Albumin for the Prevention of OHSS

In a Cochrane review of the use of intravenous albumin to prevent severe OHSS, seven randomized controlled trials were identified (Aboulghar et al., 2002). Five studies (Shoham et al., 1994; Shalev et al., 1995c; Isik et al., 1996; Gokman et al., 2001; Ben-Chetrit et al., 2001) met the inclusion criteria (Aboulghar et al., 2002). All were single-center, randomized controlled trials with parallel design. In these five clinical trials, 378 patients were enrolled, of which 193 were in the albumin-treated group and 185 in the control group (Table VII.17). The meta-analysis of the five trials showed a significant reduction in severe OHSS with an OR of 0.28 and 95% CI, 0.11–0.73. The RR was 0.35 (0.14–0.87) and the absolute RR was 5.5. Albumin infusion would save one case of OHSS for every 18 women at risk for severe OHSS. The authors concluded that intravenous albumin shows a clear benefit for the prevention of OHSS; however, whether the number needed to treat would justify the routine use of albumin in high risk patients must be judged by the clinical decision-makers and future large randomized trials (Aboulghar et al., 2002).

A recent study, published after the Cochrane review, represents the largest randomized controlled trial to date of albumin infusion vs. no treatment in IVF patients who are at risk of developing moderate–severe OHSS (Belver et al., 2003). Between March 1999 and February 2002, women undergoing IVF with more than 20 retrieved oocytes were included. A total of 988 patients were involved. Immediately after retrieval, patients were allocated to one of two groups based on computer randomization. The first group received intravenous albumin (40 g) and the second group received no treatment. In women who developed moderate–severe ($n = 66$) or severe ($n = 46$) OHSS, there was no difference based on prior albumin administration between blood parameters or body weight on the day of oocyte retrieval or seven days later. Furthermore, the number of patients with paracentesis, hospital admissions, complications and days of OHSS until resolution did not differ. The authors concluded that albumin infusion on the day of oocyte retrieval is not a useful means for preventing the development of moderate–severe OHSS.

It is my impression that if a new meta-analysis is performed taking into account the more recently published trials, it is possible that the role of intravenous albumin at the time of follicular aspiration for the prevention of OHSS would be nonsignificant.

Table VII.16 Intravenous albumin for the prevention of OHSS
Reproduced with permission from Delvigne and Rozenberg (2002b). Hum Reprod Update **8**:559–77

Study	Study design (n)	Control group	Risk patients	OHSS incidence with albumin use	OHSS incidence in controls	Comment
Asch et al. (1993)	not controlled (36)	historical high-risk patients	E_2* >6000 pg/ml and >30 oocytes	0%	80%	in 21 patients no transfer occurred
Shoham et al. (1994)	prospective randomized controlled (31)	placebo of NaCl	E_2 >1906 pg/ml and multiple follicular development	0/16	4/15 severe OHSS ($p < 0.05$)	no information about moderate forms
Shahata et al. (1994)	retrospective (200)	historical whole IVF population	E_2 >2997 pg/ml and >20 oocytes or >30 follicles	0/104	8/96	only 18% of controls had E_2 >2997 pg/ml
Ng et al. (1995)	prospective controlled (207)	placebo of ringer's solution	E_2 >2724 pg/ml and >15 follicles	2/49	10/158 NS*	albumin blunted the severity of OHSS
Mukherjee et al. (1995)	case report (2)	–	E_2 >4500 pg/ml and >20 oocytes	2 severe OHSS (1 early and 1 late)	–	–
Orvieto et al. (1995)	case report (1)	–	E_2 2293 pg/ml and 46 oocytes	early severe OHSS	–	–
Ben-Rafael et al. (1995b)	case report (1)	–	E_2 >2293 pg/ml, >35 oocytes	early severe OHSS	–	–
Halme et al. (1995)	case report (1)	–	1 oocyte donor, E_2 2400 pg/ml, 15 oocytes	early severe OHSS	–	–
Shalev et al. (1995b)	prospective randomized (40)	no treatment	E_2 >2500 pg/ml and >20 follicles	0/22	4/18	no transfer in 5.5% of controls and 13.6% of study group
Shaker et al. (1996)	prospective randomized controlled (26)	cryopreservation	E_2 >3540 pg/ml or >2745 pg/ml and >15 oocytes	4/13 moderate OHSS, no severe	3/13 moderate OHSS, not severe NS	pregnancy significantly higher in controls
Isik et al (1996)	prospective randomized controlled (55)	no treatment	E_2 >3000 pg/ml	0/27	1/28 severe and 4/28 moderate, $p < 0.05$	–

Reference	Study design (n)	Comparison	Criteria	Result	Result	Comments
Lewit et al. (1996)	retrospective cases review (5)	–	previous OHSS, E$_2$ >3600 pg/ml and large number of follicles	2/5 early severe, 2/5 moderate	–	the most severe received 75 g and had no transfer
Orvieto and Ben-Rafael (1996)	retrospective review (30)	–	–	2/30 early severe OHSS	–	–
Chen et al. (1997)	prospective (72)	historical controls	E$_2$ >3600 pg/ml and >20 oocytes	4/30; 0/16 not pregnant, 4/14 pregnant	14/42; $p = 0.047$, 5/23 not pregnant, 9/19 pregnant	prevention is effective in non-pregnancies and singleton pregnancies
Egbase et al. (1997)	uncontrolled (31)	–	E$_2$ >3269 pg/ml and >12 follicles >12 mm per ovary	9.7% severe	–	early follicular aspiration before hCG was also performed ($n = 16$)
Ndukwe et al. (1997)	retrospective (60)	–	E$_2$ >4086 pg/ml and >20 follicles	5/60 severe (1 early, 4 late); 8/60 moderate	–	no preventive effect, especially in pregnant patients
Koike et al. (1999)	prospective randomized controlled (98)	no treatment	>20 oocytes	11/43 early, 2/43 late severe OHSS	15/55 early, 6/55 late severe OHSS	–
Panay et al. (1999)	prospective randomized (86)	no treatment	E$_2$ >3541 pg/ml or >20 follicles	2/37 mild, 2/37 moderate	4/49 mild	Pregnancy rate per cycle significantly higher in controls
Costabile et al. (2000)	prospective randomized controlled (96)	200 mg/day progesterone from 1 day post-retrieval	E$_2$ >2452 pg/ml and >20 follicles	4/42 moderate (no severe)	0/54 moderate (no severe)	high progesterone dose is effective in preventing OHSS and better for pregnancy rate
Gokmen et al. (2001)	prospective randomized placebo (168)	placebo	E$_2$ >3000 pg/ml or >20 follicles	0/85 severe and 4/85 moderate	4/83 severe and 12/83 moderate $p < 0.05$	–

* E$_2$ = 17β-estradiol
** NS = not significant

Hydroxyethyl Starch Solution Administration

Rizk (2002) reviewed the role of synthetic macromolecules used to prevent OHSS and avoid the potential risks from using human products such as albumin. Hydroxyethyl starch (HES) is a synthetic colloid, glycogen-like polysacharride which is derived from amylopectin. It has been used as an effective volume expander and is available in several molecular weights with different chemical properties. Graf et al. (1997) used 1000 ml of 6% HES at the time of oocyte retrieval and an additional 500 ml 48 h later in 100 patients considered at high risk of OHSS (estradiol > 11 000 pm/l and 20 follicles or more). They compared the outcome to an historical control group of 82 patients without any prophylactic measures. Seven cases of severe OHSS and 32 cases of moderate OHSS occurred in the control group compared with two cases of severe and 10 cases of moderate OHSS in the HES group ($p < 0.05$ and $p < 0.001$, respectively).

Konig et al. (1998) in a prospective, randomized trial evaluated HES and placebo in patients with estradiol levels > 1500 pg/ml and with 10 follicles on the day of hCG. The dose of HES was 1000 ml after the oocyte retrieval. In the HES group, there was one case of moderate OHSS and no severe cases compared with six cases of moderate OHSS and one case of severe OHSS in the control group.

Gokman et al. (2001) performed a prospective randomized placebo-controlled trial on 253 patients considered at risk of OHSS. They compared the efficacy of 500 ml of 6% HES ($n = 85$) and 50 ml 20% human albumin ($n = 85$) or placebo ($n = 83$). In high-risk patients whose estradiol was > 3000 pg/ml, or ultrasound showed more than 20 follicles, all the treatments were administered

Table VII.17 Intravenous albumin for the prevention of OHSS included in the Cochrane database review
*Reproduced with permission from Aboulghar and Monsour (2003). Hum Reprod Update **9**:275–89*

Study	Type	No. patients Total	Albumin (IV)	Control	Albumin dose	E_2 level on day of hCG (pg/ml)	No. OHSS (albumin)	No. OHSS (control)
Shoham et al. (1994)	prospective randomized	31	16	15	50 g	1906	0	4
Shalev et al. (1995c)	prospective randomized	40	22	18	20 g	>2500	0	4
Isik et al. (1996)	prospective randomized	55	27	28	10 mg	≥3000	0	4
Ben Chetrit et al. (2001)	prospective randomized	87	46	41	50 g	2724	4	1
Ng et al. (1995)	cohort controlled	207	49	158	50 g	2724	2	10
Chen et al. (1997)	prospective historical control	72	30	42	according to BMI*	≥3600	4	14

Odds ratio $= 0.42$; 95% CI 0.21–0.88 ($p = 0.012$)
* BMI = body mass index

during oocyte retrieval. No severe OHSS cases were observed in the albumin and HES groups while four patients developed severe OHSS in the placebo group. Moderate OHSS was observed in four patients in the albumin group, five patients in the HES group and 12 patients in the placebo group ($p < 0.05$). Gokman (2001) recommended HES for the prevention of OHSS, since it is as efficient as but safer and cheaper than albumin.

These three studies provide consistent results suggesting a beneficial effect of HES in decreasing OHSS. Although the patient cohort was too small to draw definitive conclusions, these studies suggest that HES rather than albumin should be further investigated (Delvigne and Rozenberg, 2002b).

Glucocorticoid Administration

Rizk (1993) has found no protective effect of intravenous glucocorticoid. The pathophysiology suggests the involvement of an inflammatory mechanism during the development of the fluid leakage associated with the syndrome. Therefore, investigators hypothesized that glucocorticoids could possibly prevent OHSS in patients at high risk. Tan et al. (1992) in a prospective randomized trial investigated the usefulness of glucocorticoids in the reduction of the rate of OHSS. Thirty-one patients, who were stimulated with hMG and who were desensitized with GnRH agonists and developed more than 20 follicles > 12 mm and/or had serum estradiol of $> 10\,000$ pmol/l on the day of hCG administration, were recruited. The patients were randomized into two groups. Group A ($n = 17$) were administered intravenous hydrocortisone immediately after transvaginal ultrasound oocyte recovery. Prednisolone 10 mg three times daily was given for five days, starting on the day of oocyte recovery, followed by prednisolone 10 mg twice daily for three days and 10 mg once daily for two days. Group B ($n = 14$) did not have any intravenous or oral glucocorticoid treatment. Luteal phase support was given in the form of intramuscular Gestone 100 mg/day. Seven of the 17 patients (41.2%) who received glucocorticoids developed OHSS compared with six of the 14 patients (42.9%) who did not. The authors concluded that the administration of glucocorticoids to high-risk patients did not diminish the risk of developing OHSS.

In contrast, Lainas (2002) reported that methylprednisolone 16 mg/day, starting on the 6th day of controlled ovarian hyperstimulation and tapered to day 13 after embryo transfer, was effective in reducing OHSS significantly to 10%, compared with 43.9% in the control group.

Intramuscular Progesterone vs. Intravenous Albumin

Costabile et al. (2000) compared the use of intramuscular progesterone versus intravenous albumin for the prevention of OHSS. Progesterone was administered at the time of oocyte retrieval and continued throughout the luteal phase. The OHSS rates in this interesting study do not permit a conclusion to be drawn. The authors suggested that progesterone appears likely to be safer than albumin, with a possible benefit to pregnancy rates.

FOLLICULAR ASPIRATION

Does follicular aspiration protect against OHSS? The first case of severe OHSS in an IVF program was reported by Friedman et al. (1984). The incidence of moderate and severe OHSS in the major IVF series varied from 0.6% to 14%. Rabinowitz et al. (1987) postulated that multiple follicular aspirations, which empty most of the follicles of follicular fluid granulosa cells, may have a protective effect against OHSS. Four of the 81 patients in the series who developed OHSS during a cycle where egg retrieval was cancelled did not develop the syndrome in cycles when multiple follicular punctures and aspiration were performed.

Follicular Aspiration at the Time of Oocyte Retrieval

In a retrospective study, the incidence of OHSS was compared in IVF to intrauterine insemination (IUI) patients who had undergone similar controlled ovarian hyperstimulation (Aboulghar et al., 1991). At that point, the incidence of OHSS was thought to be lower in those who had undergone IVF. This was attributed to the effect of follicular aspiration. However, when the results were analyzed according to the cause of infertility in 182 patients who underwent follicular aspiration compared with 137 patients who did not, it became apparent that OHSS was significantly higher in patients with PCOS regardless of whether they had undergone IVF or IUI procedures (Aboulghar et al., 1992). There was no difference in OHSS whether follicular aspiration occurred or not in each group independently.

Follicular Aspiration Prior to hCG

In a prospective randomized study, Egbase et al. (1997) performed unilateral follicular aspiration prior to administration of hCG for the prevention of severe OHSS. The authors recruited 31 patients who were considered to be at risk of OHSS. This was defined by a serum estradiol of $>12\,000\,pmol/l$ and with a total of >12 follicles, each larger than 12 mm in diameter per ovary. These patients were randomized into two groups: unilateral ovarian follicular aspiration was performed in Group I patients ($n = 16$) 6–8 h prior to hCG administration under conscious sedation using midazolam 5 mg IV and fentanyl 100 μg IV. In 15 patients (Group II), no aspiration was performed prior to hCG. All patients in both groups had transvaginal ultrasound-guided oocyte recovery 35–36 h after the administration of 10 000 IU of hCG, pro-phylactic human albumin was administered to patients in all groups in the form of 100 ml of 20% human albumin during oocyte recovery, and this was repeated every 12 h for 48 h. The mean number of oocytes retrieved from patients in Group I was significantly lower than from Group II (14.9 vs. 22.6, $p < 0.001$). The incidence of OHSS was 25% in Group I and 33.3% in Group II. Two patients in Group I and one patient in Group II developed severe OHSS. The clinical pregnancy rate was 37.5% in Group I and 46.6% in Group II.

They concluded that unilateral follicular aspiration 6–8 h prior to hCG fails to protect against the incidence of severe OHSS in women at risk. They postulated that the hCG induced mediators of OHSS in the contralateral ovary, and they may have reached too high a level of activity to be modified by intervention in the ipsilateral ovary. They also noted that prophylactic human albumin administration does not protect against the development of severe OHSS.

Follicular Aspiration of One Ovary 12 h after hCG

Tomazevic and Meden-Vrtovec (1996) investigated whether follicular aspiration 12 h after hCG administration would prevent OHSS. In the first group, 106 patients at high risk of developing OHSS underwent follicular aspiration of one ovary, 12 h after hCG administration. In the control group, 92 patients, also at high risk of developing OHSS, underwent normally timed follicular aspiration of both ovaries. No cases of severe OHSS occurred in the aspiration group compared to 16 cases in the control group ($p < 0.0005$).

LUTEAL PHASE SUPPORT

Luteal Phase Support with Progesterone

GnRH agonist long protocols became the standard of care for IVF protocols in the 1980s. It became apparent that the prolonged pituitary recovery from downregulation during the luteal phase resulted in luteal phase deficiency (Smitz et al., 1992; Donderwinkel et al., 1993; Stoufer, 1990). Corpus luteum could be rescued by the administration of hCG which became the standard of care for luteal support during the late 1980s (Fauser and Macklon, 2004). A meta-analysis by Soliman et al. (1994) combining results from 18 randomized trials demonstrated an increase in IVF pregnancy rates with supplementation. While the outcome was better than compared with progesterone, OHSS developed in 5% of patients receiving hCG supplementation. Because of the association between hCG and OHSS, luteal phase progesterone supplementation replaced hCG support in patients at high risk of developing OHSS (Rizk and Smitz, 1992), and over the years, for all patients undergoing IVF (Penzias, 2002). A recent meta-analysis (Pritts and Atwood, 2002) concluded that intramuscular hCG or intramuscular progesterone are equally efficacious in improving IVF outcome compared with no treatment. Furthermore, intramuscular progesterone was slightly more effective than oral or vaginal administration, and implantation rates were slightly improved with the addition of oral estrogens to progesterone (Pritts and Atwood, 2002; Fauser and Macklon, 2004).

Luteal Phase Progesterone and Estradiol vs. hCG

In a prospective, randomized trial including 945 IVF cycles, the efficiency of high-dose progesterone and estradiol administration during the luteal phase was evaluated for the prevention of OHSS (Schwarzler et al., 2003). After ovulation induction, patients were allocated by a series of computer-generated random numbers to receive either 5000 IU of hCG, four and eight days after embryo transfer ($n = 534$), or 500 mg hydroxyprogesterone caproate and 10 mg estradiol valerate on days 2, 6, 10 and 14 after embryo transfer ($n = 411$) by intramuscular injection. A total of 163 women (30.5%) in the hCG group and 22 women (5.4%) in the estradiol–progesterone group developed signs of OHSS ($p < 0.0001$). The authors suggested that steroidal ovarian suppression during the luteal phase is a promising tool to reduce the incidence and severity of OHSS in patients at high risk of developing this syndrome, without compromising the pregnancy rate.

CRYOPRESERVATION OF EMBRYOS AND SUBSEQUENT REPLACEMENT

The availability of cryopreservation has made it possible not to lose the cycle and to achieve pregnancy by replacement of the frozen-thawed embryos at a later cycle (Table VII.18). In one of the first reports, Amso et al. (1990) presented four cases in which cryopreservation and later replacements resulted in pregnancies and avoided hyperstimulation. Salat-Baroux et al. (1990) electively deferred fresh embryo transfer in 33 high-risk patients monitored for the development of OHSS. Embryo transfer was performed in 87% of the cycles and there was only one severe case of OHSS.

Wada et al. (1991; 1992a, b; 1993a, b) performed a series of studies to address the relevance of cryopreservation as a secondary prevention method. In the first study, the authors collected all IVF cycles with ($n = 203$) and without ($n = 38$) embryo transfer. The groups were classified according to their estradiol level and whether or not pregnancy occurred. No cases of OHSS occurred in the non-embryo transfer group when estradiol levels were below 3500 pg/ml. However, in the cycles when embryo transfer occurred, OHSS was observed in 12% of pregnant patients and 2.3% of non-pregnant patients with estradiol levels <3500 pg/ml. When estradiol levels were >3500 pg/ml, OHSS occurred in 60% (8%, severe) in the non-transfer group but was 11% and 57% (28%, severe) in non-pregnant and pregnant women with embryo transfer. Wada et al. (1992a) suggested that withholding transfer does not reduce the incidence of OHSS in women with estradiol levels >3500 pg/ml. The same investigators (Wada et al., 1992a) reported a series of 78 cases of elective cryopreservation for estradiol levels >3500 pg/ml on the day of hCG. OHSS occurred in 27%, of which severe OHSS was detected in 8%. Frozen-thawed embryo replacement was performed subsequently with 71.8% of embryos surviving, a pregnancy rate of 26% and an implantation rate of 11.7%. This pregnancy rate was comparable to the pregnancy rate of IVF patients in Manchester during that period of time.

In the third study, the authors compared two periods (Wada et al., 1993a). During the first period no cryopreservation of embryos was done and, furthermore, hCG was given for luteal phase supplementation (Wada et al., 1993a). During the second period cryopreservation was employed. OHSS occurred in 9.5% in the first period and 8.8% in the second period. More importantly, OHSS in its severe form occurred in 6% when cryopreservation was performed compared with 60% when pregnancy occurred in women with estradiol levels > 3500 pg/ml. Wada et al. (1993a) concluded that cryopreservation of all embryos from women with high estradiol levels would reduce the severity of OHSS but not its incidence.

Pattinson et al. (1994) in a retrospective study of 69 patients at risk of OHSS cryopreserved all embryos and delayed embryo transfer, resulting in a low incidence of severe OHSS (1.8%). The subsequently replaced embryos resulted in a 25% pregnancy rate.

Queenan et al. (1997) reported that cryopreservation of all prezygotes in patients at risk of severe hyperstimulation did not eliminate the syndrome, but the chances of pregnancy were excellent with subsequent frozen-thawed transfers. In their series of 15 patients, two patients (13%) developed severe OHSS and two others developed moderate OHSS. Subsequent transfer of the cryopreserved embryos resulted in a 58% pregnancy rate.

Ferraretti et al. (1999) performed a prospective randomized study on 125 patients at risk of OHSS. All the patients had serum estradiol ≥1500 pg/ml on the day of hCG, and 15 or more oocytes were retrieved. One group of patients had all their embryos cryopreserved at pronucleate stage ($n = 58$) and the control group had fresh embryo transfers ($n = 67$). No cases of OHSS occurred in the group with cryopreservation, while four patients developed the syndrome in the group that had fresh embryo transfers. The implantation rate was slightly but not significantly lower in the cryopreserved group. Ferraretti et al. (1999) suggested that elective cryopreservation of all zygotes might prevent the risk of OHSS.

Is Continuation of GnRH Agonist Necessary to Prevent OHSS?

Studies addressing the issue of continuation of GnRH agonist have given conflicting results. Wada et al. (1992b) studied 28 women undergoing IVF using hMG and buserelin for stimulation. Group I consisted of 17 women given hCG (10 000 IU) to trigger ovulation, and the resulting embryos were cryopreserved because of the high risk of OHSS since their serum estradiol was > 3500 pg/ml. Six women continued buserelin therapy in the luteal phase and 11 did not. In the second group, consisting of 11 patients, the hMG injections were discontinued because of their exaggerated ovarian response and the hCG was cancelled. Six of these 11 women continued the buserelin until the onset of menses and five did not. In both groups, the ovarian response to the induction of ovulation, as judged by the number of follicles and the serum estradiol concentration, was similar for those who did or did not continue buserelin therapy. There was no difference in the rate of ovarian quiescence, as judged by the fall in the serum estradiol concentration following the stimulation, between those women who did or did not continue the buserelin

Table VII.18 Cryopreservation as a prevention of OHSS
Reproduced with permission from Delvigne and Rozenberg (2002). Hum Reprod Update **8**:559–77

Study	Design	Control group (n)	Risk factors (n)	Pregnancy with thawed embryos	OHSS with cryo-preservation (vs. control)	Comments
Amso et al. (1990)	observational	–	25 to 45 follicles, abdominal	100%/trsf*	10% moderate	–
Salat-Baroux et al. (1990)	observational	–	E_2 4722 ± 1190 pg/ml the day	27%/trsf	3% severe	–
Wada et al. (1991)	retrospective observational	pregnant (49) and non-pregnant (154)	NA (38)	–	18% all grades, only if $E_2 > 3500$ pg/ml (18 and 4%)	0% if $E_2 < 3500$ pg/ml; 1 with cryopreservation
Wada et al. (1992b)	retrospective observational	–	$E_2 > 3500$ pg/ml (78)	26%/trsf	27% all grades (8% severe)	–
Wada et al. (1993a)	retrospective observational	historical group without prevention (105)	$E_2 > 3500$ pg/ml (136)	21%/trsf	8.8%, only 6% severe, (9.5%, 60% severe)	7.8% survival embryos
Pattinson et al. (1994)	retrospective	general IVF without risk	$E_2 \geq 4086$ pg/ml and >50 follicles (69)	25.2%/trsf 40%/patient	1.4% (1.8% severe)	84% survival embryos; 14% canceling
Tiitinen et al. (1995)	prospective	general IVF without risk	$E_2 > 2724$ pg/ml and/or >20 oocytes (33)	32.6%/trsf 65.2%/patient	4.3% moderate (vs. 0.5%)	22.7% implantation rate
Awonuga et al. (1996)	retrospective controlled	$E_2 > 2724$ pg/ml and/or >15 oocytes (52)	$E_2 > 2724$ pg/ml and/or >15 oocytes (65)	17%/trsf	3% severe; 3% moderate; (3.8% severe and moderate) NS**	significantly higher PR in controls (35%; $p < 0.05$)
Queenan et al. (1997)	prospective, noncontrolled	–	$E_2 > 4500$ pg/ml and >15 oocytes (15)	58%/trsf, 67% delivery/patient	13% severe, 13% moderate	–
Benavida et al. (1997)	retrospective controlled	coasting group (22)	$E_2 > 3000$ pg/ml (26)	25.6%/trsf	7.6% (4.5%) NS	–
Ferraretti et al. (1999)	prospective randomized	$E_2 > 1500$ pg/ml and >15 oocytes (67)	$E_2 > 1500$ pg/ml and >15 oocytes (58)	35.4%/trsf, 48.3% per patient	0% (versus 6%)	–

* Trsf = embryo transfer
** NS = non significant

therapy in either group. The serum LH concentrations remained low in all women in both groups. The authors concluded that the omission of buserelin after the discontinuation of hMG in women at risk of developing OHSS does not affect subsequent ovarian quiescence.

Endo et al. (2002) designed an open-controlled clinical trial at three infertility centers in Sapporo, Japan to determine the impact of continuation of GnRH agonist for one week after hCG injection on the prevention of OHSS following cryopreservation of all pronuclear embryos. A total of 138 patients at risk of OHSS during IVF were assigned either to Group I with elective cryopreservation of all pronuclear embryos ($n=68$), or to Group II with continuation of GnRH agonist administration for one week after hCG injection following elective cryopreservation ($n=70$). The embryos were transferred in subsequent hormone replacement cycles. A total of 10% of patients developed severe OHSS, requiring hospitalization because of the remarkable increase of ascites in the upper abdomen and hemoconcentration in the elective-cryopreservation-alone group. At the same time, no patients developed severe OHSS in the GnRH agonist continuation group. Endo et al. (2002) concluded that GnRH agonist continued one week after hCG injection prevented severe early OHSS following elective cryopreservation of all embryos. In addition, they concluded that this treatment is safe and cost-beneficial, and also recommended that this treatment should be performed in patients at risk of developing OHSS.

In a Cochrane review, D'Angelo and Amso (2002b) identified studies, two of which met the inclusion criteria. In one of the two studies (Shaker et al., 1996), cryopreservation was compared with intravenous albumin, and in the other study, cryopreservation of all embryos was compared with fresh embryo transfer and intravenous albumin was administered to all the patients which may have influenced the severity of OHSS. When elective cryopreservation was compared with fresh embryo transfer, no difference was found between the two groups. This Cochrane review suggests that there is insufficient evidence at present to support routine cryopreservation, and also insufficient evidence to be able to determine the relative merits of intravenous albumin and cryopreservation.

Cryopreservation: Conclusion

Cryopreservation would significantly decrease late-onset OHSS and the overall incidence of severe cases. However, OHSS will not be completely prevented if cryopreservation is the only tool applied in patients at high risk.

SELECTIVE OOCYTE RETRIEVAL IN SPONTANEOUS CONCEPTION CYCLES

Selective oocyte retrieval was used for prevention of OHSS and multiple pregnancies in spontaneous conception, by puncturing most of the ovarian follicles 35 h after hCG administration, as in IVF programs. The remaining intact follicles may still result in singleton or twin pregnancy (Belaish-Allart et al., 1988).

COMBINED APPROACH FOR THE PREVENTION OF SEVERE OHSS

Clinicians faced with an over-responsive patient should be prepared to employ more than one method at the same time for prevention. It would be advisable to decrease the dose of gonadotrophin followed by coasting. A lower dose of hCG to trigger ovulation and progesterone for luteal phase support should be employed in sequence to avert the serious consequences of severe cases. Isik and Vicdan (2001) compared the results of a combined approach in 87 patients considered at high risk to those in 274 low-risk patients. Their combined approach consisted of step-down administration of gonadotrophins, a lower dose of hCG, intravenous albumin at the time of oocyte retrieval and progesterone usage for luteal phase support. There was only one moderate and no severe cases of OHSS in the high-risk group, while five moderate and one severe case of OHSS developed in the control group of low-risk patients. The authors concluded that the combined approach is an effective approach for the prevention of OHSS in high-risk patients. I cannot overemphasize this message, as the final objective is complete prevention of severe cases, and not testing the efficiency of one or another method of prevention.

VEGF RECEPTOR BLOCKADE

Rizk and Nawar (2004) critically evaluated the place of VEGF receptor blockade in the management and prevention of OHSS. Since VEGF is a mediator of the OHSS cascade, receptor blockade could prove to be a wise step in the prevention of this syndrome. In an ASRM prize-winning presentation, Gomez et al. (2001) investigated the release and production of VEGF by human granulosa cells and luteal cells in experimental animals who developed OHSS. In a second series of experiments, the authors investigated whether VEGF receptor 2 blockade would prevent OHSS. They concluded that the ovary is the major source of VEGF in hyperstimulated animals. VEGF-121 and 164 isoforms were differentially expressed. The increased vascular permeability through the VEGF receptor 2 and its specific inhibition prevents increased vascular permeability.

REFERENCES

Abdalla HI, Ahmoye NM, Brinsden P et al. (1987). The effect of the dose of human chorionic gonadotrophin and the type of gonadotrophin stimulation on oocyte recovery rates in an in-vitro fertilization program. *Fertil Steril* **48**:958–63.

Abdel Gadir A, Khatim MS, Mowafi RS et al. (1990a). Hormonal changes in patients with polycystic ovarian disease after ovarian electrocautery or pituitary desensitization. *Clin Endocrinol* **32**:749–54.

Abdel Gadir A, Mowafi RS, Alnaser HM et al. (1990b). Ovarian electrocautery, human menopausal gonadotropins and pure follicle stimulating gormone therapy in the treatment of patients with polycystic ovary disease. *Clin Endocrinol (Oxford)* **33**:585–92.

Abdul-Jalil AK, Child TJ, Phillips S et al. (2001). Ongoing twin pregnancy after ICSI of PESA-retrieved spermatozoa into in-vitro matured oocytes: case report. *Hum Reprod* **16**:1424–6.

Aboulghar M & Al-Inany H (2005). Triggering ovulation for IVF: Letter to the Editor. *Reprod Biomed Online* **10**:142.

Aboulghar MA & Mansour RT (2003). Ovarian hyperstimulation syndrome: classification and critical analysis of preventive measures. *Hum Reprod Update* **9**:275–89.

Aboulghar MA, Mansour RT, Serour GI et al. (1991). The impact of follicular aspiration and luteal phase support on the incidence of ovarian hyperstimulation. *Hum Reprod* **6**(Suppl):174–5.

Aboulghar MA, Mansour RT, Serour GI et al. (1992). Follicular aspiration does not protect against the development of ovarian hyperstimulation syndrome. *J Assist Reprod Genet* **9**:238–43.

Aboulghar MA, Mansour RT, Serour GI et al. (1996a). Ovarian hyperstimulation syndrome: modern concepts in pathophysiology and management. *Middle East Fertil Soc J* **1**:3–16.

Aboulghar MA, Mansour RT, Serour GI et al. (1996b). Recombinant follicle-stimulating hormone in the treatment of patients with history of severe ovarian hyperstimulation syndrome. *Fertil Steril* **66**:757–60.

Aboulghar MA, Mansour RT, Serour GI et al. (1997). Oocyte quality in patients with severe ovarian hyperstimulation syndrome. *Fertil Steril* **68**:17–21.

Aboulghar MA, Mansour RT, Serour GI et al. (2000). Reduction of human menopausal gonadotrophin dose before coasting prevents severe ovarian hyperstimulation syndrome with minimal cycle cancellation. *J Assist Reprod Genet* **17**:298–301.

Aboulghar M, Evers JH, and Al-Inany H (2002). Intravenous albumin for preventing severe ovarian hyperstimulation syndrome. *Hum Reprod* **17**:3027–32; and *Cochrane Database Syst Rev* **2**:CD001302.

Adamson G, Lancaster P, De Mouzon J et al. (2005). ICMART world collaborative report on in vitro fertilization 2000. *Fertil Steril* **84**(suppl 1):S107–259.

Adashi EY, Rock JA, Guzick D et al. (1981). Fertility following bilateral ovarian wedge resection: a critical analysis of 90 consecutive cases of the polycystic ovary syndrome. *Fertil Steril* **36**:320–5.

Albano C, Felberbaum RE, Smitz J et al. (2000). Ovarian stimulation with hMG: results of a prospective randomized phase III European study comparing the luteinizing hormone-releasing hormone (LHRH)-antagonist, cetrorelix and the LHRH-agonist buserelin. *Hum Reprod* **15**:526–31.

Al-Inany H & Aboulghar M (2002). GnRH antagonist in assisted reproduction: a Cochrane review. *Hum Reprod* **17**:874–85.

Almeida OD Jr & Rizk B (1998). Microlaparoscopic ovarian drilling under local anesthesia. *Middle East Fertil Soc J* **3**:189–91.

Al-Shawaf T, Zosmer A, Hussain S et al. (2001). Prevention of severe ovarian hyperstimulation syndrome in IVF with or without ICSI and embryo transfer: a modified 'coasting' strategy based on ultrasound for identification of high-risk patients. *Hum Reprod* **16**:24–30.

Al-Shawaf T, Zosmer A, Tozer A et al. (2002). Value of measuring serum FSH in addition to serum estradiol in a coasting programme to prevent severe OHSS. *Hum Reprod* **17**:1217–21.

Amso NN, Ahuga KK, Morris N et al. (1990). The management of predicted OHS involving gonadotrophin-releasing analogue with elective cryopreservation of all pre-embryos. *Fertil Steril* **53**:1087–90.

Armar NA & Lachelin GC (1993). Laparoscopic ovarian diathermy: an effective treatment for antiestrogen resistant anovulatory infertility in women with polycystic ovary syndrome. *Br J Obstet Gynaecol* **100**:161–4.

Asch RH, Ivery G, Goldsman M et al. (1993). The use of intravenous albumin in patients at high risk for severe ovarian hyperstimulation syndrome. *Hum Reprod* **8**:1015–20.

Awonuga AO, Pittrof RF, Zaidi J et al. (1996). Elective cryopreservation of all embryos in women at risk of developing ovarian hyperstimulation syndrome may not prevent the condition but reduces the live birth rate. *J Assist Reprod Genet* **13**:401–6.

Balasch J, Fabregues F, Tur R et al. (1995). Further characterizaion of the luteal phase inadequacy after gonadotrophin-releasing hormone agonist-induced ovulation in gonadotrophin-stimulated cycles. *Hum Reprod* **10**:1377–81.

Balasch J, Tur R, Creus M, Buxaderas R et al. (1994). Triggering of ovulation by a gonadotrophin releasing hormone agonistin gonadotrophin-stimulated cycles for prevention of ovarian hyperstimulation syndrome and multiple pregnancy. *Gynecol Endocrinol* **8**:7–9.

Balen AH (1999). Ovarian hyperstimulation syndrome. Letter to the Editor. *Hum Reprod* **14**:1138.

Balen AH & Jacobs HS (1991). Gonadotropin surge attenuating factor: a missing link in the control of LH secretion? *Clin Endocrinol (Oxford)* **35**:399–402.

Balen AH & Jacobs HS (1994). Prospective study comparing unilateral and bilateral laparoscopic ovarian diathermy in women with polycystic ovary syndrome. *Fertil Steril* **62**:921–5.

Balen AH, Braat DD, West C et al. (1994). Cumulative conception and live birth rates after the treatment of anovulatory infertility: safety and efficacy ovulation induction in 200 patients. *Hum Reprod* **9**:1563–70.

Barnes F, Crombie A, Gardner D et al. (1995). Blastocyst development and birth after in vitro maturation of human primary oocytes, intracytoplasmic sperm injection and assisted hatching. *Hum Reprod* **10**:3243–7.

Barnes FL, Kausche A, Tiglias J et al. (1996). Production of embryos from in vitro-matured primary human oocytes. *Fertil Steril* **65**:1151–6.

Barroso G, Barrionuevo M, Rao P et al. (1999). Vascular endothelial growth factor, nitric oxide, and leptin follicular fluid levels correlate negatively with embryo quality in IVF patients. *Fertil Steril* **72**:1024–6.

Bayram N, van Wely M & van der Veen F (2001). *Recombinant FSH versus urinary gonadotrophins or recombinant FSH for ovulation induction in subfertility associated with polycystic ovary syndrome* (Review). Cochrane Database, Issue 1. The Cochrane Collaboration, Chichester: John Wiley & Sons, Ltd.

Belaisch-Allart J, Balaisch J, Hazout A et al. (1988). Selective oocyte retrieval: a new approach to ovarian hyperstimulation. *Fertil Steril* **50**:654–6.

Belver J, Munoz EA, Ballesteros A et al. (2003). Intravenous albumin does not prevent moderate-severe ovarian hyperstimulation syndrome in high-risk IVF patients: a randomized controlled study. *Hum Reprod* **18**:2283–8.

Benadiva CA, Davis O, Kligman I et al. (1997). Withholding gonadotropin administration is an effective alternative for the prevention of ovarian hyperstimulation syndrome. *Fertil Steril* **67**:724–7.

Ben-Chetrit A, Eldar-Geva T & Gal M (2001). The questionable use of albumin for the prevention of ovarian hyperstimulation syndrome in an IVF programme: a randomized placebo-controlled trial. *Hum Reprod* **16**:1880–4.

Ben-Nun I, Shulman A, Ghetler Y et al. (1993). The significance of 17 beta estradiol levels in highly responding women during ovulation induction in IVF treatment: its impact and prognostic value with respect to oocyte maturation and treatment outcome. *J Assist Reprod Genet* **10**:213–15.

Ben-Rafael Z, Orvieto R, Dekel A et al. (1995). Intravenous albumin and the prevention of severe ovarian hyperstimulation syndrome [comment]. *Hum Reprod* **10**:2750–2.

Blankstein J, Shalev J, Saadon T et al. (1987). Ovarian hyperstimulation syndrome prediction by number and size of preovulatory follicles. *Fertil Steril* **47**:597–602.

Bracero MW, Jurema MN, Posada JG et al. (2001). Triggering ovulation with leuprorelide acetate (LA) instead of human chorionic gonadotrophin (hCG) after the use of ganirelix for in-vitro fertilization-embryo transfer (IVF-ET) does not compromise cycle outcome and may prevent ovarian hyperstimulation syndrome. *Fertil Steril* **S-93**, Abstract O-245. American Society for Reproductive Medicine 57th Annual Meeting, Orlando, FL, General Program Prize, Abstracts of the scientific oral and poster sessions program supplement.

Buvat J, Buvat-Herbaut M, Marcolin G et al. (1989). Purified follicle stimulating hormone in polycystic ovary syndrome: slow administration is safer and more effective. *Fertil Steril* **51**:553–9.

Cha K, Koo JJ, Choi DH et al. (1991). Pregnancy after in vitro fertilitzation of human follicular oocytes collected from non stimulated cycles, their culture in vitro and their transfer in a donor oocyte program. *Fertil Steril* **55**:103–20.

Cha KY & Chian RC (1998). Maturation in vitro of immature human oocytes for clinical use. *Hum Reprod Update* **4**:103–20.

Cha KY, Han SY, Chung HM et al. (2000). Pregnancies and deliveries after in vitro maturation culture followed by in vitro fertilization and embryo transfer without stimulation in women with polycystic ovary syndrome. *Fertil Steril* **73**:978–83.

Chang P, Kenley S, Burns T et al. (2001). Recombinant human chorionic gonadotrophin (rhCG) in assisted reproductive technology: results of a clinical trial comparing two doses of rhCG (Ovidrel) to urinary hCG (Profasi) for induction of final follicular maturation in in vitro fertilization embryo transfer. *Fertil Steril* **76**:67–74.

Chang RJ (2004). Polycystic ovary syndrome and hyperandrogenic states. In (Strauss, Barbieri, Eds), *Yen and Jaffe's Reproductive Endocrinology: Pathophysiology and Clinical Management*, 5th edition. Philadelphia: Elsevier & Saunders, Chapter 19, p. 600.

Chen CD, Wu MY, Yang JH et al. (1997). Intravenous albumin does not prevent the development of severe ovarian hypertimulation syndrome. *Fertil Steril* **68**:287–91.

Chian RC & Tan SL (2002). Maturational and developmental competence of cululus-free immature human oocytes derived from stimulated and intracytoplasmic sperm infection cycles. *Reprod Biomed Online* **5**:125–32.

Chian RC, Buckett WM, Too LL et al. (1999a). Pregnancies resulting from in vitro matured oocytes retrieved from patients with polycystic ovary syndrome after priming with human chorionic gonadotropin. *Fertil Steril* **72**:639–42.

Chian RC, Gulekli B, Buckett WM et al. (1999b). Priming with human chorionic gonadotropin before retrieval of immature oocytes in women with infertility due to the polycystic ovary syndrome. *New Eng J Med* **341**:1624–6.

Chian RC, Buckett WM, Tulandi T et al. (2000). Prospective randomized study of human chorionic gonadotrophin priming before immature oocyte retrieval from unstimulated women with polycystic ovarian syndrome. *Hum Reprod* **15**:165–70.

Chian RC, Gulekli B, Buckett WM et al. (2001). Pregnancy and delivery after cryopreservation of zygotes produced by in-vitro matured oocytes retrieved from a woman with polycystic ovarian syndrome. *Hum Reprod* **16**:1700–2.

Child TJ, Abdul-Jalil AK, Gulekli B et al. (2000). In vitro maturation and fertilization of oocytes from unstimulated normal ovaries, polycystic ovaries, and women with polycystic ovary syndrome. *Fertil Steril* **76**:936–42.

Child TJ, Phillips SJ, Abdul-Jalil AK et al. (2002). A comparison of in vitro maturation and in vitro fertilization for women with polycystic ovaries. *Obstet Gynecol* **100**:665–70.

Christin-Maitre S & Hughes JN (2003). A comparative randomized multicentric study comparing the step-up versus the step-down protocol in polycystic ovary syndrome. *Hum Reprod* **18**:1626–31.

Costabile L, Unfer V, Manna C et al. (2000). Use of intramuscular progesterone versus intravenous albumin for the prevention of ovarian hyperstimulation syndrome. *Gynecol Obstet Invest* **50**:182–5.

D'Angelo A & Amso N (2002a). 'Coasting' (withholding gonadotrophins) for preventing ovarian hyperstimulation syndrome. *Cochrane Database Syst Rev* **3**:CD002811.

D'Angelo A & Amso NN (2002b). Embryo freezing for preventing ovarian hyperstimulation syndrome: a Cochrane review. *Hum Reprod* **17**:2787–94.

Daniell JF & Miller W (1989). Polycystic ovaries treated by laparoscopic laser vaporization. *Fertil Steril* **51**:232–6.

Dechaud H, Anahory T, Aligier N et al. (2000). Coasting: a response to excessive ovarian stimulation. *Gynecol Obstet Fertil* **28**:115–19.

DeJonge D, Macklon NS & Mannaerts BMJ et al. (1998). High dose gonadotrophin-releasing hormone antagonist (ganirelix) may prevent ovarian hyperstimulation syndrome caused by ovarian stimulation for in-vitro fertilization. *Hum Reprod* **13**:573–5.

De Leo V, la Marca A, Ditto A et al. (1999). Effects of metformin on gonadotrophin-induced ovulation in women with polycystic ovary syndrome. *Fertil Steril* **72**:282–5.

Delvigne A (2004). Epidemiology and pathophysiology of ovarian hyperstimulation syndrome. In (Gerris J, Olivennes F, de Sutter P, Eds), *Assisted Reproductive Technologies: Quality and Safety*, New York: Parthenon Publishing, Chapter 12, pp. 149–62.

Delvigne A & Rozenberg S (2001). Preventive attitude of physicians to avoid OHSS in IVF patients. *Hum Reprod* **16**:2491–5.

Delvigne A & Rozenberg S (2002a). A qualitative systematic review of coasting, a procedure to avoid ovarian hyperstimulation syndrome in IVF patients. *Hum Reprod Update* **8**:291–6.

Delvigne A & Rozenberg S (2002b). Epidemiology and prevention of ovarian hyperstimulation syndrome (OHSS): a review. *Hum Reprod Update* **8**:559–77.

Delvigne A, Demoulin A, Smitz J et al. (1993). The ovarian hyperstimulation syndrome in in-vitro fertilization: a Belgian multicentric study. I. Clinical and biological features. *Hum Reprod* **8**:1353–60.

Delvigne A, Carlier C & Rozenberg S (2001). Is coasting effective for preventing ovarian hyperstimulation syndrome in patients receiving a gonadotropin-releasing hormone antagonist during an in vitro fertilization cycle? *Fertil Steril* **76**:844–6.

Delvigne A, Manigart Y, Kostyla et al. (2002). Oocyte quality after coasting for ovarian hyperstimulation syndrome prevention. *Hum Reprod.* **17** (Abstract book 1, p. 450):153.

Dhont M, Van der straiten F, De Sutter P (1998). Prevention of severe ovarian hyperstimulation by coasting. *Fertil Steril* **70**:847–50.

Donderwinkel PF, Schoot DC, Pache TD et al. (1993). Luteal function following ovulation induction in polycystic ovary syndrome patients using exogenous gonadotrophins in combination with a gonadotrophin-releasing hormone agonist. *Human Reprod* **8**:2027–32.

Driscoll GL, Tyler JP, Hangan JT et al. (2000). A prospective, randomized, controlled, double-blind, double-dummy comparison of recombinant and urinary HCG for inducing oocyte maturation and follicular luteinization in ovarian stimulation. *Hum Reprod* **15**:1305–10.

Edwards R (1965). Maturation in vitro of mouse, sheep, cow, pig, rhesus monkey and human ovarian oocytes. *Nature* **20**:349–51.

Edwards R, Bavister B & Steptoe P (1969). Early stages of fertilization in vitro of human oocytes matured in vitro. *Nature* **221**:632–5.

Egbase PE, Makhseed M, Al Sharhan M et al. (1997). Timed unilateral ovarian follicular aspiration prior to administration of human chorionic gonadotrophin for the prevention of severe ovarian hyperstimulation syndrome in in-vitro fertilization: a prospective randomized study. *Hum Reprod* **12**:2603–6.

Egbase P, Al-Awadi S, Al-sharhan M et al. (1998). Unilateral ovarian diathermy prior to successful in-vitro fertilisation: a strategy to prevent ovarian hyperstimulation syndrome? *J Obstet Gynaecol* **18**:171–3.

Egbase PE, Sharhan MA & Grudzinskas JG (1999). Early unilateral follicular aspiration compared with coasting for the prevention of severe ovarian hyperstimulation syndrome: a prospective randomized study. *Hum Reprod* **14**:1421–5.

Egbase PE, Al-Sharhan M & Grudzinskas JG (2002). Early coasting in patients with polycystic ovarian syndrome is consistent with good clinical outcome. *Hum Reprod* **17**:1212–16.

El-Sheikh MM, Hussein M, Fouad S et al. (2001). Limited ovarian stimulation (LOS) prevents the recurrence of severe forms of ovarian hyperstimulation syndrome in polycystic ovarian disease. *Eur J Obstet Gynecol Reprod Biol* **94**:245–9.

Emperaire JC (2005). Triggering ovulation with LH. *Reprod Biomed Online* **11**:270.

Emperaire JC & Ruffie A (1991). Triggering ovulation with endogenous luteinizing hormone may prevent ovarian hyperstimulation syndrome. *Hum Reprod* **6**:506–10.

Emperaire JC & Edwards RG (2004). Time to revolutionize the triggering of ovulation. *Reprod Biomed Online* **9**:480–3.

Endo T, Honnma H, Hayashi T et al. (2002). Continuation of GnRH agonist administration for 1 week, after hCG injection, prevents ovarian hyperstimulation syndrome following elective cryopreservation of all pronucleate embryos. *Hum Reprod* **17**:2548–51.

European Orgalutran Study Group (2000). Treatment with the gonadotrophin-releasing hormone antagonist ganirelix in women undergoing ovarian stimulation with recombinant follicle stimulation hormone is effective, safe and convenient: results of a controlled, randomized, multicenter trial. *Hum Reprod* **15**:1490–98.

European Recombinant LH Study Group (2001). Recombinant human leuteinizing hormone is as effective as, but safer than, urinary human chorionic gonadotrophin in inducing final follicular maturation and ovulation in in-vitro fertilization procedures: results of a multi-center double blind study. *J Clin Endocrinol* **86**:2607–16.

European-Middle East Orgalutran Study Group (2001). Comparable clinical outcome using the GnRH antagonist ganirelix or a long protocol of the GnRH agonist triptorelin for the prevention of premature LH surges in women undergoing ovarian stimulation. *Hum Reprod* **16**:644–51.

The European Recombinant Human Chorionic Gonadotropin Study Group (2000). Induction of final follicular maturation and early luteinization in women undergoing superovulation for ART–recombinant human chorionic gonadotropin (rhCG; Ovidrel) versus urinary hCG (Profasi). *Hum Reprod* **15**:1446–51.

Farquhar C, Vandederckhove P & Lilford R (2001). Laparoscopic "drilling" by diathermy or laser for ovulation induction in anovulatroy polycystic ovary syndrome. *Cochrane Database Syst Rev* **4**:CD001122.

Fatemi HM, Platteau P, Albano C et al. (2002). Rescue IVF and coasting with the use of a GnRH antagonist after ovulation induction. *Reprod Biomed Online* **5**:273–5.

Fauser B & Macklon N (2004). Medical approaches to ovarian stimulation for infertility. In (Strauss, Barbieri, Eds), *Reproductive Endocrinology: Physiology, Pathophysiology and Clinical Management*, 5th edition. Philadelphia: Elsevier, Chapter 31, pp. 965–1012.

Felberbaum RE & Diedrich K (2003). Gonadotrophin-releasing hormone antagonists: will they replace the agonists? *Reprod Biomed Online* **6**:43–53.

Felberbaum RE, Reissmann T, Kupker W et al. (1995). Preserved pituitary response under ovarian stimulation with hMG and GnRH antagonists (Cetrorelix) in women with tubal infertility. *Eur J Obstet Gynecol Reprod Biol* **61**:151–5.

Ferraretti AP, Gianaroli L, Magli C et al. (1999). Elective cryopreservation of all pronucleate embryos in women at risk of ovarian hyperstimulation syndrome: efficiency and safety. *Hum Reprod* **14**:1457–60.

Ferraretti AP, Gianaroli L, Magli C et al. (2001). Transvaginal ovarian drilling: a new surgical treatment for improving the clinical outcome of assisted reproductive technologies in patients with polycystic ovary syndrome. *Fertil Steril* **76**:812–46.

Feste JR (1990). General aspects of CO_2 laser laparoscopy. In (Baggish MS, Ed.), *Endoscopic Laser Surgery*, New York: Elsevier, pp. 67–8.

Fluker MR, Hooper WM & Yuzpe AA (1999). Withholding gonadotrophins ('coasting') to minimize the risk of ovarian hyperstimulation during superovulation and in-vitro fertilization-embryo transfer cycles. *Fertil Steril* **71**:294–301.

Fluker M, Grifo J, Leader A et al. (2001). Efficacy and safety of ganirelix acetate versus leuprolide acetate in women undergoing controlled ovarian hyperstimulation. *Fertil Steril* **75**:38–45.

Forman RG, Frydman R, Egan D et al. (1990). Severe ovarian hyperstimulation syndrome using agonists of gonadotropin-releasing hormone for in vitro fertilization: a European series and a proposal for prevention. *Fertil Steril* **53**:503–9.

Fountain S, Rizk B, Avery S et al. (1995). An evaluation of the effect of pentoxifylline on sperm function and treatment outcome of male-factor infertility: a preliminary study. *J Assist Reprod Genet* **12**:704–9.

Friedman CI, Schmidt GE, Chang FE et al. (1984). Severe ovarian hyperstimulation syndrome following follicular aspiration. *Am J Obstet Gynecol* **150**:436–7.

Friedman CI, Seifer DB, Kennard EA et al. (1998). Elevated level of follicular fluid vascular endothelial growth factor is a marker of diminished pregnancy potential. *Fertil Steril* **64**:268–72.

Fukaya T, Murakami T, Tamura M et al. (1995). Laser vaporization of the ovarian surface in polycystic ovary disease results in reduced ovarian hyperstimulation and improved pregnancy rates. *Am J Obstet Gynecol* **173**:119–25.

Garcia-Velasco JA, Zuniga A & Pacheco A (2004). Coasting acts through downregulation of VEGF gene expression and protein secretion. *Hum Reprod* **19**:1530–8.

Gerris J & Van Royen E (2000). Avoiding multiple pregnancies in ART: a plea for single embryo transfer. *Hum Reprod* **15**:1884–8.

Gerris J, De Vits A, Joostens M et al. (1995). Triggering of ovulation in human menopausal gonadotrophin-stimulated cycles: comparison between intravenously administered gonadotrophin-releasing hormone (100 and 500 micrograms), GnRH agonist (buserelin, 500 micrograms) and human chorionic gonadotrophin (10,000 IU). *Hum Reprod* **10**:56–62.

Gerris J, de Neubourg D, Van Royen E et al. (2002). Elective single day 3 embryo transfer halves the twinning rate without decrease in the ongoing pregnancy rate of an IVF/ICSI program. *Hum Reprod* **17**:2626–31.

Gerris J, de Sutter P, de Neuberg D et al. (2004). A real-life prospective health economic study of elective single embryo transfer versus two-embryo transfer in first IVF/ICSI cycles. *Hum Reprod* **19**:917–23.

Gjönnaess H (1984). Polycystic ovarian syndrome treated by ovarian electrocautery through the laparoscope. *Fertil Steril* **41**:20–5.

Gjönnaess H (1994). Ovarian electrocautery in the treatment of women with the polycystic ovary syndrome (PCOS). Factors affecting the results. *Acta Obstet Gynecol Scan* **73**:407–12.

Gjönnaess H & Norman N (1987). Endocrine effects of ovarian electrocautery in patients with polycystic ovarian disease. *Br J Obstet Gynaecol* **94**:779–82.

Goldberg JM & Falcone T, Eds (2000). *Atlas of Endoscopic Techniques in Gynecology*, Edinburgh: W. B. Saunders, Chapter 13, p. 61.

Gokman O, Ugur M, Ekin M et al. (2001). Intravenous albumin versus hydroxyethyl starch for the prevention of ovarian hyperstimulation in an in-vitro fertilisation programme: a prospective randomized placebo controlled study. *Eur J Obstet Gynecol Reprod Biol* **96**:187–92.

Gomez R, Simon G, Remohi J et al. (2001). Vascular endothelial growth factor 121 and 164 isoforms increase vascular permeability in hyperstimulation rats. *Fertil Steril* **76**(Suppl 3):4339–48.

Gomez R, Lima I, Simon C et al. (2004). Administration of low-dose LH induces ovulation and prevents vascular hyperpermeability and vascular endothelial growth factor expression in superovulated rats. *Reproduction* **127**:483–9.

Gonen Y, Balakier H, Powell W et al. (1990). Use of gonadotrophin-releasing hormone agonist to trigger follicular maturation for in-vitro fertilization. *J Clin Endocrinol Metab* **71**:918–22.

Grace J, Rizk B, Mulekar M (2005). Coasting decreases ovarian hyperstimulatin syndrome in patients at risk. Is the quality of oocytes, embryos and pregnancy rate the price to pay? *Fertil Steril* **84**(Suppl I)s300: 416.

Graf MA, Fischer R, Naether OG et al. (1997). Reduced incidence of ovarian hyperstimulation syndrome by prophylactic infusion of hydroxyethyl starch solution in an in-vitro fertilization programme. *Hum Reprod* **12**:2599–602.

Grochowski D, Wolczynski S, Kuczynski W et al. (2001). Correctly timed coasting reduces the risk of ovarian hyperstimulation syndrome and gives good cycle outcome in an in vitro fertilization program. *Gynecol Endocrinol* **15**:234–8.

Gurgan T, Urman B, Aksu T et al. (1992). The effect of short-interval laparoscopic lysis of adhesions on pregnancy rates following Nd-Yag laser photocoagulation of polycystic ovaries. *Obstet Gynecol* **30**:45–7.

Halme J, Toma SK & Talbert LM (1995). A case of severe ovarian hyperstimulation in a healthy oocyte donor. *Fertil Steril* **64**:857–9.

Hamilton-Fairley D, Kiddy D, Watson H et al. (1991). Low-dose gonadotrophin therapy for induction of ovulation in 100 women with polycystic ovary syndrome. *Hum Reprod* **6**:1095–9.

Haning RV Jr, Austin CW, Carlson IH et al. (1983). Plasma estradiol is superior to ultrasound and urinary estriol glucuronide as a predictor of ovarian hyperstimulation during induction of ovulation with menotropins. *Fertil Steril* **40**:31–6.

Hedon B, Hughes JN, Emperaire JC et al. (1998). A comparative prospective study of a chronic low dose versus a conventional ovulation stimulation regimen using recombinant human follicle stimulating hormone in anovulatory women. *Hum Reprod* **13**:2688–92.

Heylen SM, Puttemans PJ & Brosens IA (1994). Polycystic ovarian disease treated by laparoscopic argon laser capsule drilling: comparison of vaporization versus perforation technique. *Hum Reprod* **9**:1038–42.

Hoeger KM, Kochman L, Wixom N et al. (2004). A randomized, 48-week, placebo-controlled trial of intensive lifestyle modification and/or metformin therapy in over-weight women with polycystic ovary syndrome: a pilot study. *Fertil Steril* **82**:421–9.

Homburg R, Armar NA, Eshel J et al. (1988). Influence of serum luteinizing hormone concentrations on ovulation, conception and early pregnancy loss in polycystic ovary syndrome. *Br Med J* **297**:1024–6.

Homburg R, Levy T & Ben-Rafael Z (1995). A comparative prospective study of conventional regimen with chronic low-dose administration of follicle-stimulating hormone in polycystic ovary syndrome: slow administration is safer and more effective. *Fertil Steril* **63**:729–33.

Hornnes P, Giroud D, Howles C et al. (1993). Recombinant human follicle-stimulating hormone treatment leads to normal follicular growth, estradiol secretion, and pregnancy in a World Health Organization group II anovulatory woman. *Fertil Steril* **60**:724–6.

Howles CM (2002). The place of gonadotrophin-releasing hormone antagonists in reproductive medicine. *Reprod Biomed Online* **4**(Suppl 3):64–71.

Humaidan O, Bredkjaer HE, Bungum I et al. (2005). GnRH agonist (buserelin) or hCG for ovualtion induction in GnRH antagonist IVF/ICSI cycles: a prospective randomized study. *Hum Reprod* **20**:1213–20.

Imoedemhe DAG, Chan RCW, Signe AB et al. (1991). A new approach to the management of patients at risk of ovarian hyperstimulation in an in-vitro fertilization program. *Hum Reprod* **6**:1088–91.

International Recombinant Human Chorionic Gonadotropin Study Group (2001). Induction of ovulation in World Health Organization group II anovulatory women undergoing follicular stimulation with recombinant human follicle-stimulating hormone: a comparison of recombinant human chorionic gonadotropin (rhCG) and urinary hCG. *Fertil Steril* **75**:1111–18.

Isaza V, Garcia-Velasco JA, Aragones M et al. (2002). Oocyte and embryo quality after coasting: the experience from oocyte donation. *Hum Reprod* **17**:1737–58.

Isik AZ & Vicdan K (2001). Combined approach as an effective method in the prevention of severe ovarian hyperstimulation syndrome. *Eur J Obstet Gynecol Reprod Biol* **97**:208–12.

Isik AZ, Gokmen A, Zeyneloglu HB et al. (1996). Intravenous albumin prevents moderate-severe ovarian hyperstimulation in in vitro fertilisation patients: a prospective randomized and controlled study. *Eur J Obstet Gynecol Reprod Biol* **70**:170–83.

Itskovitz J, Boldes R, Levron J et al. (1991). Induction of pre-ovulatory luteinizing hormone surge and prevention of hyperstimulation syndrome by gonadotrophin-releasing hormone agonist. *Fertil Steril* **56**:213–20.

Itskovitz-Eldor J, Kol S & Mannaerts B (2000). Use of a single bolus of GnRH agonist triptorelin to trigger ovulation after GnRH antagonist ganirelix treatment in women undergoing ovarian stimulation for assisted reproduction, with special reference to the prevention of ovarian hyperstimulation syndrome: preliminary report: short communication. *Hum Reprod* **15**:1965–8.

Jewelewicz R, James SL, Finster M et al. (1972). Quintuplet gestation after ovulation induction with menopausal gonadotropins and pituitary luteinizing hormone. *Obstet Gynecol* **40**:1–5.

Keckstein J, Rossmanith W, Spatzier K et al. (1990). The effect of laparoscopic treatment of polycystic ovarian disease by CO_2 laser or Nd:YAG laser. *Surg Endoscopy* **4**:103–7.

Kinget K, Nijs M, Cox AM et al. (2002). A novel approach for patients at risk for ovarian hyperstimulation syndrome: elective transfer of a single zona free blastocyst on day 5. *Reprod Biomed Online* **4**:51–5.

Koike T, Araki S, Ogawa S et al. (1999). Does i.v. albumin prevent ovarian hyperstimulation syndrome? *Hum Reprod* **14**:1920.

Kolibianakis EM, Schultze-Morgan A, Schroer A et al. (2005). A lower ongoing pregnancy rate can be expected when GnRH agonist is used for triggering final oocyte maturation instead of HCG in patients undergoing IVF with GnRH antagonists. *Hum Reprod* **20**:2887–92.

Konig E, Bussen S, Sitterlin M & Steck T (1998). Prophylactic intravenous hydroxyethyl starch solution prevents moderate–severe ovarian hyperstimulation in in-vitro fertilization patients: a prospective, randomized, double-blind and placebo-controlled study. *Hum Reprod* **13**:2421–4.

Kovacs GT (1998). Polycystic ovaries, surgical management. In (Sutton C, Diamond M, Eds), *Endoscopic Surgery for Gynecologists*, London: W.B. Saunders, Chapter 23, pp. 233–40.

Kovacs G, Buckler H, Bangah M et al. (1991). Treatment of anovulation due to polycystic ovarian syndrome by laparoscopic ovarian electrocautery. *Br J Obstet Gynecol* **98**:30–5.

Kulikowski M, Wolczynski S, Kuczynski W et al. (1995). Use of GnRH analog for induction of the ovulatory surge of gonadotropins in patients at risk of the ovarian hyperstimulation syndrome. *Gynecol Endocrinol* **9**:97–9.

Kyono K, Fukunaga N, Haigo K et al. (2002). Successful delivery following cryopreservation of zygotes produced by in vitro matured oocytes retrieved from a woman with polycystic ovarian syndrome-like disease: a case report. *J Assisted Reprod Genetics* **19**:390–3.

Lainas T, Petsas G, Stavropoulou G et al. (2002). Administration of methylprednisolone to prevent severe ovarian hyperstimulation syndrome in patients undergoing in-vitro fertilization. *Fertil Steril* **78**:529–33.

Lanzone A, Fulghesu AM, Apa R et al. (1989). LH surge induction by GnRH agonist at the time of ovulation. *Gynecol Endocrinol* **3**:213–15.

Le Du A, Kadoch IJ, Bourcigaux N et al. (2005). In vitro oocyte maturation for the treatment of infertility associated with polycystic ovarian syndrome: the French experience. *Hum Reprod* **20**:420–4.

Lee C, Tummon I, Martin J et al. (1998). Does withholding gonadotrophin administration prevent severe ovarian hyperstimulation syndrome? *Hum Reprod* **13**:1157–8.

Levinsohn-Tavor S, Friedler M, Schachter A et al. (2003). Coasting – what is the best formula? *Hum Reprod* **18**:937–40.

Lewit N, Kol S, Manor D et al. (1995). The use of GnRH analogues for induction of the pre-ovulatory gonadotrophin surge in assisted reproduction and prevention of the ovarian hyperstimulation syndrome. *Gynecol Endocrinol* **4**(Suppl):13.

Lewit N, Kol S, Ronene N et al. (1996). Does intravenous administration of human albumin prevent severe ovarian hyperstimulation syndrome? *Fertil Steril* **66**:654–6.

Liu J, Lu G, Qian Y et al. (2003). Pregnancies and births achieved from in vitro matured oocytes retrieved from poor responders undergoing stimulation in in vitro fertilization cycles. *Fertil Steril* **80**:447–9.

Lin YH, Hwang JL, Huang LW et al. (2003). Combination of PSH priming and hCG priming for in-vitro maturation of human oocytes. *Hum Reprod* **18**:1632–6.

Lord JM, Flight IHK & Norman RJ (2005). *Insulin-sensitizing drugs (metformin, troglitazone, rosiglitazone, pioglitazone, D-chiro-inositol) for polycystic ovary syndrome (Review).* In: The Cochrane Library, Chichester: John Wiley & Sons Ltd, Issue 1, pp. 1–90.

Ludwig M, Felberbaum RE, Devroey P et al. (2000). Significant reduction of the incidence of ovarian hyperstimulation syndrome (OHSS) by using the LHRH antagonist Cetrorelix (Cetrotide®) in controlled ovarian stimulation for assisted reproduction. *Arch Gynecol Obstet* **264**:29–32.

Ludwig M, Katalinic A & Diedrich K (2001). Use of GnRH antagonists in ovarian stimulation for assisted reproductive technologies compared to the long protocol. Meta-analysis. *Arch Gynecol Obstet.* **265**:175–82.

Lukaszuk J, Liss B, Orpel J (2005). New method of ovarian hyperstimulation syndrome prevention. *Fertil Steril* **84**(Suppl 1):S95–232.

MacDougall JM, Tan SL, Balen AH et al. (1993). A controlled study comparing patients with and without polycystic ovaries undergoing in-vitro fertilization and the ovarian hyperstimulation syndrome. *Hum Reprod* **8**:233–7.

Marci R, Senn A, Dessole S et al. (2001). A low-dose stimulation protocol using highly purified follicle-stimulation hormone can lead to high pregnancy rates in in vitro fertilization patients with polycystic ovaries who are at risk of a high ovarian response to gonadotropins. *Fertil Steril* **75**:1131–5.

Mathur RS, Akeane AV, Keay SD et al. (2000). Distinction between early and late ovarian hyperstimulation syndrome. *Fertil Steril* **73**:901–7.

McNatty KP, Makris A, DeGrazia C et al. (1979). The production of progesterone, androgens and estrogens by granulosa cells, thecal tissue, and stromal tissue from human ovaries in vitro. *J Clin Endocrinol Metab* **49**:687–99.

Mikkelsen A (2004). In vitro maturation of human ova. *Int Congr Ser 1266* 160–6.

Mikkelsen AL & Lindenberg S (2001). Benefit of FSH priming of women with PCOS to the in vitro maturation procedure and the outcome: a randomized prospective study. *Reproduction* **122**:587–92.

Mitwally MFM & Casper RF (2000). Aromatase inhibition: a novel method of ovulation induction in women with polycystic ovarian syndrome. *Reprod Technol* **10**:244–7.

Mitwally MFM & Casper RF (2001). Use of an aromatase inhibitor for induction of ovulation. *Fertil Steril* **75**:305–9.

Mitwally MF, Biljan M & Casper RF (2005). Pregnancy outcome after the use of an aromatase inhibitor for ovarian stimulation. *Am J Obstet Gynecol* **192**:381–6.

Moreno L, Diaz I, Pacheco A et al. (2004). Extended coasting duration exerts a negative impact on IVF cycle outcome due to premature luteinization. *Reprod Biomed Online* **9**:500–4.

Morris RS, Karande VC, Dudkiewicz A et al. (1999). Octreotide is not useful for clomiphene cetrate resistance in patients with polycystic ovary syndrome but may reduce the likelihood of ovarian hyperstimulation syndrome. *Fertil Steril* **71**:452–6.

Mukherjee T, Copperman AB, Sandler B et al. (1995). Severe ovarian hyperstimulation despite prophylactic albumin at the time of oocyte retrieval for in-vitro fertilization and embryo transfer. *Fertil Steril* **64**:641–3.

Naether OGJI & Fischer R (1993). Adhesion formation after laparoscopic electrocoagulation of the ovarian surface in polycystic ovary patients. *Fertil Steril* **60**:95–8.

Nagele F, Sator MO, Juza J et al. (2002). Successful pregnancy resulting from in-vitro matured oocytes retrieved at laparoscopic surgery in a patient with polycystic ovary syndrome: case report. *Hum Reprod* **17**:373–4.

Ndukwe G, Thornton S, Fishel S et al. (1997). Severe ovarian hyperstimulation syndrome: is it really preventable by prophylactic intravenous albumin? *Fertil Steril* **68**:851–4.

Ng E, Leader A, Claman P et al. (1995). Intravenous albumin does not prevent the development of severe ovarian hyperstimulation syndrome in an in-vitro fertilization programme. *Hum Reprod* **10**:107–10.

Ohata Y, Harada T, Ito M et al. (2000). Coasting may reduce the severity of the ovarian hyperstimulation syndrome in patients with polycystic ovary syndrome. *Gynecol Obstet Invest* **50**:186–8.

Olivennes F, Fanchin R, Bouchard P et al. (1996). Triggering of ovulation by a gonadotrophin-releasing hormone (GnRH) agonist in patients pretreated with GnRH antagonist. *Fertil Steril* **66**:151–3.

Olivennes F, Belaisch-Allart J, Emeraire JC et al. (2000). Prospective, randomized, controlled study of in vitro fertilization-embryo transfer with a single dose of a luteinizing hormone-releasing hormone (LH-RH) antagonist (Cetrorelix) or a depot formula of an LH-RH agonist (triptorelin). *Fertil Steril* **73**:314–20.

Olivennes F, Fanchin R, Bertrand C et al. (2001). GnRH antagonist in single dose applications. *Infertility and Reproductive Medicine Clinics of North America* **12**:119–28.

Orvieto R & Ben-Rafael Z (1996). Prophylactic intravenous albumin for the prevention of severe ovarian hyperstimulation syndrome. *Hum Reprod* **11**:460–1.

Orvieto R, Dekel A, Dicker D et al. (1995). A severe case of ovarian hyperstimulation syndrome despite the prophylactic administration of intravenous albumin. *Fertil Steril* **64**:860–2.

Ostrzenski A (1992). Endoscopic carbon dioxide laser ovarian wedge resection in resistant polycystic ovarian disease. *Int J Fertil* **37**:295–9.

Panay N, Iammarrone E, Zosmer A et al. (1999). Does the prophylactic use of intravenous albumin prevent ovarian hyperstimulation syndrome? A randomized prospective study. *Hum Reprod* **14**:105.

Parsanezhad ME, Alborzi S, Pakniat M et al. (2003). A double-blind, randomized, placebo-controlled study to assess the efficacy of ketoconazole for reducing the risk of ovarian hyperstimulation syndrome. *Fertil Steril* **80**:1151–5.

Pasetto N & Montanino G (1964). Induction of ovulation by human gonadotrophins. *Acta Endocrinologica* **47**:1–9.

Pattinson HA, Hignett M, Dunphy BC et al. (1994). Outcome of thaw embryo transfer after cryopreservation of all embryos in patients at risk of ovarian hyperstimulation syndrome. *Fertil Steril* **62**:1192–6.

Penarrubia J, Balasch J, Fabregues F et al. (1998). Human chorionic gonadotrophin luteal support overcomes luteal phase inadequacy after gonadotrophin-releasing hormone agonist-induced ovulation in gonadotrophin-stimulated cycles. *Hum Reprod* **13**:3315–8.

Penzias AL (2002). Luteal phase support. *Fertil Steril* **77**:318–23.

Polson DW, Mason HD, Saldahna MB et al. (1987). Ovulation of a single dominant follicle during treatment with low dose pulsatile follicle stimulation hormone in women with polycystic ovary syndrome. *Clin Endocrinol (Oxford)* **26**:205–12.

Pritts EA & Atwood AK (2002). Luteal phase support in infertility treatment: a meta-analysis of the randomized trials. *Hum Reprod* **147**:2287–99.

Queenan JT Jr, Veeck LL, Toner JP et al. (1997). Cryopreservation of all prezygotes in patients at risk of severe hyperstimulation does not eliminate the syndrome, but chances of pregnancy are excellent with subsequent frozen-thaw transfers. *Hum Reprod* **12**:1573–6.

Rabau E, Serr DM, David A et al. (1967). Human menopausal gonadotrophin for anovulation and sterility. *Am J Obstet Gynecol* **98**:92–8.

Rabinovici J, Kushnir O, Shalev J et al. (1987). Rescue of menotropin cycles prone to develop ovarian hyperstimulation. *Br J Obstet Gynecol* **94**:1098–102.

Rabinowitz R, Laufer N, Lewin A et al. (1987). Rate of ovarian hyperstimulation syndrome after high dose hMG for the induction of ovulation in IVF cycles. *Hum Reprod* **2**(Suppl 1)(Abst 63):48.

Ragni G, Vegetti W, Riccaboni A et al. (2005). Comparison of GnRH agonists and antagonists in assisted reproduction cycles of patients at high risk of ovarian hyperstimulation syndrome. *Hum Reprod* **20**:2421–5.

Revel A & Casper RF (2001). The use of LHRH agonists to induce ovulation. In (Devroey P, Ed.), *Infertility and Reproductive Medicine Clinics of North America: GnRH Analogues.* Philadelphia: W.B. Saunders and Company, pp. 105–18.

Rimington MR, Walker SM & Shaw RW (1997). The use of laparoscopic ovarian electrocautery in preventing cancellation of in-vitro fertilization treatment cycles due to risk of ovarian hyperstimulation syndrome in women with polycystic ovaries. *Hum Reprod* **12**:1443–7.

Risquez F, Pennehouat G, Fernandez R et al. (1993). Microlaparoscopy: a preliminary report. *Hum Reprod* **8**:1701–5.

Rizk B (1992). Ovarian hyperstimulation syndrome. In (Brinsden PR, Rainsbury PA, Eds), *A Textbook of in Vitro Fertilization and Assisted Reproduction.* Carnforth, UK: Parthenon Publishing, Chapter 23, pp. 369–84.

Rizk B (1993a). Ovarian hyperstimulation syndrome. In (Studd J, Ed.), *Progress in Obstetrics and Gynecology*, Volume 11. Edinburgh: Churchill Livingtone, Chapter 18, pp. 311–49.

Rizk B (1993b). Prevention of ovarian hyperstimulation syndrome: the Ten Commandments. Presented at the European Society of Human Reproduction and Embryology Symposium, Tel Aviv, Israel, 1–2.

Rizk B (2001). Ovarian hyperstimulation syndrome: prediction, prevention and management. In (Rizk B, Devroey P, Meldrum DR, Eds), *Advances and Controversies in Ovulation Induction.* 34th ASRM Annual Postgraduate Program, Middle East Fertility Society Precongress Course. ASRM, 57th Annual Meeting, Orlando, FL, Birmingham, Alabama: the American Society for Reproductive Medicine, pp. 23–46.

Rizk B (2002). Can OHSS in ART be eliminated? In (Rizk B, Meldrum D, Schoolcraft W, Eds), *A Clinical Step-by-Step Course for Assisted Reproductive*

Technologies. 35th ASRM Annual Postgraduate Program, Middle East Fertility Society Precongress Course. ASRM, 58th Annual Meeting, Seattle, WA, Birmingham, Alabama: The American Society for Reproductive Medicine, pp. 65–102.

Rizk B (in press). The role of coasting in the prevention of threatening OHSS: an American perspective. In (Gerris J, Olivennes F, Delvigne A, Eds), *Ovarian Hyperstimulation Syndrome.* London: Taylor and Francis.

Rizk B & Aboulghar M (1991). Modern management of ovarian hyperstimulation syndrome. *Hum Reprod* **6**:1082–7.

Rizk B & Abdalla H (2006). Ovulatory dysfunction and ovulation induction. In (Rizk B, Abdalla H, Eds), *Infertility and assisted reproduction.* Oxford, UK: Health Press, Chapter I.4, pp. 39–59.

Rizk B & Aboulghar MA (2005). Classification, pathophysiology and management of ovarian hyperstimulation syndrome. In (Brinsden P, Ed.), *A Textbook of In-vitro Fertilization and Assisted Reproduction.* London: Parthenon, Chapter 12, pp. 217–58.

Rizk B & Nawar MG (2001). Laparoscopic ovarian drilling for surgical induction of ovulation in polycystic ovarian syndrome. In (Allahbadia G, Ed.), *Manual of Ovulation Induction.* Mumbai, India: Rotunda Medical Technologies, Chapter 18, pp. 140–4.

Rizk B & Nawar MG (2004). Ovarian hyperstimulation syndrome. In (Serhal P, Overton C, Eds), *Good Clinical Practice in Assisted Reproduction.* Cambridge, UK: Cambridge University Press, Chapter 8, pp. 146–66.

Rizk B & Smitz J (1992). Ovarian hyperstimulation syndrome after superovulation for IVF and related procedures. *Hum Reprod* **7**:320–7.

Rizk B & Thorneycroft IH (1996). Does recombinant follicle stimulating hormone abolish the risk of severe ovarian hyperstimulation syndrome? *Fertil Steril* **65**:S151–2.

Rizk B, Aboulghar MA, Mansour RT et al. (1991a). Severe ovarian hyperstimulation syndrome: analytical study of twenty-one cases. *Hum Reprod* **6**:S368–9.

Rizk B, Vere M, Martin R et al. (1991b). Incidence of severe ovarian hyperstimulation syndrome after GnRH agonist/HMG super-ovulation for in-vitro fertilization. *Hum Reprod* **6**:S368.

Rizk B, Tan SL, Morcos S et al. (1991c). Heterotopic pregnancies after in-vitro fertilizations and embryo transfer. *Am J Obstet Gynecol* **164**:161–4.

Rizk B, Fountain S, Avery S et al. (1995). Successful use of pentoxifylline in male-factor infertility and previous failure of in vitro fertilization: a prospective randomized study. *J Assist Reprod Genet* **12**:710–14.

Rizk B, Aboulghar MA, Smitz J et al. (1997). The role of vascular endothelial growth factor and interleukins in the pathogenesis of severe ovarian hyperstimulation syndrome. *Hum Reprod Update* **3**:255–66.

Romeu A, Monzo A, Peiro T et al. (1997). Endogenous LH surge versus hCG as ovulation trigger after low-dose highly purified FSH in IUI: a comparison of 761 cycles. *J Assist Reprod Genet* **14**:518–24.

Rongieres-Bertrand C, Olivennes F, Gighini C et al. (1999). Revival of the natural cycles in in-vitro fertilization with the use of a new gonadotrophin-releasing hormone antagonist (Cetrorelix): a pilot study with minimal stimulation. *Hum Reprod* **14**:683–8.

Rosenwaks Z (2003). Ovarian hyperstimulation syndrome (OHSS): strategies for prevention. In (Muasher SJ, Rizk B, Eds), *American Society for Reproductive Medicine 59th Ann Mtg. 36th Annual Post Graduate Program.* San Antonio, Texas: Published by the American Society for Reproductive Medicine, Birmingham, AL, pp. 153–73.

Salat-Baroux J, Alvarez S, Antoine JM et al. (1990). Treatment of hyperstimulation during in-vitro fertilization. *Hum Reprod* **5**:36–9.

Schenker JG & Weinstein D (1978). Ovarian hyperstimulation syndrome: a current survey. *Fertil Steril* **30**:255–68.

Schmidt-Sarosi C, Kaplan DR, Sarosi P et al. (1995). Ovulation triggering in clomiphene citrate-stimulated cycles: human chorionic gonadotrophin versus a gonadotrophin releasing hormone agonist. *J Assist Reprod Genet* **12**:167–74.

Schwarzler P, Abendstein BJ, Klingler A et al. (2003). Prevention of severe ovarian hyperstimulation syndrome (OHSS) IVF patients by steroidal ovarian suppression – a prospective randomized study. *Hum Fertil* **6**:125–9.

Scott RT, Bailey SA, Kost ER et al. (1994). Comparison of leuprolide acetate and human chorionic gonadotrophin for the induction of ovulation in clomiphene citrate-stimulated cycles. *Fertil Steril* **61**:872–4.

Segal S & Casper RF (1992). Gonadotrophin-releasing hormone agonist versus human chorionic gonadotrophin for triggering follicular maturation in in-vitro fertilization. *Fertil Steril* **57**:1254–8.

Seibel MM, Kamrava MM, McArdle C et al. (1984). Treatment of polycystic ovarian disease with chronic low dose follicle stimulating hormone: biochemical changes and ultrasound correlation. *Int J Fertil* **29**:39–43.

Serin IS, Ozcelik B, Bekyurek T et al. (2002). Effects of pentoxifylline in the prevention of ovarian hyperstimulation syndrome in a rabbit model. *Gynecol Encocrinol* **5**:355–9.

Shahata M, Yang D, al-Natsha SD et al. (1994). Intravenous albumin and severe ovarian hyperstimulation. *Hum Reprod* **9**:2186.

Shaker AG, Zosmer A, Dean N et al. (1996). Comparison of intravenous albumin and transfer of fresh embryos with cryopreservation of all embryos for subsequent transfer in prevention of ovarian hyperstimulation syndrome. *Fertil Steril* **65**:992–6.

Shalev E, Geslevich Y & Ben-Ami M (1994). Induction of pre-ovulatory luteinizing hormone surge by gonadotrophin-releasing hormone agonist for women at risk for developing the ovarian hyperstimulation syndrome. *Hum Reprod* **9**:417–19.

Shalev E, Geslevich Y, Matilsky M et al. (1995a). Gonadotrophin-releasing hormone agonist compared with human chorionic gonadotrophin for ovulation induction after clomiphene citrate treatment. *Hum Reprod* **10**:2541–4.

Shalev E, Geslevich Y, Matilsky M et al. (1995b). Induction of pre-ovulatory gonadotrophin surge with gonadotrophin-releasing hormone agonist compared to pre-ovulatory injection of human chorionic gonadotrophins for ovulation induction in intrauterine insemination. *Hum Reprod* **10**:2244–7.

Shalev E, Giladi Y, Matilsky M et al. (1995c). Decreased incidence of severe ovarian hyperstimulation syndrome in high risk in-vitro fertilization patients receiving intravenous albumin: a prospective study. *Hum Reprod* **10**:1373–6.

Sher G, Salem R, Feinman M et al. (1993). Eliminating the risks of life-endangering complications following over-stimulation with menotropin fertility agents: a report on women undergoing in-vitro fertilization and embryo transfer. *Obstet Gynecol* **81**:1009–11.

Sher G, Zouves C, Feinman M et al. (1995). Prolonged coasting: an effective method. *Hum Reprod* **10**:3107–9.

Shoham Z, Patel A & Jacobs HS (1991). Polycystic ovarian syndrome: safety and effectiveness of stepwise and low-dose administration of purified follicle-stimulating hormone. *Fertil Steril* **55**:1051–6.

Shoham Z, Weissman A, Barash A et al. (1994). Intravenous albumin for the prevention of severe ovarian hyperstimulation syndrome in an in vitro fertilization program: a prospective, randomized, placebo controlled study. *Fertil Steril* **62**:137–42.

Smitz J, Gerard P, Camus M et al. (1992). Pituitary gonadotrophin secretory capacity during the luteal phase in superovulation using GnRH-agonists and hMG in a desensitization or flare-up protocol. *Hum Reprod* **7**:1225–9.

Soliman S, Daya S, Collins J et al. (1994). The role of luteal phase support in infertility treatment: a meta-analysis of randomized trials. *Fertil Steril* **61**:1068–76.

Son WY, Yoon SH, Park SJ et al. (2002). Ongoing twin pregnancy after virification of blastocysts produced by in-vitro matured oocytes retrieved from a woman with polycystic ovary syndrome: case report. *Hum Reprod* **17**:2963–6.

Stein FI (1964). Duration of fertility following ovarian wedge resection – Stein–Leventhal syndrome. *Western J Surg, Obstet Gynecol* **78**:237–40.

Stein FI & Leventhal ML (1935). Amenorrhea associated with bilateral polycystic ovaries. *Am J Obst Gynecol* **29**:181–91.

Tan SL & Child TJ (2002). In-vitro maturation of oocytes from unstimulated polycystic ovaries. *Reprod Biomed Online* **4**:18–23.

Tan SL, Balen A, El Hussein E et al. (1992). The administration of glucocorticoids for the prevention of ovarian hyperstimulation syndrome in in-vitro fertilization: a prospective randomized study. *Fertil Steril* **58**:378–83.

Tomazevic T & Meden-Vrtovec H (1996). *J Assist Reprod Genet* **13**:282–6.

Tortoriello DV, McGovern PG, Colon JM et al. (1998a). 'Coasting' does not adversely affect cycle outcome in a subset or highly responsive in-vitro fertilization patients. *Fertil Steril* **69**:454–60.

Tortoriello DV, McGovern PG, Colon JM et al. (1998b). Critical ovarian hyperstimulation syndrome in coasted in-vitro fertilization patients. *Hum Reprod* **13**:3005–8.

Tozer AJ, Al-Shawaf T, Zosmer A et al. (2001). Does laparoscopic ovarian diathermy affect the outcome of IVF-embryo transfer in women with polycystic ovarian syndrome: a retrospective comparative study. *Hum Reprod* **16**:91–5.

Tozer AJ, Iles RK, Iammarrone E et al. (2004a). Characteristics of populations of granulosa cells from individual follicles in women undergoing 'coasting' during controlled ovarian stimulation (COS) for IVF. *Hum Reprod* **19**:2561–8.

Tozer AJ, Iles RK, Iammarrone E et al. (2004b). The effects of 'coasting' on follicular fluid concentrations of vascular endothelial growth factor in women at risk of developing ovarian hyperstimulation syndrome. *Hum Reprod* **19**:522–8.

Trounson A, Wood C & Kausche A (1994). In vitro maturation and the fertilization and developmental competence of oocytes recovered from untreated polycystic ovarian patients. *Fertil Steril* **62**:353–62.

Tulchinsky D, Nash H, Brown K et al. (1991). A pilot study of the use of gonadotrophin-releasing hormone analog for triggering ovulation. *Fertil Steril* **55**:644–6.

Tütinen A, Husa LM, Tulppala M et al. (1995). The effect of cryopreservation in prevention of ovarian hyperstimulation syndrome. *Br J Obstet Gynaecol* **102**:326–9.

Ulug U, Bahceci M, Erden HF et al. (2002). The significance of coasting duration during ovarian stimulation for conception in assisted fertilization cycles. *Hum Reprod* **17**:310–13.

Urman B, Pride SM & Ho Yuen B (1992). Management of over-stimulated gonadotrophin cycles with a controlled drift period. *Hum Reprod* **7**:213–17.

Van Blerkom J, Antczak M & Schrader R (1997). The developmental potential of the human oocyte is related to the dissolved oxygen content of follicular fluid: association with vascular endothelial growth factor levels and perifollicular blood flow characteristics. *Hum Reprod* **12**:1047–55.

Vande Wiele RL, Bogumil J, Dyrenfurth I et al. (1970). Mechanisms regulating the menstrual cycle in women. *Hormone Res* **26**:63–103.

Van der Meer S, Gerris J, Joostens M et al. (1993). Triggering of ovulation using a gonadotrophin-releasing hormone agonist does not prevent ovarian hyper-stimulation syndrome. *Hum Reprod* **8**:1628–31.

Van Santbrink EJ & Fauser BC (1997). Urinary follicle-stimulating hormone for normogonadotropic clomiphene-resistant anovulatory infertility: prospective, randomized comparison between low-dose step-up and step-down regimen. *J Clin Endocrinol Metab* **82**:3597–602.

Van Santbrink EJ, Donderwinkel PF, van Dessel TJ et al. (1995). Gonadotrophin induction of ovulation using a step-down dose regimen: single-centre clinical experience in 82 patients. *Hum Reprod* **10**:1043–53.

Veek L, Wothman J, Witmyer J et al. (1983). Maturation and fertilization of morphologically immature human oocytes in a program of in vitro fertilization. *Fertil Steril* **39**:694–6.

Verhelst J, Gerris J, Joostens M et al. (1993). Clinical and endocrine effects of laser vaporization in patients with polycystic ovarian disease. *Gynecol Endocrinol* **7**:49–55.

Wada I, Matson PI, Burslem RM et al. (1991). Ovarian hyperstimulation syndrome in GnRH/Hmg stimulated cycles for IVF or GIFT. *J Obstet Gynecol* **11**:88–9.

Wada I, Matson PL, Troup SA et al. (1992a). Outcome of treatment subsequent to the elective cryopreservation of all embryos from women at risk of developing the ovarian hyperstimulation syndrome. *Hum Reprod* **7**:962–6.

Wada I, Matson PL, Horne G et al. (1992b). Is continuation of a gonadotrophin releasing hormone agonist (GnRH-a) necessary for women at risk of developing ovarian hyperstimulation syndrome? *Hum Reprod* **7**:1090–3.

Wada I, Matson PL, Troup SA et al. (1993a). Does elective cryopreservation of all embryos from women at risk of ovarian hyperstimulation syndrome reduce the incidence of the condition? *Br J Obstet Gynaecol* **10**:265–9.

Wada I, Matson PL, Horne G et al. (1993b). Assisted conception using buserelin and human menopausal gonadotrophins in women with polycystic ovary syndrome. *Br J Obstet Gynaecol* **100**:365–9.

Waldenstrom U, Kahn J, Marsk L et al. (1999). High pregnancy rates and successful prevention of severe ovarian hyperstimulation syndrome by 'prolonged coasting' of very hyperstimulated patients: a multi-centre study. *Hum Reprod* **14**:294–7.

Yovich JL (1993). Pentoxyfylline: actions and applications in assisted reproduction. *Hum Reprod* **8**:1786–91.

Zelinski-Wooten MB, Lanzendorf SE, Wolf DO et al. (1991). Titrating luteinizing hormone surge requirements for ovulatory changes in the primate follicle. I. Oocyte maturation and corpus luteum function. *J Clin Endocrin Metab* **73**:577–83.

VIII

TREATMENT OF OVARIAN HYPERSTIMULATION SYNDROME

The clinical course of OHSS depends on its severity, whether complications already occurred and the presence or absence of pregnancy (Rizk, 2002). Clinical management involves dealing with electrolyte imbalance, neurohormonal and haemodynamic changes, pulmonary manifestations, liver dysfunction, hypoglobulinaemia, febrile morbidity, thromboembolic phenomena and neurological manifestations (Delvigne and Rozenberg, 2003). Despite the increased prevalence of severe OHSS, the management of critical cases presents a unique challenge to the reproductive endocrinologist and fertility specialist (Rizk et al., 1991a). The general approach will be adapted to the severity. Specific approaches such as paracentesis and pleural puncture should be carefully performed when necessary. Medical management requires familiarity with the condition, and many of the problems that occur happen as a result of lack of realization by intensivists and medical specialists that the syndrome is different from similarly presenting medical syndromes. A better understanding of the underlying pathophysiological mechanisms will help to refine management (Rizk, 1992; Rizk and Smitz, 1992). Novel treatment options for OHSS are currently being investigated (Rizk and Nawar, 2004; Rizk and Aboulghar, 2005; Gomez-Gallego et al., 2005).

OUTPATIENT MANAGEMENT FOR MODERATE AND SEVERE OHSS

Based on our classification, moderate OHSS will be followed up by regular telephone calls at least daily, and by twice-weekly office visits (Rizk and Aboulghar, 1999). Assessment at the office includes pelvic ultrasound, complete blood count, liver function tests and coagulation profile (Rizk and Nawar, 2004). Fluker et al. (2000) suggested that active outpatient intervention in the early stages of OHSS, including paracentesis and albumin administration, can avoid hospitalization while minimizing the progression and complications of OHSS. Lincoln et al. (2002) assessed the effectiveness of outpatient treatment of 48 patients diagnosed with OHSS. The patients were treated with outpatient transvaginal culdocentesis and rehydration with intravenous crystalloids and albumin every one to three days until resolution of symptoms or hospitalization was required. No complications occurred from outpatient treatment, and 91.6% of patients avoided hospitalization. The authors concluded that outpatient treatment, consisting of culdocentesis, intravenous rehydration and albumin, minimized the need for hospitalization in these patients. The patient should be instructed to report to the hospital if she develops dyspnea, if the volume of urine is diminished or upon development of any unusual symptoms, such as leg swelling, dizziness, numbness and neurological problems.

The question whether severe OHSS should be managed on an outpatient basis depends on the classification and definition of severity, comfort of the physician, and compliance and reliability of patients. Severe OHSS grade A is managed on an outpatient basis by the aspiration of ascitic fluid, administration of intravenous fluids and the evaluation of all biochemical parameters. Shrivastav et al. (1994) reviewed their experience in the management of 18 patients who developed severe OHSS. The first group of eight patients was managed conservatively with hospitalization, intravenous hydration and supportive therapy. The average duration of hospitalization was seven days and the patients were uncomfortable throughout. The second group, which consisted of 10 patients, was managed on an outpatient basis with early ultrasound guided paracentesis. While the patients were hydrated intravenously, 1—3 liters were removed over 2—3 hours. The original hospitalization was for 6—7 h and no inpatient stay was required. The patient's symptoms were promptly relieved and none of the patients in this series required retapping. Shrivastav et al. (1994) suggested that day care management with abdominal paracentesis is a simple, safe and effective method, and is more acceptable for patients. However, I have to emphasize that each center should adopt the policies that best serve their patients and take into account their facilities' expertise and resources.

A more recent report included 139 patients who developed severe OHSS during 8311 IVF cycles from 1998 to 2004 (Gustofson et al., 2005). Aggressive outpatient management of severe OHSS with early paracentesis, intravenous fluid hydration, antiemetics, and DVT prophylaxis minimized the need for hospital admission. Therefore, there has been a trend toward the use of outpatient management that has gradually increased over the last decade.

HOSPITALIZATION OF PATIENTS WITH SEVERE OHSS

Patients with severe OHSS grade B and C are admitted to hospital for treatment (Rizk and Aboulghar, 1999) (Figure VIII.1). Hospitalization should

Fig. VIII.1: Indications for hospitalization in OHSS

- **Severe abdominal pain or peritoneal signs**
- **Intractable nausea and vomiting that prevents ingestion of food and adequate fluids**
- **Severe oliguria or anuria**
- **Tense ascites**
- **Dyspnea or tachypnea**
- **Hypotension (relative to baseline), dizziness, or syncope**
- **Severe electrolyte imbalance (hyponatremia, hyperkalemia)**

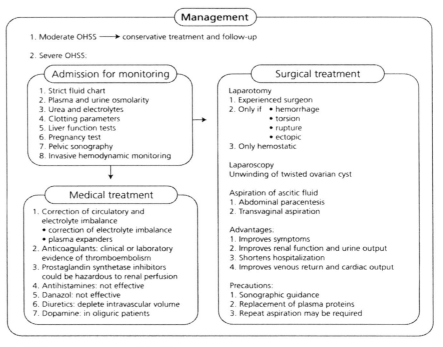

Fig. VIII.2: Management of OHSS

be considered if one or more of these symptoms or signs are present (Practice Committee for the American Society for Reproductive Medicine, 2003) (Figure VIII.2).

Clinical and Biochemical Monitoring in Hospital

The patient's general condition requires regular assessment, with documentation of vital signs, together with daily weight and girth measurement (Rizk, 1993). Strict fluid balance recording is needed, particularly of urine output.

Biochemical monitoring should include serum and electrolytes, renal and liver function tests, a coagulation profile and blood count (Rizk, 2001, 2002). Serum and urinary osmolarity and urinary electrolyte estimation may be required as the severity of the disease increases. Respiratory compromise and/or significant deterioration in renal function require evaluation of blood gases and acid-base balance. The frequency of these investigations will depend on the severity of the condition.

Ultrasonographic examination provides accurate assessment of ovarian size and the presence or absence of ascites, as well as pleural or pericardial effusions (Rizk and Aboulghar, 1991). In addition, it will help in the diagnosis of intra- or extrauterine pregnancy as well as multiple or heterotopic pregnancy (Rizk and Nawar, 2004). Chest X-ray will also provide information on the presence of hydrothorax. Assay of β-hCG will help to diagnose pregnancy as early as possible.

MEDICAL TREATMENT

Circulatory Volume Correction

The main line of treatment is correction of the circulatory volume and electrolyte imbalance (Rizk and Aboulghar, 1999). Every effort should be directed towards restoring a normal intravascular volume and preserving adequate renal function (Rizk and Nawar, 2004). Whelan and Vlahos (2000) recommended starting with 1 l of IV normal saline and assessing change in urine output and hematocrit response after 1 h. If urine output response is adequate and hematocrit normalizes, switch to dextrose 5% normal saline and maintain at the rate of 125 to 150 ml per hour while monitoring very closely every 4 h. If urine output is inadequate in response to fluid bolus and the hematocrit does not reflect a change toward euvolumia, IV crystalloid may be stopped and IV albumin administered; 200 ml of a 25% solution administered at 50 ml/h over 4 h. One concern with using plasma expanders is that the beneficial effect is transitory before their redistribution into the extravascular space, further exacerbating ascites formation (Rizk and Aboulghar, 1991; Kissler et al., 2001). Dextran, mannitol and fresh frozen plasma have also been used.

Hydryoxyethyl starch (HES) has the advantage of a non-biologic origin and high molecular weight 200–1000 kDa vs. 69 kDa for albumin. Abramov et al. (2001) compared the efficacy and safety of 6% HES and human albumin as colloid solutions for treatment of 16 patients with severe OHSS. They observed a higher urine output, fewer paracenteses and shorter hospital stays with HES (Table VIII.1). Gamzu et al. (2002) compared HES 10% and Haemaccel and found no clinical advantage for the HES (Table VIII.2). A recent case report in which a patient experienced rapid recovery following treatment with 10% HES was reported by Rabinerson et al. (2001). We agree with Delvigne and Rozenberg (2003) that larger prospective randomized controlled studies are needed before definite conclusions can be drawn.

Electrolyte Replacement

Delvigne et al. (1993) observed electrolyte disorders in 54.6% of 128 cases of OHSS; 24.2% of these were related to potassium and 22.2% were related to sodium. Similarly, hyponatremia was observed in 56% of patients (Fabregues et al., 1999). Appropriate intravenous solutions administered according to protocol in the previous section will correct most electrolyte imbalances; if hypokalemia is significant, a cation exchange resin may be needed (Rizk and Aboulghar, 2005). Sodium and water restriction were advocated by Shapiro et al. (1977) and Haning et al. (1985), but Thaler et al. (1981) found no change

Table VIII.1 Controlled cohort study to compare the efficacy of 6% hydroxyethyl starch and human albumin for treatment of severe OHSS
*Reproduced with permission from Abramov et al. (2001). Fertil Steril **75**:1228–30*

Variable	Human albumin (n = 10)	Hydroxyethyl starch group (n = 6)
Baseline characteristics		
age (years)	28.1 ± 8.9	29.4 ± 7.4
Estradiol level on day of HCG	6164 ± 1418	9.080 ± 2450
Administration (pg/ml)	10 (100)	6 (100)
ascites (%)	2 (20)	1 (17)
pleural effusion (%)	4 (40)	6 (100)
gastrointestinal symptoms (%)	10.7 ± 3.4	10.5 ± 3.8
ovarian diameter	1 (10)	1 (16)
oliguria	42 ± 3.6	43 ± 7
hematocrit (%)	3300 ± 310	3150 ± 270
daily fluid intake (ml)*		
Patient outcome	2557 ± 1032	3580 ± 1780
daily urine output (ml)**	8 (80)	2 (33)
abdominal paracentesis (%)	2300 ± 230	1930
total fluid aspirated per patient (ml)	2 (20)	0
pleurocentesis (%)		
hospital stay (days)	19.0 ± 8.2	15.7 ± 5.7
conception	7 (70)	4 (67)
miscarriage	2 (28)	1 (17)
congenital malformation	0	0

Values are means ± SD or percentages of patients
* Including oral and intravenous hydration
** During the first five days of hospitalization

in the patient's weight, abdominal circumference or peripheral edema when sodium and water were restricted. Therefore, salt and water restriction are not widely advocated.

Anticoagulant Therapy

Anticoagulant therapy is indicated if there is clinical evidence of thrombo-embolic complications (Rizk et al., 1990a) or laboratory evidence of hyper-coagulability (Rizk, 1993a). Arterial and venous thromboses are the most common serious complications of OHSS.

Table VIII.2 Hydroxyethyl starch and Haemaccel for the correction of circulatory volume depletion in OHSS
Reproduced with permission from Gamzu et al. (2002). Fertil Steril. **77**:*1302–03*

Characteristic	Hydroxyethyl starch (n = 20)	Haemaccel (n = 20)
Reduction in body weight (g)	1020 ± 390	960 ± 650
Reduction in hematocrit (%)	7 ± 0.8	7 ± 1.1
Reduction in leukocyte (×10 000 cells µl)	4.7 ± 0.6	4.4 ± 0.6
Increase in urine volume (ml)	1336 ± 226	1217 ± 187
Duration of hospitalization	5.4 ± 0.6	5.1 ± 0.3

Values are the mean ($\pm$ SD). There were no statistically significant differences between the values for the two groups of women

Duration of Anticoagulation

The duration of anticoagulant administration is also debatable (Delvigne, 2004; Rizk and Aboulghar, 2005). Some investigators have reported late thrombosis up to 20 weeks post transfer, and many investigators are in favor of maintaining heparin therapy for some weeks (Serour et al., 1998; Delvigne, 2004).

Anticoagulant Prophylaxis

Preventative treatment with heparin should be used whenever there is a thromboembolic risk (Delvigne and Rozenberg, 2003; Rizk and Aboulghar, 2005; Rizk et al., 1991a). However, what constitutes high risk for thrombo-embolism? In cases of severe OHSS, the following situations are recognized as indicating an increased risk of thromboembolism: immobilization, compression of pelvic vessels by large ovaries or ascites, thrombophilias and hyperestrogenemia (Rizk, 2001, 2002). Prevention using mobilization and antithrombosis stockings are insufficient, as thrombosis may occur at all locations and may be systemic in nature.

Prophylaxis with heparin remains debatable for two reasons (Delvigne and Rozenberg, 2003). First, there are no randomized studies proving its efficacy in preventing thromboembolic complications during severe OHSS. Furthermore, in some clinical scenarios, thromboembolism still occurs despite giving heparin (Hortskamp et al., 1996; Todros et al., 1999; Cil et al., 2000). Despite these important reservations from Delvigne and Rozenberg (2003), I recommend giving heparin or Lovenox for patients with severe OHSS.

I would like to separate the issue of severity of OHSS from thromboem-bolism because of the prevalence of intrinsic coagulopathy that triggers the problem even in moderate cases. While I have advocated a more liberal policy for prophylaxis, others have followed that lead but, unfortunately, had to operate on ruptured ectopic pregnancies in anticoagulated patients.

Therefore, thromboembolism will remain a difficult complication to prevent and may complicate the outcome.

Antibiotic Treatment

Infections are not uncommon in the treatment of OHSS because of frequent catheterizations, venipuncture, transvaginal aspiration of ascitic fluid and pleural drainage (Abramov et al., 1998a, 1999b). Furthermore, hypoglobuline-mia is present in severe cases. Preoperative antibiotic prophylaxis is highly recommended.

Immunoglobulin Replacement Therapy

Immuonoglobulin concentrations, specifically IgG and IgA, are significantly lower in the plasma of patients with severe OHSS. Both IgG and IgA levels increase as patients clinically improve. Ascitic fluid contains high levels of IgG but moderate levels of IgA and negligible IgM levels. Severe OHSS is characterized by hypogammaglobulinemia that is attributed to leakage of medium molecular weight immunoglobulins such as IgG and IgA into the peritoneal cavity (Abramov, 1999a). Patients with nephrotic syndrome that have hypogammaglobulinemia tend to develop infections that progress rapidly and may result in death despite antibiotic treatment. Immunoglobulin replacement therapy decreases bacterial infections in such patients. In light of these favorable results, Abramov et al. (1999a) recommend prophylactic immunoglobulin replacement therapy in patients with severe OHSS. However, this intervention still awaits further evaluation (Delvigne and Rozenberg, 2003).

Diuretics

Diuretic therapy without prior volume expansion may prove detrimental, by further contracting the intravascular volume, thereby worsening hypotension and its sequelae (Rizk et al., 1990a; Rizk and Aboulghar, 1991). Diuretics will increase blood viscosity and increase the risk of venous thrombosis (Rizk and Nawar, 2004; Rizk and Abdalla, 2006). Diuretics should used in the management of pulmonary edema. Other authorities have used an albumin-lasix chase protocol with success (Navot et al., 1992). I have not used that protocol but their published experience should be consulted by the interested clinician.

Dopamine

The use of dopamine has been successful in the treatment of oliguria associated with severe OHSS (Ferraretti et al., 1992; Tsounado et al., 2003). This is usually carried out in the intensive care setting, which will be discussed below.

Indomethacin

Indomethacin has been investigated as an inhibitor of prostaglandin synthesis that might play a role in the pathophysiology of OHSS. Schenker and Polishuk (1976) demonstrated that indomethacin could prevent fluid shifts in ascites and pleural effusion. However Pride et al. (1986) demonstrated that ascites formation is not suppressed by indomethacin in experimental animal studies (in the rabbit). In clinical practice, Katz et al. (1984) observed clinical improvement by using indomethacin; however, a few years later, Borenstein et al. (1989) from the same group found no clinical improvement in ascites formation by using indomethacin in severe OHSS patients. Furthermore, oliguria and renal failure have been attributed to indomethacin in cases of OHSS in the absence of hypovolemia, due to its interference with renal perfusion (Balasch et al., 1990).

INTENSIVE CARE TREATMENT OF PATIENTS WITH SEVERE OHSS

Patients with renal failure, thromboembolism or adult respiratory distress syndrome should be admitted to intensive care for treatment (Rizk and Nawar, 2004; Rizk and Aboulghar, 1999, 2005).

Patients with Renal Compromise

Dopamine

Dopamine has been used in oliguric patients with severe OHSS, resulting in significant improvement in renal function (Ferraretti, 1992; Tsunoda et al., 2003). Dopamine produces its renal effect by increasing renal blood flow and glomerular filtration. This is accomplished via stimulation of the dopaminergic receptors present in the vascular kidney (Felder et al., 1984). The rationale for treating oliguric patients with dopamine is to avoid fluid and salt retention and to prevent acute renal failure. Dopamine therapy should be given cautiously and under strict observation.

Ferraretti et al. (1992) reported on the treatment of seven patients with severe OHSS following gonadotrophin stimulation for IVF or GIFT using low doses of dopamine by peripheral infusion. Management of the seven patients consisted of bed rest, restriction of fluid intake to 500 ml/day, and daily monitoring of urine output, abdominal girth and weight. In addition, biochemical and hematological clotting factors were measured daily in the pregnant women. Serum hCG was measured every two days and the patients were given a protein z- and salt-rich diet in order to increase oncotic and osmotic blood pressure. Dopamine treatment commenced within 10 h of hospital admission using an intravenous infusion pump, which strictly controlled the dosage of dopamine. The dopamine dosage used by the authors was 4.32 mg/kg per 24 h. The reason for choosing this dosage was to produce dilatation of renal vessels and increased renal blood flow without affecting the systemic blood pressure and pulse rate (Kirshon et al., 1988). Dopamine treatment was continued until there was complete resolution of ascites. In the five patients who were pregnant, dopamine treatment was required for 9 to 22 days. The duration of treatment was related to the magnitude of the increase of hCG. It was longest (18−22 days) in patients with triplets, shortest (9−10 days) in patients with a singleton pregnancy and intermediate (14 days) for patients with twins. In the two non-pregnant women, dopamine was only required for seven days. Albumin or plasma expanders were only administered if required, and anticoagulants were given to prevent thromboembolism if clotting factors were abnormal.

Tsunoda et al. (2003) reported on 27 patients, hospitalized because of OHSS and refractory to the initial therapy with intravenous albumin, who were treated with docarpamine. A 750-mg tablet of docarpamine was taken every 8 h. In 19 (86.4%) out of 22 patients, clinical symptoms associated with ascites gradually improved after administrating docarpamine. Moreover, there were no major adverse effects of docarpamine in this study. These findings indicate that oral docarpamine administration could be one of the options in the management of patients with OHSS using dopamine therapy.

Invasive Hemodynamic Monitoring

Invasive hemodynamic monitoring (of central venous pressure and pulmonary artery pressures) may be needed in critical cases in which volume expanders are being employed (Kirshon et al., 1988; Navot et al., 1992). The contracted intravascular volume has been associated with a low central venous pressure (Kirshon et al., 1988). Hemodialysis may be necessary once frank renal failure ensues.

Pleurocentesis and Treatment of Pulmonary Complications

Pleural effusion was observed in 21% of 128 cases in a Belgian multi-center conducted by Delvigne et al. (1993). Evaluation and treatment of patients with severe OHSS complaining of dyspnea includes physical examination, chest ultrasound, X-ray and arterial blood gases. It is essential to evaluate accurately any pulmonary complications that may result in hypoxia. Serial arterial blood gas measurements should be monitored, and if a pulmonary embolus is suspected, a spiral CT scan or ventilation perfusion scan should be performed. Pulmonary compromise should be treated with oxygen supplementation, and the criteria for assisted ventilation should be reviewed (Whelan and Vlahos, 2000). A dramatic improvement in the clinical status of these patients is seen after paracentesis. Thoracocentesis may be necessary for patients with significant hydrothorax. Interestingly, placement of a chest drainage tube for bilateral pleural effusion has facilitated resolution of abdominal ascites without the need for paracentesis (Rinaldi and Spirtos, 1995).

Conversely, Whelan and Vlahos (2000) treated a woman with severe OHSS complicated by complete right-sided hydrothorax that resolved almost completely within 48 h of transvaginal paracentesis and evacuation of ascites. I find these two cases very interesting and they complement each other.

Adult Respiratory Distress Syndrome

ARDS is encountered after fluid overload (Abramov et al., 1999b). Delvigne and Rozenberg (2003) stressed the importance of a strict fluid input/output balance in patients with moderate complications of OHSS and suggested the optimum management would be in an intensive care unit. ARDS subsides after three to six days with fluid restriction, forced diuresis and dopamine therapy (Delvigne and Rozenberg, 2003).

At the present time there is no therapeutic modality that would reverse the pathophysiologic changes that occur in OHSS that produce ARDS. The first priority is to reverse the life-threatening hypoxemia (Schenker, 1995). Positive end-expiratory pressure (PEEP) is the most supportive therapy (Zosmer et al., 1987).

Pericardiocentesis

Pericardial effusion was observed in 3% of 128 cases in the Belgian multi-center study (Delvigne et al., 1993). Drainage by specialists has been suggested (Brinsden et al., 1995; Delvigne and Rozenberg, 2003).

Thromboembolic Complications

Patients with evidence of thromboembolism will need therapeutic anti-coagulation with clinical monitoring of potential complications and laboratory adjustment of their anticoagulation therapy (Rizk, 1992, 1993).

ANESTHESIA CONSIDERATIONS IN OHSS PATIENTS

It is likely that patients admitted with severe OHSS may require surgery, such as laparoscopy, to treat large ovarian cysts or ectopic pregnancy, and paracentesis may even require intravenous sedation. There are several features of prime importance for the anesthesiologist (Table VIII.3) before treating such patients (Reed et al., 1990; Whelan and Vlahos, 2000). Careful positioning of the patients during surgery is important, as the Trendelenberg position may further compromise the residual pulmonary functional capacity. Establishment of access lines may be necessary in patients with contracted vascular volume. Drainage of pleural effusions may assist in improving the pulmonary status.

Table VIII.3 Challenges to the anesthesiologist in OHSS

- Pulmonary compromise
- Severe hemoconcentration
- Pleural effusions
- Restricted IV access
- Infections and febrile morbidity
- Difficult positioning in surgery
- Thrombophilia
- Pelvic masses
- Ascites
- Electrolyte disturbances

Table VIII.4 Indications for aspiration of ascites in OHSS

- Severe abdominal pain
- Pulmonary compromise
- Renal compromise resulting in oliguria
- Renal compromise resulting in an increase in creatinine concentration

ASPIRATION OF ASCITIC FLUID AND PLEURAL EFFUSION IN SEVERE OHSS

The presence of ascites is indeed the hallmark of ovarian hyperstimulation syndrome. In fact, symptoms resulting from ascites are often the most common reason for hospitalization. Aspiration is not indicated in every patient. Paracentesis by the transabdominal or transvaginal route is indicated for severe abdominal pain, pulmonary compromise as demonstrated by low pulsoximetry, and tachypnea and renal compromise as demonstrated by oliguria and increased creatinine concentration (Table VIII.4). Navot et al. (1992) suggested that paracentesis constitutes the single most important treatment modality in life-threatening OHSS not controlled by medical therapy. Familiarity with transabdominal and transvaginal ultrasound guided procedures is a prerequisite for the safe accomplishment of the removal of ascitic fluid (Rizk et al., 1990c).

Abdominal Paracentesis

Rabau et al. (1967) reported the first treatment with paracentesis of ascites associated with OHSS. Abdominal paracentesis has been considered controversial in the past but is no longer so. Thaler et al. (1981), in a case report, showed that paracentesis was followed by increased urinary output shortly after the procedure, with a concomitant decrease in the patient's weight, leg edema and abdominal circumference. They also showed that there was an increase of 50% in creatinine clearance rate following the procedure.

Bider et al. (1989a) treated 12 patients with severe OHSS, accompanied by a pleural effusion or ascites causing respiratory discomfort and dyspnea, by abdominal puncture. Drainage of abdominal or pleural effusion improved the symptoms in all patients. The amount of fluid aspirated ranged between 200 and 1400 ml. The risk of injury to an ovarian cyst was minimized by ultrasonographic guidance. Paracentesis offered temporary relief of respiratory distress, but, since the fluid tended to recur, some patients needed repeated paracentesis and drainage of effusions before spontaneous improvement ensued. The experience with this group of patients indicates that the actual risk of paracentesis is negligible. However, a possible drawback is the loss of fluid that is rich in proteins.

Levin et al. (2002) studied the effect of paracentesis of ascitic fluids on urinary output and blood indices in patients with severe OHSS. Paracentesis of ascitic fluids in women with severe OHSS had an isolated effect in improving renal function, as is evident by the increased urinary output and reduced blood urea nitrogen.

Padilla et al. (1990) demonstrated that abdominal paracentesis is a well-tolerated treatment to relieve severe pulmonary compromise caused by severe ascites and pleural effusion in OHSS. The improvement in renal function may be another benefit that deserves further investigation.

Peritoneal Catheter for the Drainage of Ascitic Fluid

Al-Ramahi et al. (1997) reported three cases in which an indwelling peritoneal catheter was used to decrease the need for repeated paracentesis. Under ultrasound guidance, a closed system Dawson—Mueller catheter with 'simp-loc' locking design was inserted to allow continuous drainage of the ascitic fluid. A total of 23, 20 and 28 l were subsequently aspirated from the three patients. There was a significant decrease in abdominal discomfort and improvement of urine output, with no complications. The only possible drawback to this technique would be depletion of a huge amount of plasma protein. We believe that monitoring of plasma proteins is essential if this treatment is applied, and human albumin should be infused whenever necessary. Abuzeid et al. (2003) studied the efficacy and safety of percutaneous pigtail catheter drainage for the management of ascites complicating severe OHSS. A pigtail catheter was inserted under transabdominal ultrasound guidance and kept in place until drainage ceased. Percutaneous placement of a pigtail catheter is a safe and effective treatment modality for severe OHSS. It may represent an attractive alternative to multiple vaginal or abdominal paracentesis.

Transvaginal Ultrasound-guided Aspiration

The aspiration of ascitic fluid by the transvaginal route was popularized by Aboulghar et al. (1990, 1992a, 1993). In a prospective randomized clinical trial, Aboulghar (1990) investigated the effects of transvaginal aspiration of ascitic fluid under sonographic guidance in patients with severe OHSS (Table VIII.5). The average hospital stay and the period with severe symptoms and disturbed electrolyte balance was much shorter in the group in which aspiration of ascitic fluid was performed, when compared with the group that underwent conservative treatment. Rizk and Aboulghar (1991) found that aspiration of the ascitic fluid immediately relieved the patients' symptoms, improved their general condition and increased urinary output. A marked improvement in the symptoms was noted after drainage of as little as 900 ml of ascitic fluid. There were no adverse hemodynamic effects as a result of the aspiration of large volumes of ascitic fluid (Table VIII.6). Replacement of the plasma proteins was mandatory because of the high protein content of ascitic fluid. This is essential, as repeated aspiration was required in 30% of patients. The rate of accumulation of ascitic fluid varied significantly. However, reaccumulation of a large volume of ascitic fluid sufficient to cause discomfort would require, on average, 3–5 days.

Rizk and Abdalla (2006) urged early and prompt management of ascitic fluid. Aboulghar et al. (1993) assessed the value of intravenous fluid therapy and ascitic fluid aspiration in the management of severe OHSS. Forty-two women with severe OHSS were treated by ultrasonically guided transvaginal aspiration of ascitic fluid and intravenous fluid infusion. Ten women with the same condition treated conservatively constituted a comparison group. The main outcome measures included percentage change in hematocrit, creatinine clearance and urine output before and after aspiration. The duration of hospital stay was

Table VIII.5 Clinical characteristics of 21 patients hospitalized for severe OHSS
Reproduced with permission from Aboulghar et al. (1990). Fertil Steril **53**:933–5

	Group A	Group B
Total no. patients	10	11
Age*	29.8 ± 4.1	31.9 ± 5.5
Indication for ovulation induction		
polycystic ovarian disease	3	4
IVF**	5	6
amenorrhea	2	1
Stimulation protocol		
CC/hMG/hCG**	5	7
Serum estradiol on admission* (pg/ml)	6400 ± 2100	6900 ± 4500

* Values are expressed as means ± SD
** IVF-in vitro fertilization; CC = clomiphene citrate; hMG = human menopausal gonadotropin; hCG = human chorionic gonadotropin

Table VIII.6 Analysis of aspirated ascitic fluid.
Clinical characteristics of 21 patients hospitalized
for severe OHSS.
Reproduced with permission from Aboulghar et al.
(1990). Fertil Steril **53***:933–5*

Total proteins (mg/100 ml)	4.7 ± 2.2 (3.2 – 5.1)
Estradiol (pg/ml)	6500 ± 1554 (5400 – 9500)
Sodium (mEq/l)	132 ± 11 (120 – 145)
Potassium (mEq/l)	4.1 ± 1.2 (3.8 – 4.7)

compared between the groups. Marked improvement of symptoms and general condition followed soon after aspiration. Hematocrit readings decreased by 22%, creatinine clearance increased by 79.3% and urine output increased by 220.7%. The average volume of aspirated fluid was 3900 ml. The average duration of hospital stay was 3.8 days for the treated women. In the comparison group, severe symptoms and electrolyte imbalance continued for an average of nine days, and the average hospital stay was 11 days. Intensive intravenous fluid therapy and transvaginal aspiration of ascitic fluid are safe and effective in improving symptoms, preventing complications and shortening the hospital stay in severe OHSS.

Transvaginal ultrasound-guided aspiration is an effective and safe procedure. Injury to the ovary is easily avoided by puncture under ultrasonic visualization. No anesthesia is required for the procedure, and better drainage of the ascitic fluid is accomplished because the pouch of Douglas is the most dependent part (Rizk and Aboulghar, 1991; Rizk et al., 1990b, c).

Autotransfusion of Ascitic Fluid

Autoreinfusion of aspirated ascitic fluid has been suggested by several investigators (Aboulghar et al., 1992a; Fukaya et al., 1994; Splendiani et al., 1994; Beck et al., 1995). Aboulghar et al. (1992a) reported three cases of severe OHSS treated by transvaginal aspiration of the ascitic fluid and autotransfusion of the aspirated fluid. Marked improvement of the symptoms, general condition and urine output followed shortly after the aspiration. No reactions were noted during or after the autotransfusion. The blood parameters were corrected, and the general condition and urine output continued to improve. The procedure is simple, safe and straightforward, and shows a striking physiological success in correcting the maldistribution of fluid and proteins without the use of heterogenous biological material. To avoid transfusion of concentrated large volumes and bacteria and cells, Fukaya et al. (1994) used ultrafiltration with two filters: a cellulose acetate hollow fiber filter that removes the cells and bacteria, and a polyacrylonitrile hollow fiber ultra filter that concentrates the protein before the infusion. The protein concentration obtained is increased two-fold and albumin five-fold. Fluid is reinfused

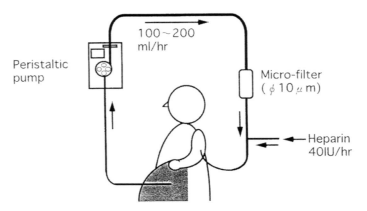

Fig. VIII.3: The continuous autotransfusion system of ascites (CATSA)
Reproduced with permission from Koike, Araki, Minakami et al. (2000).
Hum Reprod **15**:113–7

intravenously at the rate of 300–500 ml every 6 h. However, we do not recommend autotransfusion of ascitic fluid because of the possible reinjection of cytokines into the circulation.

Peritoneovenous Shunting of Ascitic Fluid in Severe OHSS

Peritoneovenous shunting has been performed in patients with ascites as a result of liver cirrhosis (Gines et al., 1991) and has also been reported in isolated cases of severe OHSS by Splendiani et al. (1994) and Beck et al. (1995). Koike et al. (2000) investigated prospectively the clinical efficacy of a newly developed continuous autotransfusion system of ascites (CATSA, Figure VIII.3) without protein supplement in patients with severe OHSS. CATSA was performed for 5 h at a rate of 100–200 ml/h once a day. Eighteen patients were treated with the CATSA (CATSA group) and 36 were treated with an intravenous 37.5 g/day of albumin supplement (albumin group). Hospital stay was significantly shorter in the CATSA group than in the albumin group (10.0 ± 5.7 vs 13.9 ± 6.2 days, $p < 0.01$). Using a single procedure, haemo-concentration, urinary output and pulse pressure were markedly improved in the CATSA group compared with the albumin group. Discomfort due to massive ascites diminished promptly and did not recur in nine of 18 CATSA group patients, whereas it persisted in all 36 patients in the albumin group. The serum concentration of protein was maintained in the CATSA group, whereas it did not increase in the albumin group despite daily supplementation with 37.5 g of albumin. The mean values of several parameters in the serum pertinent to the coagulation-fibrinolysis system did not change significantly in either group after the procedure. It was concluded that the CATSA procedure expanded circulating plasma volume without exogenous albumin and appeared to lead to a prompt recovery from severe conditions of OHSS.

Cytokine levels in a patient with severe OHSS before and after the ultrafiltration and reinfusion of ascitic fluid showed that cytokine concentrations decline in parallel with the improvement of clinical conditions and resolution of OHSS.

SURGICAL TREATMENT

Surgery for Ruptured Cysts

Rizk (1993) stated that laparotomy, in general, should be avoided in OHSS. The ovaries are enlarged, cystic and friable (Figure VIII.4). If deemed necessary, in cases of hemorrhage, it should be performed by an experienced gynecologist and only hemostatic measures undertaken to preserve the ovaries (Rizk, 1992, 1993a). Bider et al. (1989a) reported operative procedures in 16 patients with severe OHSS because of torsion, rupture and bleeding in the ovarian cysts. Amarin (2003) reported two cases of severe OHSS that did not respond to conservative treatment. Bilateral partial oophorectomy was performed at

Fig. VIII.4: Rupture of follicular and corpus luteal cysts in a case of severe OHSS
Reproduced with permission from Wallach, Zacur, Eds (1995). Reproductive Medicine and Surgery. St. Louis: Mosby, Chapter 35, p. 654

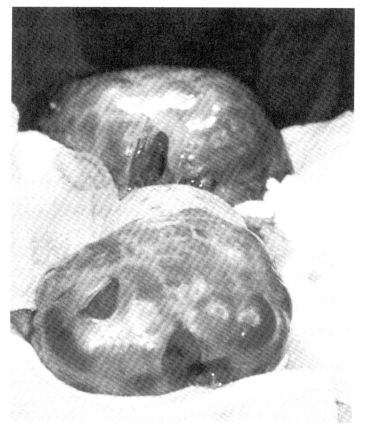

14 and 16 days respectively from oocyte retrieval. The patient made a rapid recovery. The author proposed this seemingly aggressive prodedure as a potential useful treatment when faced with patients who are severely or critically affected with OHSS. We and others believe that this is a very unfavorable approach and should be avoided (Rizk, 1993).

Unwinding of Twisted Ovary

Torsion of the ovary may be encountered by the gynecologist in cases of acute abdominal pain in patients with an ovarian cyst, in pregnancy or in the puerperium. Most general gynecologists used to remove the ovary and avoid untwisting the ovarian pedicles because of concern about thromboembolism, while most reproductive endocrinologists and reproductive surgeons attempt unwinding of the twisted ovary.

Adnexal torsion was encountered in two cases in 2945 IVF cycles in a Dutch transport IVF group (Roest et al., 1996). Hurwitz et al. (1983) reported the first case of unwinding of a cystic ovary which had undergone torsion in a patient with OHSS. The patient was admitted 10 days after hCG complaining of lower abdominal distension and pain accompanied by nausea and vomiting. On the fourth day following admission, the patient developed signs of a surgical abdomen and the diagnosis of twisted ovary was made at laparotomy. The pregnancy continued to term, resulting in a normal twin delivery. Since then, several reports have shown that unwinding of the ischemic and apparently nonviable ovary by laparotomy (Bider et al., 1989b; Mashiach et al., 1990) or laparoscopy (Mage et al., 1989; Ben-Rafael et al., 1990) can restore the blood supply to the ovary.

Ovarian Torsion in Pregnancy

Mashiach et al. (1990) reported twelve pregnant women who presented with torsion of hyperstimulated ovaries. Although the adnexa appeared dark, hemorrhagic and ischemic, they suggested that it could be saved by simply unwinding it. Professor Mashiach's team has now performed over 100 cases with success (Mashiach, personal communication). During the second trimester of pregnancy, Levy et al. (1995) reported successful unwinding of large, hyperstimulated ischemic—hemorrhagic adnexa by laparoscopy in three women.

Surgery for Ectopic, Bilateral Ectopic and Abdominal Pregnancy and OHSS

The association between OHSS and ectopic, bilateral ectopic, heterotopic and abdominal pregnancies are not commonly encountered (Rizk et al., 1990d, e, 1991b). Abnormal hCG levels may occur in early pregnancy in patients with ovarian hyperstimulation syndrome. However, these abnormal levels do not predict poor outcome in pregnancies complicated by OHSS (Abramov et al.,

1998b; Samuel and Grosskinsky, 2004), therefore they are not helpful in diagnosing ectopic pregnancy or otherwise compromised pregnancies.

Chotiner (1985) reported the non-surgical management of ectopic pregnancy associated with severe OHSS. Aboulghar et al. (1992b) treated surgically a case of severe OHSS complicated by ectopic pregnancy. The diagnosis of ectopic pregnancy in this case was difficult because internal bleeding occurred when the patient was already complaining of severe OHSS and the amount of blood loss was not severe enough to be reflected in her general condition. Diagnosis of tubal pregnancy by vaginal ultrasound examination at this stage is not always possible. The presence of large ovaries filling the pelvis makes ultrasound scanning of other structures difficult. Fluid in the pouch of Douglas is a sign of the presence of ascites. Shiau et al. (2004) described a case of severe OHSS coexisting with a bilateral ectopic pregnancy. A rare case of primary abdominal pregnancy that was detected after rapid resolution of OHSS has been reported by Nakamura et al. (2001). While we have rarely encountered OHSS associated with tubal, bilateral ectopic, ovarian, heterotopic or abdominal pregnancies, we caution that all IVF pregnancies should be screened carefully for these rare combinations (Rizk et al., 1990d, e, 1991b).

Gastrointestinal Surgery

Mesenteric resection after massive arterial infarction has been reported (Aurousseau et al., 1995). Perforated duodenal ulcer attributed to *Helicobacter pylori* in connection with the intense stress linked to critical OHSS has also been reported (Uhler et al., 2001). Perforated appendicitis and peritonitis has also been documented (Fujimoto et al., 2002).

Vascular Surgery

Vascular surgery is rarely required to treat thromboses that are complicated by recurrent emboli or resistant to medical intervention. Posterolateral thoracotomy and subclavian arteriotomy and thromboarterectomy by the Fogarthy technique have been reported (Aurousseau et al., 1995; Choktanasiri and Rojanasakul, 1995; Germond et al., 1996). Inferior vena cava interruption to prevent massive thromboembolism has been used by Mozes et al. (1965).

Pregnancy Termination

Pregnancy termination has been paradoxically performed in extreme cases and has improved the clinical picture of neurological, hematological and vascular complications (Dumont et al., 1980; Neau et al., 1989; Aurousseau et al., 1995; Choktanasiri and Rozanasakul, 1995; Ryo et al., 1999; Southgate et al., 1999; Yoshii et al., 1999; Shan Tang et al., 2000).

NOVEL MEDICAL TREATMENT FOR OHSS

A wide array of novel ideas for the treatment of OHSS are currently being investigated (Rizk and Nawar, 2004; Rizk and Aboulghar, 2005; Rizk et al., 1997).

Blocking VEGFR-2

VEGF plays a central role in the pathogenesis of OHSS. Therefore, the role of VEGF function inhibitors as potential drugs for the treatment of the syndrome has been explored. The initial studies in this area came from the field of oncogenesis, where it has been demonstrated that the inhibition of VEGF signal transduction can inhibit tumor progression (Kim et al., 1993). These studies were followed by other investigations that indicated that inhibition of VEGF signaling inhibits many types of tumors (Neufeld et al., 1999).

Gomez et al., (2002) developed an in-vivo murine model to induce OHSS and considered the two main characteristics of ovarian enlargement and increased vascular permeability leading to ascites. They investigated the hormonal conditions leading to OHSS, the involvement of VEGF in the development of the syndrome, the tissue sources of VEGF and specific VEGF isoforms involving OHSS. They tested a new strategy for the prevention and treatment of OHSS by blocking VEGFR-2 to inhibit vascular permeability.

SU5416 is a novel synthetic compound that was developed to inhibit KDR signaling in different cancers by avoiding the initial VEGFR-2 phosphorylation. SU5416 treatment does not affect surface expression or the affinity of the receptor for VEGF. In fact, the durability of the SU5416 activity is attributed to its long-lasting ability to inhibit VEGF-dependent phosphorylation of flk-1/KDR and subsequent downstream signaling. SU5416 is not an irreversible inhibitor of flk-1/KDR tyrosine kinase (Mendel et al., 2000). The authors observed that, although the flk-1/KDR is upregulated in the gonadotropin-treated animals, the massive doses of SU5416 administered prevented the possibility of any effect due to upregulation (Fong et al., 1999).

The authors observed that the administration of SU5416 during ovarian stimulation with PMSG but not after the hCG injection was unable to block increasing permeability (Figure VIII.5). This finding agrees with the observation that OHSS appears during the luteal phase after hCG administration. It also suggests that the temporary inhibition of VEGFR-2 previous to hCG injection is not a valid strategy to avoid the onset of OHSS. Its injection after hCG effectively reversed the increased vascular permeability (Figure VIII.5), and their observations not only support the role of VEGF in OHSS but also provide new insights and strategies to prevent and treat the syndrome based on pathophysiologic mechanisms.

Anti-VEGF antibody

A novel potential approach is the anti-VEGF antibody available as a recombinant human monoclonal antibody from Genentech in San Francisco, CA,

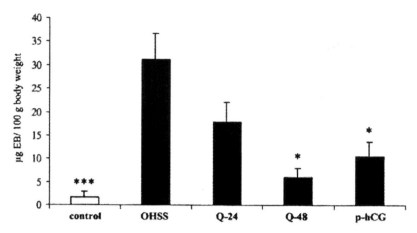

Fig. VIII.5: Vascular permeability is significantly inhibited after SU5416 administration after hCG injection
Reproduced with permission from Gomez, Simon, Remohi et al. (2002). Endocrinology ***143****:4339– 48*

under the brand name Avastin (Meldrum, 2002; Jain, 2002; McDonough, 2003).

Cabergoline for Treatment of OHSS

Dopamine (D_2) has been thought to be able to block VEGFR-2 phosphorylation which is the first step in VEGFR-2 downstream signaling. Gomez-Gallego et al. (2005) investigated whether the dopamine (D_2) agonist cabergoline could block vascular permeability in OHSS and if these inhibitory effects were related to decreased VEGFR-2 phosphorylation. They have utilized the same protocol for ovarian stimulation used to study OHSS in rats (see Chapter III, the role of progesterone in OHSS): hCG was given on day 26, and prolactin pellets 5 mg were implanted in OHSS rats to avoid functional luteolysis by the administration of cabergoline 3 μg and 6 μg, 24 h later on day 27. Vascular permeability was measured and quantified as the extravasation of a previously injected dye and expressed as μg extravased dye per 100 g body weight. The presence of functional luteolysis was evaluated by the assessment of progesterone by ELISA and prolactin by radioimmunoassay. To study VEGFR-2 phosphorylation, VEGFR-2 was previously immunoprecipitated from whole ovarian extracts and then Western blot testing was performed using a phosphotyrosine antibody to detect phosphorylated VEGFR-2. The receptor phosphorylation was expressed as phosphorylated VEGFR-2/VEGFR-2(total). Vascular permeability in the cabergoline-treated rats was significantly lower compared with the cabergoline-untreated rats. In fact, the vascular permeability factors corresponded to the decrease in VEGFR-2 phosphorylation in the cabergoline treated rats compared with the untreated rats (63% and 83% in the 3 μg and 6 μg cabergoline groups). There were no luteolytic effects observed. Gomez-Gallego et al. (2005) concluded that cabergoline is able to inhibit vascular permeability in OHSS. These inhibitory effects are related to VEGFR-2 downstream signaling blockade and not to luteolytic effects. Gomez-Gallego et al. (2005) suggested that cabergoline is a non-toxic as well as a specific approach to effectively treat OHSS.

REFERENCES

Aboulghar MA, Mansour RT, Serour GI et al. (1990). Ultrasonically guided vaginal aspiration of ascites in the treatment of ovarian hyperstimulation syndrome. *Fertil Steril* **53**:933–5.

Aboulghar MA, Mansour RT, Serour GI et al. (1992a). Autotransfusion of the ascitic fluid in the treatment of severe ovarian hyperstimulation syndrome (OHSS). *Fertil Steril* **58**:1056–9.

Aboulghar MA, Mansour RT, Serour GI et al. (1992b). Severe ovarian hyperstimulation syndrome complicated by ectopic pregnancy. *Acta Obstet Gynecol Scand* **70**:371–2.

Aboulghar MA, Mansour RT, Serour GI et al. (1993). Management of severe ovarian hyperstimulation syndrome by ascitic fluid aspiration and intensive intravenous fluid therapy. *Obstet Gynecol* **81**:108–1.

Abramov Y, Elchalal U & Schenker JG (1998a). Febrile morbidity in severe and critical ovarian hyperstimulation syndrome: a multicentre study. *Hum Reprod* **13**:2088–91.

Abramov Y, Elchalal U & Schenker JG (1998b). Obstetric outcome of in-vitro fertilized pregnancies complicated by severe ovarian hyperstimulation syndrome: a multicenter study. *Fertil Steril* **70**:1070–6.

Abramov Y, Naparstek Y, Elchalal U et al. (1999a). Plasma immunoglobulins in patients with severe ovarian hyperstimulation syndrome. *Fertil Steril* **71**:102–5.

Abramov Y, Elchalal U & Schenker JG (1999b). Pulmonary manifestations of severe ovarian hyperstimulation syndrome: a multicenter study. *Fertil Steril* **71**:645–51.

Abramov Y, Fatum M, Abrahomov D et al. (2001). Hydroxyethyl starch versus human albumin for the treatment of severe ovarian hyperstimulatin syndrome: a preliminary report. *Fertil Steril* **75**:1228–30.

Abuzeid MI, Nassar Z, Massaad Z et al. (2003). Pigtail catheter for the treatment of ascites associated with ovarian hyperstimulation syndrome. *Hum Reprod* **18**:370–3.

Al-Ramahi M, Leader A, Claman P et al. (1997). A novel approach to the treatment of ascites associated with ovarian hyperstimulation syndrome. *Hum Reprod* **12**:2614–16.

Amarin ZO (2003). Bilateral partial oophorectomy in the management of severe ovarian hyperstimulation syndrome. An aggressive, but perhaps life-saving procedure. *Hum Reprod* **4**:659–64.

Aurousseau MH, Samama MM, Belhassen A et al. (1995). Risk of thromboembolism in relation to an in-vitro fertilization programme: three case reports. *Hum Reprod* **10**:94–7.

Balasch J, Carmona F, Llach J et al. (1990). Acute prerenal failure and liver dysfunction in a patient with severe ovarian hyperstimulation syndrome. *Hum Reprod* **5**:348–51.

Beck DH, Massey S, Taylor BL et al. (1995). Continuous ascitic recirculation in severe ovarian hyperstimulation syndrome. *Intensive Care Med* **21**:590–3.

Ben-Rafael Z, Bider D & Mashiach S (1990). Laparoscopic unwinding of twisted ischemic hemorrhagic adnexa after in vitro fertilization. *Fertil Steril* **53**:569–71.

Bider D, Menashe Y, Oelsner G et al. (1989a). Ovarian hyperstimulation syndrome due to exogenous gonadotrophin administration. *Acta Obstet Gynecol Scand* **68**:511–14.

Bider D, Ben-Rafael Z, Goldenberg M et al. (1989b). Pregnancy outcome after unwinding of twisted ischemic-hemorrhagic adnexa. *Br J Obstet Gynaecol* **96**:428–30.

Borenstein R, Elhalah U, Lunenfeld B & Schwartz ZS (1989). Severe ovarian hyperstimulation syndrome: a reevaluated therapeutic approach. *Fertil Steril* **51**:791−5.

Brinsden PR, Wada I, Tan SL et al. (1995). Diagnosis, prevention and management of ovarian hyperstimulation syndrome. *Br J Obstet and Gynecol* **102**:767−72.

Choktanasiri W & Rojanasakul A (1995). Acute arterial thrombosis after gamete intrafallopian transfer: a case report. *J Assist Reprod Genet* **12**:335−7.

Chotiner HC (1985). Nonsurgical management of ectopic pregnancy associated with severe hyperstimulation syndrome. *Obstet Gynecol* **66**:740−3.

Cil T, Tummon IS, House AA et al. (2000). A tale of two syndromes: ovarian hyperstimulation syndrome and abdominal compartment. *Hum Reprod* **15**:1058−60.

Delvigne A (2004). Epidemiology and pathophysiology of ovarian hyperstimulation syndrome. In (Gerris J, Olivennes F, de Sutter P, Eds), *Assisted Reproductive Technologies.* New York: Parthenon Publishing, Chapter 12, pp. 149−62.

Delvigne A & Rozenberg S (2003). Review of clinical course and treatment of ovarian hyperstimulation syndrome (OHSS). *Hum Reprod Update* **9**:77−96.

Delvigne A, Demoulin A, Smitz J et al. (1993). The ovarian hyperstimulation syndrome in in-vitro fertilization: a Belgian multicentric study. I. Clinical and biological features. *Hum Reprod* **8**:1353−60.

Dumont M, Combet A & Domenichini Y (1980). Cerebral arterial thrombosis following ovarian hyperstimulation and sextuple pregnancy. Therapeutic abortion. *Nouv Presse Med* **13**:3628−9.

Fabregues F, Balasch J, Gines P et al. (1999). Ascites and liver test abnormalities during severe ovarian hyperstimulation syndrome. *Am J Gastroenterol* **94**:994−9.

Felder RA, Blecher M & Eisner GM (1984). Cortical tubular and glomerular dopamine receptors in the rat kidney. *Am J Physiol* **246**:557−61.

Ferraretti AP, Gianaroli L, Diotallevi L et al. (1992). Dopamine treatment for severe hyperstimulation syndrome. *Hum Reprod* **7**:180−3.

Fluker MR, Copeland JE & Yuzpe AA (2000). An ounce of prevention: outpatient management of the ovarian hyperstimulation syndrome. *Fertil Steril* **73**:821−4.

Fong TA, Shawver LK, Sun L et al. (1999). SU5416 is a potent and selective inhibitor of the vascular endothelial growth factor receptor (Flk-1/KDR) that inhibits tyrosine kinase catalysis, tumor vascularization, and growth of multiple tumor types. *Cancer Res* **59**:99−106.

Fujimoto A, Osuga Y, Yano T et al. (2002). Ovarian hyperstimulation syndrome complicated by peritonitis due to perforated appendicitis: Case Report. *Hum Reprod* **17**:966−7.

Fukaya T, Chida S, Terada Y et al. (1994). Treatment of severe ovarian hyperstimulation syndrome by ultrafiltration and reinfusion of ascitic fluid. *Fertil Steril* **61**:561−4.

Gamzu R, Almog B, Levin Y et al. (2002). Efficacy of hydroxyethyl starch and Haemaccel for the treatment of severe ovarian hyperstimulation syndrome. *Fertil Steril* **77**:1302−3.

Germond M, Wirthner D, Thorin D et al. (1996). Aorto-subclavian thromboembolism: a rare complication associated with moderate ovarian hyperstimulation syndrome. *Hum Reprod* **11**:1173−6.

Gines P, Arroyo V, Vargas V et al. (1991). Paracentesis with intravenous infusion of albumin as compared with peritoneovenous shunting in cirrhosis with refractory ascites. *N Engl J Med* **325**:829−35.

Gomez R, Simon C, Remohi J & Pellicer A (2002). Vascular endothelial growth factor receptor-2 activation induces vascular permeability in hyperstimulated rats and this effect is prevented by receptor blockade. *Endocrinol* **143**:4339−48.

Gomez-Gallego R, Gonzalez M, Alonso-Muriel I et al. (2005). Cabergoline administration is a non-toxic and specific approach to effectively treat OHSS. *J Soc Gyn Invest* **12**(Suppl) Abstract 324: 188A−9A.

Gustofson P, Browne RL & Van Nest KS (2005). Aggressive outpatient management of severe ovarian hyperstimulation syndrome avoids complications and prolonged disease course. *Fertil Steril* **84**(Suppl 1):S95—230.

Haning RV, Strawn EY & Nolten WE (1985). Pathophysiology of the ovarian hyperstimulation syndrome. *Obstet Gynecol* **66**:220—4.

Hortskamp B, Lubke M, Kentenich H et al. (1996). Internal jugular vein thrombosis caused by resistance to activated protein C as a complication of ovarian hyperstimulation after in-vitro fertilization. *Hum Reprod* **11**:280—2.

Hurwitz A, Milwidsky A, Yagel S et al. (1983). Early unwinding of torsion of an ovarian cyst as a result of hyperstimulation syndrome. *Fertil Steril* **40**:393—4.

Ito M, Harada T, Iwabe T et al. (2000). Cytokine levels in a patient with severe ovarian hyperstimulation syndrome before and after the ultrafiltration and reinfusion of ascitic fluid. *J Assist Reprod Genet* **17**:118—20.

Jain RK (2002). Tumor angiogenesis and accessibility: role of vascular endothelial growth factor. *Semin Oncol* **29**(Suppl 16):3—9.

Katz Z, Lancet M, Borenstein R et al. (1984). Absence of teratogenicity of indomethacin in ovarian hyperstimulation syndrome. *Int J Fertil* **29**:186—8.

Kim KJ, Li B, Winer J et al. (1993). Inhibition of vascular endothelial growth factor induced angiogenesis suppresses tumour growth in vivo. *Nature (London)* **362**:841—4.

Kirshon B, Lee W, Mauer MB et al. (1988). Effects of low-dose dopamine therapy in the oliguric patient with preeclampsia. *Am J Obstet Gynecol* **159**:604—7.

Kissler S, Neidhardt B, Siebzehnrubl E et al. (2001). The detrimental role of colloidal volume substitutes in severe ovarian hyperstimulation syndrome: a case report. *Eur J Obstet Gynecol Reprod Biol* **99**:131—4.

Koike T, Araki S, Minakami H et al. (2000). Clinical efficacy of peritoneovenous shunting for the treatment of severe ovarian hyperstimulation syndrome. *Hum Reprod* **15**:113—17.

Levin I, Almog B, Avni A et al. (2002). Effect of paracentesis of ascitic fluids on urinary output and blood indices in patients with severe ovarian hyperstimulation syndrome. *Fertil Steril* **77**:986—8.

Levy T, Dicker D, Shalev J et al. (1995). Laparoscopic unwinding of hyperstimulated ischaemic ovaries during the second trimester of pregnancy. *Hum Reprod* **10**:1478—80.

Lincoln SR, Opasahl MS, Blauer KL et al. (2002). Aggressive outpatient treatment of ovarian hyperstimulation syndrome with ascites using transvaginal culdocentesis and intravenous albumin minimizes hospitalization. *J Assist Reprod Genet* **19**:159—63.

Mage G, Canis M, Manhes H et al. (1989). Laparoscopic management of adnexal torsion. A review of 35 cases. *J Reprod Med* **34**:520—4.

Mashiach S, Bider D, Moran O et al. (1990). Adnexal torsion of hyperstimulated ovaries in pregnancies after gonadotrophin therapy. *Fertil Steril* **53**:76—80.

McDonough P (2003). Vascular endothelial growth factor-mediator of OHSS? *Fertil Steril* **79**:1466—7.

Meldrum RD (2002). Vascular endothelial growth factor, polycystic ovary syndrome, and ovarian hyperstimulation syndrome. *Fertil Steril* **78**:1170—1.

Mendel DB, Schreck RE, West DC et al. (2000). The angiogenesis inhibitor SU5416 has long-lasting effects on vascular endothelial growth factor receptor phosphorylation and function. *Clin Cancer Res* **6**:4848—58.

Mozes M, Bogowsky H, Anteby E et al. (1965). Thrombo-embolic phenomena after ovarian stimulation with human menopausal gonadotrophins. *Lancet* **2**:1213—15.

Nakamura Y, Muso A, Toduyama O et al. (2001). Primary abdominal pregnancy associated with severe ovarian hyperstimulation syndrome. *Arch Gynecol Obstet* **265**:233—5.

Navot D, Bergh PA & Laufer N (1992). Ovarian hyperstimulation syndrome in novel reproductive technologies: prevention and treatment. *Fertil Steril* **58**:249—61.

Neau JP, Marechaud M, Guitton P et al. (1989). Occlusion of the middle cerebral artery after induction of ovulation with gonadotropins. *Rev Neurol (Paris)* **145**:859−61.

Neufeld G, Cohen T, Gengrinovitch S et al. (1999). Vascular endothelial growth factor (VEGF) and its receptors. *The FASEB Journal* **13**:9−22.

Padilla SL, Zamaria S, Baramki TA et al. (1990). Abdominal paracentesis for the ovarian hyperstimulation syndrome with severe pulmonary compromise. *Fertil Steril* **53**:365−7.

Practice Committee of the American Society for Reproductive Medicine (2003). Ovarian hyperstimulation syndrome. *Fertil Steril* **80**:1309−14.

Pride SM, Yuen BH, Moon YS & Leung PCS (1986). The relationship of gonadotrophin releasing hormone, danazol and prostaglandin blockade to ovarian hyperstimulation syndrome in the rabbit. *Am J Obstet Gynecol* **154**:1155−60.

Rabau E, Serr DM, David A et al. (1967). Human menopausal gonadotrophin for anovulation and sterility. *Am J Obstet Gynecol* **98**:92−8.

Rabinerson D, Shalev J, Roybury M et al. (2000). Severe unilateral hydrothorax as the only maifestation of the ovarian hyperstimulation syndrome. *Gynecol Obstet Invest* **49**:140−2.

Reed AP, Tausk H & Reynolds H (1990). Anesthetic considerations for severe ovarian hyperstimulation syndrome. *Anesthesiology* **73**:1275−7.

Rinaldi ML & Spirtos NJ (1995). Chest tube drainage of pleural effusion correcting abdominal ascites in a patient with severe ovarian hyperstimulation syndrome: a case report. *Fertil Steril* **63**:1114−17.

Rizk B (1992). Ovarian hyperstimulation syndrome. In (Brinsden PR, Rainsbury PA, Eds), *A Textbook of In-vitro Fertilization and Assisted Reproduction*. Carnforth, UK: Parthenon Publishing, Chapter 23, pp. 369−83.

Rizk B (1993). Ovarian hyperstimulation syndrome. In (Studd J, Ed.), *Progress in Obstetrics and Gynecology*. Edinburgh: Churchill Livingstone, Vol. 11, Chapter 18, pp. 311−49.

Rizk B (2001). Ovarian hyperstimulation syndrome: prediction, prevention and management. In (Rizk B, Devroey P, Meldrum DR, Eds), *Advances and Controversies in Ovulation Induction*. 34th ASRM Annual Postgraduate Program, Middle East Fertility Society. ASRM, 57th Annual Meeting, Orlando, FL, Birmingham, Alabama: American Society for Reproductive Medicine, pp. 23−46.

Rizk B (2002). Can OHSS in ART be eliminated? In (Rizk B, Meldrum D, Schoolcraft W, Eds), *A Clinical Step-by-Step Course for Assisted Reproductive Technologies*. 35th ASRM Annual Postgraduate Program, Middle East Fertility Society. ASRM, 58th Annual Meeting, Seattle, WA, Birmingham, Alabama: American Society for Reproductive Medicine, pp. 65−102.

Rizk B & Abdalla H (2006). Ovulatory dysfunction and ovulation induction. In (Rizk B, Abdalla H, Eds), *Infertility and Assisted Reproductive Technology*. Oxford, UK: Health Press, pp. 39−59.

Rizk B & Aboulghar M (1991). Modern management of ovarian hyperstimulation syndrome. *Hum Reprod* **6**:1082−7.

Rizk B & Aboulghar MA (1999). Classification, pathophysiology and management of ovarian hyperstimulation syndrome. In (Brinsden P, Ed.), *A Textbook of In-vitro Fertilization and Assisted Reproduction*, Second Edition. Carnforth, UK: The Parthenon Publishing Group, Chapter 9, pp. 131−55.

Rizk B & Aboulghar MA (2005). Classification, pathophysiology and management of ovarian hyperstimulation syndrome. In (Brinsden P, Ed.), *A Textbook of In-vitro Fertilization and Assisted Reproduction*. New York and London: Parthenon Publishing, Chapter 12, pp. 217−58.

Rizk B & Nawar MG (2004). Ovarian hyperstimulation syndrome. In (Serhal P, Overton C, Eds), *Good Clinical Practice in Assisted Reproduction*. Cambridge, UK: Cambridge University Press, Chapter 8, pp. 146−66.

Rizk B & Smitz J (1992). Ovarian hyperstimulation syndrome after superovulation for IVF and related procedures. *Hum Reprod* **7**:320–7.

Rizk B, Meagher S & Fisher AM (1990a). Ovarian hyperstimulation syndrome and cerebrovascular accidents. *Hum Reprod* **5**:697–8.

Rizk B, Tan SL, Kingsland CR et al. (1990b). Ovarian cyst aspiration and the outcome of in vitro fertilization. *Fertil Steril* **54**:661–4.

Rizk B, Stear C, Tan SL & Mason BA (1990c). Vaginal versus abdominal ultrasound guided retrieval in IVF. *Br J Rad* **63**:388–9.

Rizk B, Morcos S, Avery S et al. (1990d). Rare ectopic pregnancies after in-vitro fertilization: one unilateral twin and four bilateral tubal pregnancies. *Hum Reprod* **5**:1025–8.

Rizk B, Lachelin GCL, Davies MC et al. (1990e). Ovarian pregnancy following in vitro fertilization and embryo transfer. *Hum Reprod* **5**:763–4.

Rizk B, Aboulghar MA, Mansour RT et al. (1991a). Severe ovarian hyperstimulation syndrome: analytical study of twenty-one cases. Proceedings of the VII World Congress on In-vitro Fertilization and Assisted Procreations, Paris. *Hum Reprod*: S368–9.

Rizk B, Tan SL, Morcos S et al. (1991b). Heterotopic pregnancies after in-vitro fertilizations and embryo transfer. *Am J Obstet Gynecol* **164**:161–4.

Rizk B, Aboulghar MA, Smitz J & Ron-El R (1997). The role of vascular endothelial growth factor and interleukins in the pathogenesis of severe ovarian hyperstimulation syndrome. *Hum Reprod Update* **3**:255–66.

Roest J, Mous H, Zeilmaker G et al. (1996). The incidence of major clinical complications in a Dutch transport IVF programme. *Hum Reprod Update* **2**:345–53.

Ryo E, Hagino D, Yano N et al. (1999). A case of ovarian hyperstimulation syndrome in which antithrombin III deficiency occurred because of its loss into ascites. *Fertil Steril* **71**:860–2.

Salat-Baroux J, Alvarez S, Antoine JM et al. (1990). Treatment of hyperstimulation during in-vitro fertilization. *Hum Reprod* **5**:36–39.

Samuel MJ & Gjrosskinsky CM (2004). Abnormal human chorionic gonadotropin levels and normal pregnancy outcomes in the ovarian hyperstimulation syndrome. *J. Reprod Med* **49**:8–12.

Schenker JG (1995). Ovarian hyperstimulation syndrome. In (Wallach EE, Zacur HA, Eds), *Reproductive Medicine and Surgery*. St. Louis: Mosby Publishing, Chapter 35, pp. 649–79.

Schenker JG & Polishuk WZ (1976). The role of prostaglandins in ovarian hyperstimulation syndrome. *Eur J Obstet Gynecol Reprod Biol* **6**:47–52.

Serour GI, Aboulghar M, Mansour R et al. (1998). Complications of medically assisted conception in 3,500 cycles. *Fertil Steril* **70**:638–42.

Shan Tang O, Ng E, Wai Cheng P et al. (2000). Cortical vein thrombosis misinterpreted as intracranial haemorrhage in severe ovarian hyperstimulation syndrome. *Hum Reprod* **15**:1913–16.

Shapiro AG, Thomas T & Epstein M (1977). Management of hyperstimulation syndrome. *Fertil Steril* **28**:237–9.

Shiau CS, Chang MY, Chiang CH et al. (2004). Severe ovarian hyperstimulation syndrome coexisting with a bilateral ectopic pregnancy. *Chang Gung Med J.* **27**:143–7.

Shrivastav P, Nadkarni P & Craft I (1994). Daycare management of severe ovarian hyperstimulation syndrome avoids hospitalization and morbidity. *Hum Reprod* **9**:812–14.

Southgate HJ, Anderson SK, Lavies NG et al. (1999). Pseudocholinesterase deficiency: a dangerous, unrecognized complication of the ovarian hyperstimulation syndrome. *Ann Clin Biochem* **36**:256–8.

Splendiani G, Mazzarella B, Tozzo C et al. (1994). Autologous protein reinfusion in severe ovarian hyperstimulation syndrome. *J Am Coll Surg* **179**:25–8.

Thaler I, Yoffe N, Kaftory J et al. (1981). Treatment of ovarian hyperstimulation syndrome: the physiologic basis for a modified approach. *Fertil Steril* **36**:110–13.

Todros T, Carmazzi CM, Bontempo S et al. (1999). Spontaneous ovarian hyperstimulation syndrome and deep vein trombosis in pregnancy: case report. *Hum Reprod* **14**:2245–8.

Tsunoda T, Shibahara H, Hirano Y et al. (2003). Treatment of ovarian hyperstimulation syndrome using an oral dopamine prodrug, docarpamine. *Gynecol Endocrinol* **17**:281–6.

Uhler ML, Budinger GR, Gabram SG & Zinaman J (2001). Perforated duodenal ulcer associated with ovarian hyperstimulation syndrome: case report. *Hum Reprod* **16**:174–6.

Whelan JG & Vlahos NF (2000). The ovarian hyperstimulation syndrome. *Fertil Steril* **73**:883–96.

Yoshii F, Ooki N, Shinohara Y et al. (1999). Multiple cerebral infarctions associated with ovarian hyperstimulation syndrome. *Neurology* **53**:225–7.

Zosmer A, Katz Z, Lancet M et al. (1987). Adult respiratory distress syndrome complicating ovarian hyperstimulation syndrome. *Fertil Steril* **47**:524–6.

INDEX